"Several generations of counselors and physicians have had the benefit of Edmund Bourne's intensely researched and extremely handy *The Anxiety and Phobia Workbook*. I know few colleagues who do not have a copy on their bookshelves that they consult regularly when treating patients suffering with anxiety-related disorders. This book is especially important today as climate change continues to inflame the anxieties of our already-stressed social fabric. The WHO and NIH are all reporting sweeping increases in 'ecoanxiety.' The recent APA special report, *Mental Health and Our Changing Climate*, found that US-based hurricanes more than doubled rates of suicide and suicidal ideation, with nearly 50 percent of the catchment group studied developing a longer-term anxiety or mood disorder such as post-traumatic stress disorder (PTSD). If you don't already have this updated edition of the 'gold standard' in anxiety treatment, now is the time to add it to your clinical armamentarium."

—**Christian R. Komor, PsyD**, author of *Climate Deadline 2035*

"Here is the valuable and comprehensive update to a classic in our self-help field. This fast-paced guide unravels the mysteries of anxieties, phobias, and worry, then delivers action-focused 'how-to' techniques. With these powerful tools in your hands, you can more than survive, you can thrive."

—**Reid Wilson, PhD**, author of *Stopping the Noise in Your Head*

"This book is a timely and comprehensive update to a classic resource in the field of anxiety and its treatment. The latest edition is very readable, easily understandable, filled with updated information, and should be quite helpful and informative to anyone interested in treating or recovering from an anxiety disorder or a condition marked by anxiety. Many thanks to Ed Bourne for this excellent work!"

—**Jeffrey Brantley, MD**, psychiatrist; founding faculty member of Duke Integrative Medicine, and founding director of its mindfulness based stress reduction program; author of *Calming Your Anxious Mind*, and author or coauthor of several other books related to mindfulness practices for health and greater well-being in daily life

"The best gets better! Bourne refuses to be complacent, and brings his classic book up to date with new topics such as overcoming worry and preventing relapse. This is part informational, part workbook, part repository of practical steps, and part resource directory for all things to do with anxiety, phobias, and even obsessive-compulsive disorder (OCD). An astonishing resource in one volume! Those with anxiety will find much help in these pages."

—**Timothy A. Sisemore, PhD**, professor of psychology at California Baptist University, and author of *The Clinician's Guide to Exposure Therapies for Anxiety Spectrum Disorders*

"Ed Bourne has again produced a thoroughly updated revision of his classic book. Incredibly helpful to clients and clinicians, he describes symptoms and updated treatment techniques in detail, and provides plenty of exercises. He covers health conditions that may contribute to anxiety, safety behaviors that perpetuate it, and nutrition, medication, and meditations that reduce it— as well as relapse prevention. He updates descriptions of exposures according to new research. He describes genotypic testing that helps determine the best antidepressant medications for particular individuals. Finally, he has material on identifying values and setting goals, including those based on one's spiritual life."

—**Lynne Henderson, PhD**, founder of the Social Fitness Center; founder and codirector, with Philip Zimbardo, of the Shyness Institute; and author of *Improving Social Confidence and Reducing Shyness Using Compassion Focused Therapy* and *Helping Your Shy and Socially Anxious Client*

"Edmund Bourne's anxiety and phobia workbook is a must-read for anyone battling these painful afflictions. He goes beyond his six earlier editions to expand your knowledge on the causes for anxiety and phobias, and to evolve clear, step-by-step prescriptions that you can follow as written or shape into your own personalized program. In this organized, practical, reader-friendly self-help book, Bourne draws from science and his practice to map paths to positive change. Put this information to use to liberate yourself from what is among the worst of all possible feelings."

—**William Knaus, EdD**, author of *The Cognitive Behavioral Workbook for Anxiety* and *The Cognitive Behavioral Workbook for Depression*, and coauthor of *The Cognitive Behavioral Workbook for Anger*

# Praise for Previous Editions

"Edmund J. Bourne has refined and expanded on his thoughtful holistic message to those who struggle with anxiety. There are many things you can do to relieve your suffering in order to live a fuller and more meaningful life. I highly recommend this classic resource to anyone suffering with anxiety or a phobia."

> —**Michael A. Tompkins, PhD**, author of *Anxiety and Avoidance*, and codirector of the San Francisco Bay Area Center for Cognitive Therapy

"Edmund J. Bourne's book is chock-full of tested ideas and exercises that practically anyone who suffers from anxieties and fears can put to immediate use to get relief from anxiety and prevent it from coming back."

> —**William Knaus, EdD**, author of *The Cognitive Behavioral Workbook for Depression* and *The Cognitive Behavioral Workbook for Anxiety*

"Since Bourne sees anxiety as 'stress over time,' the twenty-five years of success for his book has given 'help over time.' This new sixth edition takes the best and makes it better by incorporating recent developments in understanding the nature and treatment of anxiety. Comprehensive in every way, it is a one-stop shop for persons with anxiety, and an invaluable and unparalleled resource for clinicians working with them."

> —**Timothy A. Sisemore, PhD**, director of research and professor of counseling and psychology at Richmont Graduate University, and author of *Free from OCD*

"In this updated version of a classic, Edmund J. Bourne guides us carefully through a wealth of information on anxiety, anxiety disorders, and phobias. Thorough and articulate, he covers solid fundamentals, from careful descriptions of symptoms to current treatments. He includes information on medication and nutrition, and self-help strategies for each area of difficulty. A must-read for anyone struggling with anxiety and a great resource for therapists, the book is an excellent contribution to the field."

> —**Lynne Henderson, PhD**, founder of the Social Fitness Center; and founder and codirector, with Philip Zimbardo, of the Shyness Institute

"As a person once challenged by anxiety, and as a professional, I am truly grateful for this book. It is the encyclopedia of healing from anxiety and phobias, not to read all at once, but a resource to reach for that has just what you need each day or each month… Easy and reassuring to follow… Life-changing."

—**Mani Feniger**, author of *Journey from Anxiety to Freedom*

"This is a concise, practical, and comprehensive directory on how to reduce anxiety. A highly regarded and widely known resource."

—*Authoritative Guide to Self-Help Resources in Mental Health*

"A great resource for a holistic approach."

—**Reid Wilson, PhD**, author of *Don't Panic*

"Extremely well done."

—**Christopher McCullough**, coauthor of *Managing Your Anxiety*

"Any who've struggled with panic attacks and fears will find this packed with self-help exercises and guidelines to overcoming anxiety and stress, from understanding how to assert oneself to creating a positive recovery strategy."

—*Midwest Book Review*

"This workbook offers a practical and comprehensive guide to anyone struggling to cope with the many-faceted manifestations of panic and anxiety."

—*Child and Behavior Therapy*

# The
# *Anxiety*
# *& Phobia*
# WORKBOOK

## SEVENTH EDITION

EDMUND J. BOURNE, PhD

New Harbinger Publications, Inc.

## Publisher's Note

Distributed in Canada by Raincoast Books

Copyright © 2020 by Edmund J. Bourne
              New Harbinger Publications, Inc.
              5674 Shattuck Avenue
              Oakland, CA 94609
              www.newharbinger.com

Cover design by Amy Shoup
Interior design by Michele Waters-Kermes and Tracy Carlson
Acquired by Catharine Meyers
Edited by Jean Blomquist

Library of Congress Cataloging-in-Publication Data on file

Printed in the United States of America

22    21    20

10   9   8   7   6   5   4   3   2   1                    First Printing

# Contents

# Grateful Acknowledgment

To all the staff at New Harbinger who contributed to this edition: Tracy Carlson, Vicraj Gill, Catharine Meyers, Amy Shoup, Michele Waters, and others—as well as Jean Blomquist, who served as copy editor. Thank you for the care and attention you gave to the seventh edition of this book and for your flexibility and patience in working with me over the year it took to bring the project to completion.

# Preface to the Seventh Edition

Thirty years have passed since this book was first published as a broad summary of the diverse approaches for treating anxiety disorders. Over that time, the book has been quite well received, reaching many people and undergoing many translations throughout the world.

Much has changed in the field of anxiety disorders in four decades. The 1980s and '90s saw the growth of cognitive behavioral therapy as the dominant treatment approach for all anxiety disorders. In the twenty-first century, there has been an increasing specialization in the field, with numerous books, programs, and special organizations devoted to each of the major anxiety disorders (for example, the International OCD Foundation for obsessive-compulsive disorder). In recent years, there has been a proliferation of websites relating to anxiety, with my website, Helpforanxiety.com, being one among many. The national organization representing anxiety disorders changed its name from the Anxiety Disorders Association of America to the Anxiety and Depression Association of America, recognizing the prevalence of depression among many people who struggle with anxiety.

This seventh edition differs in many ways from all previous editions. All of the existing chapters have been revised to varying degrees (sometimes substantially), and the book presents two new chapters, chapter 10, Overcoming Worry, and chapter 20, Relapse Prevention.

A summary of the content and revisions of many of the seventh edition's chapters follows. Space limitations prevent a description of all revisions for all chapters.

- Chapter 1 (Anxiety Disorders). The descriptions of the anxiety disorders in chapter 1 have been updated to make them compatible with the diagnostic manual for behavioral disorders presently used by all mental health practitioners, *The Diagnostic and Statistical Manual of Mental Disorders*, Fifth Edition, or *DSM-5*, which was published in 2013. The chapter also includes revisions on prevalence data and gender differences for several anxiety disorders, including agoraphobia, social anxiety disorder, generalized anxiety disorder (GAD), and obsessive-compulsive disorder (OCD).

- Chapter 2 (Major Causes of Anxiety Disorders). The descriptions of the biological causes of panic disorder, generalized anxiety disorder, and obsessive-compulsive disorder have been updated based on the latest research in neurobiology. A new section that provides greater detail on how antidepressant medications work to reduce anxiety has been added. Also, a new section on safety behaviors, "Maintaining Causes," has been added to the main section, "Major Causes of Anxiety Disorders."

- Chapter 6 (Coping with Panic Attacks). This chapter focuses on learning to overcome and replace catastrophic thoughts that propel panic attacks, such as "I'm going to have a heart attack," "I'm going to go crazy," or "This will never end." Strategies for disrupting panic attacks at an early stage, such as abdominal breathing, utilizing coping statements, refraining from safety behaviors, or engaging in physical activity, are described.

- Chapter 7 (Exposure for Phobias). This chapter has been rewritten to reflect recent new research on exposure. A key point is a change in understanding of how exposure works. Instead of an emphasis on exposure promoting desensitization to a phobia, the active ingredient in successful exposure appears to be *new learning* that the situation is neither as dreadful nor as threatening as you may have initially perceived it. The chapter concludes with a summary of factors that facilitate successful exposure therapy.

- Chapters 8 and 9 (Self-Talk and Mistaken Beliefs) present the key ideas and practices of cognitive-behavioral therapy, an approach used by almost all therapists who treat anxiety disorders. Chapter 8 focuses on learning to replace fearful self-talk (what you say to yourself) with more constructive and reassuring self-talk. Chapter 9 focuses on replacing mistaken core beliefs, which underlie negative self-talk, with constructive beliefs, utilizing several different strategies, including affirmations.

- Chapter 10 (Overcoming Worry) is a new chapter devoted to overcoming worry. It emphasizes a variety of strategies to deal with worry including proactive disruption techniques, defusion, worry exposure, postponement of worry, and taking constructive action to resolve worries.

- Chapter 11 (Personality Styles That Perpetuate Anxiety) describes personality traits that are common for people who struggle with anxiety disorders, such as perfectionism, excessive need for approval, or excessive need for control. The chapter offers a number of different strategies for dealing with these traits.

- Chapter 12 (Ten Common Specific Phobias). Many people contend with a single, specific phobia that limits their life in a significant way. This chapter provides both descriptions and treatments of common specific phobias such as the fear of performing, fear of flying, fear of dental procedures, and even fear of death.

- Chapters 13, 14, and 15 (Dealing with Feelings, Being Assertive, and Self-Esteem) move beyond cognitive behavioral therapy to cover three topics relevant to nearly all people who struggle with anxiety disorders: 1) expressing and communicating withheld feelings, 2) becoming assertive: standing up for what you want and saying no to what you don't want, and 3) building self-esteem through a wide range of strategies for increasing your sense of self-worth and self-respect.

- Chapter 16 (Nutrition) offers updated nutritional recommendations for people with anxiety disorders, providing general dietary guidelines for reducing anxiety and stress. The chapter also recommends certain over-the-counter supplements that can help anxiety as well as depression.

- Chapter 17 (Health Conditions That May Contribute to Anxiety). This chapter reviews several health conditions that commonly accompany anxiety disorders, such as adrenal fatigue (burnout), thyroid imbalances, PMS, menopause, and insomnia, with guidelines for dealing with each of these conditions.

- Chapter 18 (Medication for Anxiety). The chapter has been updated to include medications for anxiety and depression that have been utilized more recently, for example, the SMS (serotonin modulator and stimulator) antidepressants such as Viibryd and Trintellix. In addition, it explores the recent use of cannabidiol and ketamine to treat both anxiety and depression. A final section mentions the new, experimental field of genotypic testing, which uses DNA tests to determine which antidepressant medications might be most appropriate for a particular individual.

- Chapter 20 (Relapse Prevention). Why do people fail to get better in spite of good treatment? Why do others relapse? The first part of this chapter describes five possible reasons for not fully recovering after receiving cognitive behavioral therapy and/or medication for your anxiety disorder. The second part enumerates a number of "warning signs" that may suggest the potential possibility of a relapse.

- Chapter 21 (Personal Meaning). The section "Finding and Fulfilling Your Unique Purpose" has been expanded to include material on identifying values, setting personal goals, and taking committed action based on these goals. The concluding main section of this chapter, "Spirituality," offers new material that 1) assists you in defining your unique spiritual beliefs and 2) provides practices for developing your spiritual life.

The stressful society we live in provides a backdrop for the increasing prevalence of anxiety disorders seen in recent years. Broad societal conditions, such as the threat of economic recession, overpopulation, income inequality, political polarization, nuclear proliferation, the opioid crisis, increasing pollution, and climate change—as well as more immediate problems with the health care system, student debt, urban congestion, and technological complexity—all contribute to the stressful times in which we live. In such a society, many people feel anxious, and some go on to develop anxiety disorders.

Fortunately, good help for anxiety and its disorders is available. It is my hope that the variety of interventions offered in this book will provide you with a wide range of resources to better cope with anxiety in all the forms in which it may show up in these times of change.

# Introduction

Research conducted by the National Institute of Mental Health has shown that anxiety disorders are the number one mental health problem among American women and are second only to alcohol and drug abuse among men. Approximately 18 percent of the population of the United States, or over fifty million people, have suffered from panic attacks, phobias, or other anxiety disorders in the past year. Nearly a quarter of the adult population will suffer from an anxiety disorder at some time during their life. Yet only a small proportion of these people receive treatment. During the past twenty-five years, panic and anxiety reached epidemic proportions, with much coverage of these disorders in the media. In recent times, a trend in many developed countries toward an increase in collective anxiety has appeared in the wake of new uncertainties, such as economic instability, rapid deterioration of the environment, and global terrorism.

Why are problems with panic, phobias, and anxiety so prevalent? It has been my impression that anxiety disorders are an outcome of cumulative stress acting over time. Certainly there are numerous factors that cause a person to develop panic attacks, phobias, or obsessions—but stress over time plays a key role. Of course, each of us creates much of our own stress, yet the society in which we live also may affect us deeply. People living in Western society are currently experiencing more stress than they have in many previous times in history, and it is this stress that explains the increased incidence of anxiety disorders. While it can be argued that human beings have always had to deal with stressful societal conditions (wars, famines, plagues, economic depression, and so forth), there are three reasons for suggesting that the overall stress level is particularly high at the present time.

First, our environment and social order have changed more in the last thirty years than they have in the previous three hundred years. Digital information technology has changed our lives drastically in less than twenty years. The increased pace of modern society and the increased rate of technological change have deprived people of adequate time to adjust to these changes.

Second, to compound this situation, there are rapidly increasing uncertainties about the future of all of our lives. Beginning in late 2008, the worst economic downturn since the Great Depression affected people throughout the world, with continuing ramifications even up to the present time. Other serious problems such as overpopulation, income inequality, global terrorism, and the proliferation of weapons of mass destruction add to a context of collective global stress. Finally, future prospects for the world's environment are seriously in question, as a majority of scientists believe we have already reached a tipping point for climate change, extreme weather events, loss of biodiversity, and destruction of natural habitats all over the world. As these tipping points are crossed, it's very difficult returning to the world to which we are accustomed. The list of uncertainties could go on, but conditions such as these provide a social context for anxiety. When a society becomes more anxious and uncertain, this shows up as an increased incidence of anxiety disorders in the population.

Finally, cultural values are unclear. We lack a consistent, externally sanctioned set of values (traditionally prescribed by society, government, and religion). This leaves a vacuum in which people are left to fend for themselves. Faced with a barrage of inconsistent worldviews and standards presented by political divisions, hundreds of television channels, and multiple social media platforms, people must learn to cope with the responsibility of creating their own meaning and moral order.

All of these factors make it difficult for many individuals in modern society to experience a sense of stability or consistency in their lives. Anxiety disorders are simply one outcome of a diminished ability to cope with the resulting stress, as are addictive disorders, depression, the falling life expectancy in the US, and the increased incidence of suicide among teenagers.

Many good books on anxiety disorders have appeared during the past twenty years. Most of these popular books tend to be primarily descriptive. Although several of them have spoken of methods of treatment and offered practical recovery strategies, the emphasis has been on providing readers with a basic understanding of the anxiety disorders.

In writing this workbook, my intention has been to 1) describe specific skills that you need to overcome problems with panic, anxiety, and phobias, and 2) provide step-by-step procedures and exercises for mastering these skills. Although there is quite a bit of descriptive material, what makes this a *workbook* is its emphasis on coping strategies and skills along with exercises to foster your recovery.

There is probably little in this book that is altogether new. The chapters on relaxation, exercise, coping skills for panic attacks, exposure for phobias, countering fearful thoughts with constructive thoughts, expressing feelings, asserting yourself, self-esteem, nutrition, medications, and meditation summarize approaches that have been dealt with in greater detail in the books listed at the end of each chapter. It has been my hope to define in a single volume the *full range* of strategies necessary to overcome problems with anxiety. The more of these strategies you can incorporate into your own recovery program, the more efficient and rapid your progress will be.

The approach of this workbook is primarily holistic. It presents interventions that will affect your life on many levels: body, behavior, feelings, mind, interpersonal relations, self-esteem, and spirituality. A large number of popular approaches to panic and phobias emphasize primarily behavioral and cognitive (or mental) strategies. These are very important and still constitute the core of any successful program for treating all anxiety disorders. Such approaches are covered in five chapters of this workbook: Chapter 6 offers concepts and coping strategies that are crucial for learning to handle panic attacks. Chapter 7 details the process of exposure, which is necessary to any program for recovering from agoraphobia, social phobia, or other specific phobias. Chapters 8 and 9 present methods for learning to counter unhelpful "self-talk" and mistaken beliefs that tend to perpetuate anxiety on a day-to-day basis. Chapter 10 offers a variety of strategies for dealing with excessive worry.

Relaxation and personal wellness are of prime importance. As previously mentioned, anxiety disorders develop as the result of cumulative, long-term stress. This stress is apparent in the well-known fact that many people with anxiety disorders tend to be in a chronic state of physiological hyperarousal. Recovery depends first on adopting lifestyle changes that promote a more relaxed, balanced, and healthy approach to life: in short, changes that upgrade your level of *physical well-being*. The strategies and skills presented in the chapters on relaxation, exercise, and nutrition constitute a necessary *foundation* on which the other skills presented throughout this workbook rest. It is much easier, for example, to implement exposure if you have first learned about the benefits of relaxation and exercise. You will also find it easier to identify and change counterproductive self-talk when you are feeling physically healthy and relaxed. Just as learning habits of positive self-talk will help you feel better, improving your physical health through proper relaxation, exercise, and nutrition will reduce your *predisposition* to counterproductive attitudes and self-talk. In short, when you feel well, you will think well.

At the other end of the spectrum, a lack of direction or personal meaning in your life can lead to an increased vulnerability to anxiety disorders. Panic attacks and agoraphobia—especially when they involve a fear of being closed in or unable to escape—may symbolize a sense of having "nowhere to go" or being "stuck" within your life. Given the complexity of contemporary society and the lack of any externally prescribed set of values, it is common to feel confused and uncertain about the meaning and direction of your life. By getting more in touch with a larger sense of purpose, and, where appropriate, cultivating your own spirituality, you can gain a sense of meaning that will help diminish your problems with anxiety. This is an important area to consider in dealing with anxiety disorders and probably most other behavior disorders as well (see chapter 21).

In sum, a holistic model incorporating all of the approaches presented in this workbook is necessary for a more complete and lasting solution to anxiety disorders. Recovery from anxiety depends upon intervening at all levels of the whole person.

A final important point bears mentioning. It will take a strong commitment and consistent motivation on your part to successfully utilize the skills presented in this workbook. If you are self-motivated and disciplined, it is certainly possible to achieve recovery on your own. At the same time, it is not always preferable or even most effective to go it alone. Many readers will decide to use this workbook in conjunction with seeing a therapist who has expertise in treating anxiety disorders. A therapist can provide structure and support, and can help you fine-tune the concepts and strategies found in this workbook to your own individual situation. Some of you may also find support groups or treatment groups (especially for agoraphobia and social phobia) to be very valuable. A group format can motivate you and maintain your enthusiasm for learning the skills necessary for recovery.

Ultimately, you will need to choose the best way for yourself. If you decide to seek outside help for your problem, you will want to contact a specialist in the treatment of anxiety disorders to help you decide what treatment format is best for you. A list of such specialists in the United States and Canada is offered by the Anxiety and Depression Association of America (ADAA). Go to their website, adaa.org, click on the "Find a Therapist" link, and enter your city or zip code (see appendix 1 for further information).

It is quite possible to overcome your problem with panic, phobias, or anxiety on your own through the use of the strategies and exercises presented in this workbook. Yet it is equally valuable and appropriate, if you feel so inclined, to use this book as an adjunct to working with a therapist or group treatment program. Whatever approach you choose, know that there is much help available. Problems with anxiety can improve or be largely resolved when you make a commitment and follow through consistently with the types of approaches described in this book.

# 1

# Anxiety Disorders

Susan awakens suddenly almost every night, a couple of hours after going to sleep, with a tightness in her throat, a racing heart, dizziness, and a fear that she's going to die. Although she's shaking all over, she hasn't a clue why. After many nights of getting up and pacing her living room floor in an attempt to get a grip on herself, she decides to go see her doctor to find out whether something is wrong with her heart.

Cindy, a medical secretary, has been having attacks like Susan's whenever she's in a confined public situation. Not only does she fear losing control over herself, but she also dreads what others might think of her if that were to happen. Recently, she has been avoiding going into any kind of store other than the local 7-Eleven unless her boyfriend is with her. She has also needed to leave restaurants and movie theaters during dates. Now she is beginning to wonder whether she can cope with her job. She has been forcing herself to go in to work, yet after a few minutes among her office mates, she starts to fear that she's losing control of herself. Suddenly, she feels as though she *has* to leave.

Steve has a responsible position as a software engineer but feels he is unable to advance because of his inability to contribute in group meetings. It's almost more than he can bear just to sit in on meetings, let alone offer his opinions. Yesterday his boss asked him whether he would be available to make a presentation on his segment of a large project. At that point, Steve became extremely nervous and tongue-tied. He walked out of the room, stammering that he would let his boss know by the next day about the presentation. Privately, he thought about resigning.

Mike is so embarrassed about a peculiar fear he's had over the past few months that he can't tell anyone, not even his wife. While driving, he is frequently gripped by the fear that he has run over someone or perhaps an animal. Even though there is no "thud" suggesting that anything like this has happened, he feels compelled to make a U-turn and retrace the route he's just driven to make absolutely sure. In fact, recently, his paranoia about having hit someone has grown so strong that he has to retrace his route three or four times to assure himself that nothing has happened. Mike is a bright, successful professional and feels utterly humiliated about his compulsion to check. He's beginning to wonder if he's going crazy.

Susan, Cindy, Steve, and Mike are all confronted by anxiety. Yet it is not ordinary anxiety. Their experiences differ in two fundamental respects from the "normal" anxiety people experience in response to everyday life. First, their anxiety has gone out of control. In each case, the individual feels powerless to direct what's happening. This sense of powerlessness in turn creates even more anxiety. Second, the anxiety is interfering with the normal functioning of their lives. Susan's sleep is disrupted. Cindy and Steve may lose their jobs. And Mike has lost the ability to drive in an efficient and timely manner.

The examples of Susan, Cindy, Steve, and Mike illustrate four types of anxiety disorder: panic disorder, agoraphobia, social phobia, and obsessive-compulsive disorder. Later in this chapter, you can find detailed descriptions of the characteristics of each specific anxiety disorder. But first let's consider the common theme that runs through them all. What is the nature of anxiety itself?

# The Nature of Anxiety

You can better understand the nature of anxiety by looking at both what it is and what it is not. For example, anxiety can be distinguished from fear in several ways. When you are afraid, your fear is usually directed toward some concrete external object or situation. The event that you fear usually is within the bounds of possibility. You might fear not meeting a deadline, failing an exam, being unable to pay your bills, or being rejected by someone you want to please. Fear can be associated with a sudden surge of adrenaline, thoughts of immediate danger, and a need to escape. When you experience anxiety, on the other hand, you often can't specify what it is you're anxious about. The focus of anxiety is more internal than external. It seems to be a response to a vague, distant, or even unrecognized danger. You might be anxious about "losing control" of yourself or some situation. Or you might feel a vague anxiety about "something bad happening."

Anxiety affects your whole being. It is a physiological, behavioral, and psychological reaction all at once. On a physiological level, anxiety may include bodily reactions such as rapid heartbeat, muscle tension, queasiness, dry mouth, or sweating. On a behavioral level, it can sabotage your ability to act, express yourself, or deal with certain everyday situations.

Psychologically, anxiety is a subjective state of apprehension and uneasiness. In its most extreme form, it can cause you to feel detached from yourself and even fearful of dying or going crazy.

The fact that anxiety can affect you on a physiological, behavioral, and psychological level has important implications for your attempts to recover. A complete program of recovery from an anxiety disorder must intervene at all three levels to:

1. Reduce physiological reactivity

2. Eliminate avoidance behavior

3. Change subjective interpretations (or "self-talk"), which perpetuate a state of apprehension and worry

Anxiety can appear in different forms and at different levels of intensity. It can range in severity from a mere twinge of uneasiness to a full-blown panic attack marked by heart palpitations, disorientation, and terror. Anxiety that is not connected with any particular situation, that comes "out of the blue," is called free-floating anxiety or, in more severe instances, a *spontaneous panic attack*. The difference between an episode of free-floating anxiety and a spontaneous panic attack can be defined by whether you experience four or more of the following symptoms at the same time (the occurrence of four or more symptoms defines a panic attack):

• Shortness of breath

- Heart palpitations (rapid or irregular heartbeat)

- Trembling or shaking

- Sweating

- Choking

- Nausea or abdominal distress

- Numbness

- Dizziness or unsteadiness

- Feeling of detachment or being out of touch with yourself

- Hot flashes or chills

- Fear of dying

- Fear of going crazy or out of control

If your anxiety arises *only* in response to a specific situation, it is called *situational anxiety* or *phobic anxiety*. Situational anxiety is different from everyday fear in that it tends to be out of proportion or unrealistic. If you have a disproportionate apprehension about driving on freeways, going to the doctor, or confronting your spouse, this may qualify as situational anxiety. Situational anxiety becomes *phobic* when you actually start to *avoid* the situation: if you give up driving on freeways, going to doctors, or confronting your spouse altogether. In other words, phobic anxiety is situational anxiety that includes persistent avoidance of the situation.

Often anxiety can be brought on merely by thinking about a particular situation. When you feel distressed about what might happen when or if you have to face one of your phobic situations, you are experiencing what is called *anticipatory anxiety*. In its milder forms, anticipatory anxiety is indistinguishable from ordinary "worrying." But sometimes anticipatory anxiety becomes intense enough to be called *anticipatory panic*.

There is an important difference between spontaneous anxiety (or panic) and anticipatory anxiety (or panic). *Spontaneous anxiety* tends to come out of the blue, peaks to a high level very rapidly, and then subsides gradually. The peak is usually reached within five minutes, followed by a gradual tapering-off period of an hour or more. *Anticipatory anxiety*, on the other hand, tends to build up more gradually in response to encountering—or simply thinking about—a threatening situation and then usually falls off quickly. You may "worry yourself into a frenzy" about something for an hour or more and then let go of the worry as you find something else to occupy your mind.

## Anxiety vs. Anxiety Disorders

Anxiety is an inevitable part of life in contemporary society. It's important to realize that there are many situations that come up in everyday life in which it is *appropriate* and *reasonable* to react with some anxiety. If you didn't feel *any* anxiety in response to everyday challenges involving potential loss or failure, something would be wrong. This workbook can be of use to anyone experiencing normal, ordinary anxiety reactions (everyone, in other words). It is also intended for those of you who are dealing with specific anxiety disorders. Incorporating exercise, breathing skills, relaxation, and good nutritional habits into your daily life—as well as paying attention to self-talk, mistaken beliefs, feelings, assertiveness, and self-esteem—can all contribute to making your life more balanced and less anxious, regardless of the nature and extent of the anxiety you happen to be dealing with.

Anxiety disorders are distinguished from everyday, normal anxiety in that they involve anxiety that 1) *is more intense* (for example, panic attacks), 2) *lasts longer* (anxiety that may persist for months or longer instead of going away after a stressful situation has passed), or 3) *leads to phobias* that interfere with your life.

Criteria for diagnosing specific anxiety disorders have been established by the American Psychiatric Association and are listed in a well-known diagnostic manual used by mental health professionals. This manual is called the *DSM-5 (Diagnostic and Statistical Manual of Mental Disorders,* Fifth Edition). The following descriptions of various anxiety disorders are based on the criteria in the *DSM-5,* as is the self-diagnosis questionnaire at the end of this chapter. This workbook can help you even if your specific anxiety disorder or reaction doesn't fit any of the *DSM-5's* diagnostic categories. On the other hand, don't be unduly concerned if your reaction is perfectly described by one of the diagnostic categories. Approximately 15 percent of adults and 20 percent of adolescents in the United States would find themselves in your company.

This workbook describes anxiety disorders pertinent to adolescents and adults. Readers interested in anxiety disorders specific to children, such as separation anxiety disorder or selective mutism, should explore descriptions of them in *DSM-5* and consult books specializing in children's anxiety disorders. See the "Further Reading" section at the end of this chapter for a short list of suggested books on children's anxiety disorders.

## Panic Disorder

*Panic disorder* is characterized by sudden episodes of acute apprehension or intense fear that occur "out of the blue," without any apparent cause. Intense panic usually lasts no more than a few minutes, but, in rare instances, can return in "waves" for a period of up to two hours. During the panic itself, any of the following symptoms can occur:

- Shortness of breath or a feeling of being smothered

- Heart palpitations—pounding heart or accelerated heart rate

- Dizziness, unsteadiness, or faintness

- Trembling or shaking

- A feeling of choking

- Sweating

- Nausea or abdominal distress

- A feeling of unreality—as if you're "not all there" (depersonalization)

- Numbness or tingling in hands and feet

- Hot and cold flashes

- Chest pain or discomfort

- Fears of going crazy or losing control

- Fears of dying

At least four of these symptoms are present in a full-blown panic attack, while having two or three of them is referred to as a *limited symptom attack*.

Your symptoms would be diagnosed as panic disorder if 1) you have had two or more panic attacks and 2) at least one of these attacks has been followed by *one month (or more) of persistent concern about having another panic attack*, or worry about the possible implications of having another panic attack. It's important to recognize that panic disorder, by itself, does not involve any phobias. The panic doesn't occur because you are thinking about, approaching, or actually entering a phobic situation. However, you may develop a tendency to avoid places where panic attacks have occurred in the past. When this tendency persists, you are moving into the realm of the next disorder described in this chapter, agoraphobia.

In many cases, panic occurs spontaneously, unexpectedly, and for no apparent reason. There is no obvious cue or trigger for the attack. Also, the panic attacks are not due to the physiological effects of a drug (prescription or recreational) or a medical condition.

People vary in how frequently panic attacks occur. You may have two or three panic attacks without ever having another one again or without having another one for years. Or you may have several panic attacks followed by a panic-free period, only to have the panic return a month or two later. Sometimes an initial panic attack may be followed by recurring attacks three or more times per week unremittingly until you seek treatment. In all of these cases, there is a tendency to develop *anticipatory anxiety* or apprehension between panic attacks focusing on fear of having another one. This apprehension about having another panic attack is one of the hallmarks of panic disorder.

If you are suffering from panic disorder, you may be very frightened by your symptoms and consult with doctors to find a medical cause. Heart palpitations and an irregular heartbeat may lead to EKG and other cardiac tests, which, in most cases, turn out normal. (Sometimes mitral valve prolapse, a benign arrhythmia of the heart, may coexist with panic disorder.) Fortunately, an increasing number of physicians have some knowledge of panic disorder and are able to distinguish it from purely physical complaints.

A diagnosis of panic disorder is made only after possible medical causes—including hypoglycemia, hyperthyroidism, reaction to excess caffeine, or withdrawal from alcohol, tranquilizers, or sedatives—have been ruled out. The causes of panic disorder involve a combination of heredity, chemical imbalances in the brain, and recent personal stress. Sudden losses or major life changes may trigger the onset of panic attacks.

People tend to develop panic disorder during late adolescence or in their twenties. About half of the people who have panic disorder develop it before the age of twenty-four. In about a third of cases, panic is complicated by the development of agoraphobia (as described in the following section). Between 2 and 3 percent of the population have "pure" panic disorder, while about 5 percent, or one in every twenty people, suffer from panic attacks complicated by agoraphobia. Very few individuals develop panic disorder in childhood or after the age of sixty-five. Women are about twice as likely as men to develop panic disorder (3.8 percent versus 1.6 percent). However, this difference may largely reflect a gender difference between women and men in the tendency to disclose and seek help for panic disorder. White Americans are more likely to be diagnosed with panic disorder than other ethnic groups.

Cigarette smoking increases the risk of panic disorder (Isensee et al. 2003). About 30 percent of people with panic disorder use alcohol to self-medicate, which often worsens their symptoms when the effects of alcohol wear off. Cannabis (THC in particular) often precipitates panic in some people. About one-fourth of individuals who have panic attacks will have an occasional *nocturnal panic attack* (panic upon awakening from sleep).

Panic disorder is in part influenced by excessive activity in parts of the brain known as the amygdala and the hypothalamus. See chapter 2 for more detailed information on the neurobiology of panic disorder.

## Current Treatment

All of the following strategies are considered state-of-the-art treatments for panic disorder.

*Relaxation training.* Practicing abdominal breathing and some form of deep muscle relaxation (such as progressive muscle relaxation) on a daily basis. This helps reduce the *physical* symptoms of panic as well as anticipatory anxiety you might experience about having a panic attack. A physical exercise program may also be recommended to reduce anxiety. (See chapters 4 and 5.)

*Panic-control therapy.* Identifying and eliminating catastrophic thoughts (such as "I'm trapped!" "I'm going to go crazy!" or "I'm going to have a heart attack!") that tend to trigger panic attacks. (See chapter 6.)

*Interoceptive exposure.* Practicing voluntary exposure to the *bodily symptoms* of panic, such as rapid heartbeat, sweaty hands, shortness of breath, or dizziness. Such symptoms are created deliberately, usually in the therapist's office. For example, dizziness might be induced by spinning in a chair or rapid heartbeat by running up and down stairs. Repeated exposure to unpleasant bodily symptoms promotes a *process of desensitization*, which basically means "getting less sensitive" or getting more used to the symptoms to the point that they no longer frighten you. (See chapter 7.)

*Medication.* The antidepressant medications known as selective serotonin reuptake inhibitors, or SSRIs, such as Zoloft, Lexapro, or Celexa, or serotonin-norepinephrine reuptake inhibitors (SNRIs) such as Effexor or Cymbalta, are first-line medications of choice for treating panic disorder. Frequently the benzodiazepine class of medications—such as Xanax, Ativan, Klonopin, or Valium—may be used to reduce severity of panic symptoms in addition to antidepressant medications.

Such medications are best used in conjunction with the first three strategies above. (See chapter 18.) A downside of medication treatment for panic disorder is that more than 50 percent of people can relapse if the medication is discontinued six months to a year after beginning it.

*Lifestyle and personality changes.* Some of the lifestyle changes that can reduce your tendency to have panic attacks include stress management, regular exercise, eliminating stimulants and sugar from your diet, slowing down and creating "downtime," and altering your attitudes about perfectionism, the excessive need to please, and the excessive need to control. (Chapters 4, 5, 10, and 15 address these issues.)

## Agoraphobia

The word *agoraphobia* means "fear of open spaces"; however, the essence of agoraphobia is a fear of panic attacks. If you suffer from agoraphobia, you are afraid of being in situations from which escape might be difficult—or in which help might be unavailable—if you suddenly had a panic attack. You may avoid grocery stores or freeways, for example, not so much because of their inherent characteristics but because these are situations from which escape might be difficult or embarrassing in the event of panic. Fear of embarrassment plays a key role. Most agoraphobics fear not only having panic attacks but *what other people will think* should they be seen having a panic attack.

It is common for the agoraphobic to avoid a variety of situations. Some of the more common ones include:

- Crowded public places such as grocery stores, department stores, or restaurants

- Enclosed or confined places such as tunnels, bridges, theaters, or the hairdresser's chair

- Public transportation such as trains, buses, subways, or planes

- Standing in line or being in a crowd

- Being at home alone

Perhaps the most common feature of agoraphobia is anxiety about being far away from home or far from a "safe person" (usually your spouse, partner, a parent, or anyone to whom you have a primary attachment). You may completely avoid driving alone or may be afraid of driving alone beyond a certain short distance from home. In more severe cases, you might be able to walk alone only a few yards from home or you might be housebound altogether. Occasionally, you may confine yourself to a single room in your house.

To be diagnosed with agoraphobia, you must avoid at least two of the above types of situations, if not more. Generally, you avoid these situations altogether, but you may endure them with intense anxiety if accompanied by a companion.

If you have agoraphobia, you are not only phobic about a variety of situations but also tend to be anxious much of the time. This anxiety arises from *anticipating* that you *might* be stuck in a situation in which you would panic. What would happen, for example, if you were asked to go somewhere you ordinarily avoid and have to explain your way out of it? Or what would happen if you suddenly were left alone? Because of the severe restrictions in your activities and life, you may also be depressed. Depression arises from feeling in the grip of a condition over which you have no control or that you are powerless to change.

Agoraphobia, in many cases, appears to be engendered by panic disorder. At first, you simply have panic attacks that occur for no apparent reason (panic disorder). After a while, though, you become aware that your attacks occur more frequently in confined situations away from home or when you are by yourself. You begin to be afraid of these situations. At the point where you actually start to avoid these situations for fear of panicking, you've started to develop agoraphobia. From that point you might go on to develop a mild, moderate, or severe problem. In a mild case, you might feel uncomfortable in confined situations but not actually avoid them. You continue to work or shop on your own, but do not want to go far from home otherwise. In a moderate case, you might start to avoid some situations, such as public transportation, elevators, driving far from home, or being in restaurants. However, your restriction is only partial, and there are certain situations away from home or your safe person that you can handle on your own, even with some discomfort. Severe agoraphobia is marked by an all-inclusive restriction of activities to the point where you are unable to leave your house without being accompanied.

Just why some people with panic attacks develop agoraphobia and others do not is unknown at this time. (There are a few people who develop only agoraphobia without any panic attacks.) Nor is it understood why some people develop much more severe cases than others. What is known is that agoraphobia is caused by a combination of heredity and environment. Agoraphobics may have a parent, sibling, or other relative who also has the problem. When one identical twin is agoraphobic, the other has a high likelihood of being agoraphobic, too. On the environmental side, there are certain types of childhood circumstances that predispose a child to agoraphobia. These include growing up with parents who are 1) perfectionist and overcritical, 2) overprotective, and/ or 3) overly anxious to the point of communicating to their child that the world is a "dangerous place." The hereditary and environmental origins of agoraphobia and other anxiety disorders will be explored in greater depth in the following chapter.

Agoraphobia affects people in all walks of life and at all levels of the socioeconomic scale. About 2 percent of adults and adolescents in the United States suffer from agoraphobia at any given time. Approximately 80 percent of agoraphobics are women, although this percentage has been dropping recently. It is possible to speculate that as women are increasingly expected to hold down full-time jobs (making a housebound lifestyle less socially acceptable), the percentage of women and men with agoraphobia may tend to equalize.

Agoraphobia has a higher risk of occurring in late adolescence and young adulthood. A second period of higher risk occurs later in life, after the age of forty. Unfortunately, agoraphobia tends to be a chronic and recurrent condition unless properly treated. Complete remission without treatment is rare, approximately only 10 percent.

## Current Treatment

*Relaxation training, panic control therapy, and interoceptive exposure.* Since agoraphobia is usually based on a fear of panic attacks, the same treatments as were described for panic disorder are utilized. (See chapters 4 and 6.)

*Exposure.* Exposure therapy means you face, or expose yourself to, a feared situation. Situations that you have avoided are gradually confronted through a process of small incremental steps. Such exposures are often conducted first in imagination and then in real life (see chapter 7). For example, if you were fearful of driving far from home, you would gradually increase the distance you drive in small increments. A support person might accompany you in the same car at first, then drive in a second car behind you, and then, finally, you would practice driving alone. Or, if you were fearful of being home alone, the person who usually stays with you would leave for only a few minutes at first and then gradually increase the time away. Over time, you learn to confront and enter into all of the situations you have been avoiding.

*Cognitive therapy.* The aim of cognitive therapy is to help you replace exaggerated, fearful thinking about panic and phobias with more realistic and supportive mental habits. You learn to identify, challenge, and replace counterproductive thoughts with constructive ones. (See chapters 8 and 9.)

*Medication.* Current treatment for agoraphobia often utilizes medication. SSRIs such as Zoloft, Lexapro, or Celexa, or SNRIs such as Pristiq or Cymbalta, are especially likely to be used for more severe cases where people are housebound or highly restricted in what they are able to do. Low doses of tranquilizers such as Xanax or Klonopin may also be used to help people negotiate the early stages of exposure. Low doses of tranquilizers (for example, 0.25 mg of Xanax or Ativan) may be useful at the *onset* of undergoing exposure, to encourage a willingness to do exposure at all. However, use of these medications needs to be tapered and eventually discontinued at more advanced states of exposure to ensure complete recovery from agoraphobia (see chapter 7).

*Assertiveness training.* Since agoraphobics often have difficulty standing up for themselves and their rights, assertiveness training is frequently part of the treatment. (See chapter 14.)

*Group therapy.* Treatment for agoraphobia can be done very effectively in a group setting. There is much support available in a group, both for realizing that you are not alone and for completing week-to-week homework assignments.

# Social Anxiety Disorder

Social anxiety disorder (also known as social phobia) is one of the more common anxiety disorders. It involves fear of embarrassment or humiliation in situations where you are exposed to the scrutiny of others or you must perform. This fear is much stronger than the normal anxiety most nonphobic people experience in social or performance situations. Usually, it's so strong that it causes you to avoid the situation altogether, although some people with social phobia endure social situations, albeit with considerable anxiety. Typically, your concern is that you will say or do something that will cause others to judge you as being anxious, weak, "crazy," or stupid. This includes merely showing physical symptoms of anxiety, such as blushing or sweating. Your concern is generally out of proportion with the situation, and you recognize that it's excessive. (Children with social phobia, however, do not recognize the excessiveness of their fear.) To be diagnosed with social anxiety disorder, the fear must have been persistent for at least six months. Social anxiety disorder is associated with increased likelihood of dropping out of school, decreased satisfaction and productivity in the workplace, lower socioeconomic status, and generally poorer quality of life.

The most common social phobia is fear of public speaking. In fact, this is the most common of all phobias, affecting performers, speakers, people whose jobs require them to make presentations, and students who have to speak before their class. Public-speaking phobia affects a large percentage of the population and is equally prevalent among men and women.

Other common social phobias include:

- Fear of participating in meetings or any group setting

- Fear of being judged by others

- Fear of blushing or trembling in public situations

- Fear of choking on or spilling food while eating in public

- Fear of being watched at work

- Fear of using public toilets

- Fear of writing or signing documents in the presence of others

- Fear of crowds

- Fear of taking examinations

- Fear of talking to strangers

- Fear of being anxious around groups of people or talking to them in general (an example of *generalized social anxiety disorder*, described below)

Sometimes social phobia is less specific and involves a generalized fear of *any* social or group situation where you feel that you might be watched or evaluated. When your fear is of a wide range of social situations (for example, initiating conversations, participating in small groups, speaking to authority figures, dating, attending parties, or just being around people in general), the condition is referred to as *generalized social phobia.*

Common symptoms of social anxiety disorder include blushing, sweating, trembling, heart palpitations, and nausea. Many people who are unaware that they are socially phobic use alcohol to reduce these symptoms, which, in some cases, can lead to alcoholism. While social anxieties are common, you would be given a formal diagnosis of social phobia only if your avoidance interferes with work, social activities, or important relationships, and/or if it causes you considerable distress. As with agoraphobia, panic attacks can accompany social phobia, although your panic is related more to being embarrassed or humiliated than to being confined or trapped. Also, the panic arises only in connection with a specific type of social situation.

Social phobias tend to develop earlier than agoraphobia and can begin in late childhood or adolescence, often between ages eight and fifteen. They often develop in shy children around the time they are faced with increased peer pressure at school. Typically, these phobias persist (without treatment) through adolescence and young adulthood but have a tendency to decrease in severity later in life. Social phobia affects between approximately 7 percent of the US population. It shows a slightly higher incidence among women (almost 8 percent) versus men (about 7 percent). Again, the slightly higher incidence among women may reflect an increased tendency to disclose and seek treatment for social phobia. Historically, social phobia was believed to affect men more than women until women reached parity with men in holding jobs. Up to 13 percent of adults experience social phobia at some time in their lives.

A significant percentage of people with social anxiety disorder are clinically depressed, have another anxiety disorder such as panic disorder or generalized anxiety disorder, or are dealing with substance abuse. Up to 50 percent of people with social anxiety disorder may experience spontaneous remission within two to three years; the other 50 percent can continue to experience symptoms for much longer without treatment.

As with other anxiety disorders, there are both genetic and environmental components in the causes of social anxiety disorder. If one identical twin has the problem, the other twin is 30 to 50 percent more likely to have the problem. Heritability among first-degree relatives is five to six times higher than among unrelated people. At the same time, social anxiety in adoptive parents is significantly correlated with social anxiety in their children (Kendler, Karkowski, and Prescott 1999).

## Current Treatment

All of the following interventions are part of the current treatment for social phobia.

*Relaxation training.* Abdominal breathing and deep relaxation techniques are practiced on a regular basis to assuage physical symptoms of anxiety. (See chapter 4.)

*Cognitive therapy.* Fearful thoughts that tend to perpetuate social phobias are identified, challenged, and replaced with more realistic thoughts. (See chapter 8.) For example, the thought "I'll make a fool of myself if I speak up" would be replaced with the idea "It's okay if I'm a bit awkward at first when I speak up—most people won't be bothered." Cognitive therapists tend to focus on three specific types of cognitive distortions: an excessive focus on anxiety symptoms and how they might appear to others, distortions in self-concept about social attractiveness, and the tendency to overestimate the likelihood of a negative evaluation.

*Exposure.* Exposure involves gradually facing the social situation or situations you're phobic about. You might do this first in imagery and then in real life. For example, if you're phobic of public speaking, you might start out giving a one-minute talk to a friend and then gradually increase, through several steps, both the duration of your talk and the number of people you speak to. Or, if you have difficulty speaking up in groups, you'd gradually increase both the length and the degree of self-disclosure of remarks made in a group setting. (See chapter 7.) After each exposure, you'd review and challenge any unrealistic thinking that caused anxiety. While the treatment for social phobia can be done on an individual basis, group therapy is the ideal treatment format. This allows direct exposure to the situation and stimuli that evoke anxiety in the first place.

*Staying on task.* People with social phobia tend to focus a lot on how they are doing or try to gauge other people's reactions while speaking in a social situation. Treatment includes training yourself to focus only on the task at hand, whether conversing with a boss, speaking up in class, or presenting information to a group.

*Medication.* SSRI medications such as Zoloft, Luvox, Celexa, or Lexapro, or low doses of benzodiazepine tranquilizers such as Xanax or Klonopin, may be used as an adjunct to the cognitive and exposure-based treatments described above. Sometimes monoamine oxidase (MAO) inhibitor medications such as Nardil or Parnate are used to treat social phobia with success, though this is less common in current practice. (See chapter 18.)

*Social skills training.* In some cases, learning basic social skills, such as smiling and making eye contact, maintaining a conversation, self-disclosure, and active listening, are part of the treatment for social phobia.

*Assertiveness training.* Training in assertiveness, the ability to ask directly for what you want or to say no to what you don't want, is often included in the treatment. (See chapter 14.)

## Specific Phobia

A specific phobia typically involves a strong fear and avoidance of *one particular* type of object or situation. There are no spontaneous panic attacks, and there is no fear of panic attacks, as in agoraphobia. There is also no fear of humiliation or embarrassment in social situations, as in social phobia. Direct exposure to the feared object or situation may elicit a panic reaction, however. With specific phobia, fear is always out of proportion to the realistic danger posed by the object or situation. Typically, the fear and avoidance are strong enough to interfere with your normal routines, work, or relationships and to cause you significant distress for a period of six months or longer. Even though you recognize its irrationalities, a specific phobia can cause you considerable anxiety.

Among the most common specific phobias are the following. Note there are many lists of the most common types of phobias, and they vary in their rankings. The following list is a representative sample of common specific phobias.

**Animal phobias.** These can include fear and avoidance of snakes, bats, rats, spiders, bees, dogs, bears, and other creatures. Often these phobias begin in childhood, when they are considered normal fears. Only when they persist into adulthood and disrupt your life or cause significant distress do they come to be classified as specific phobias.

**Acrophobia (fear of heights).** With acrophobia, you tend to be afraid of high floors of buildings or of finding yourself atop mountains, hills, or high-level bridges. In such situations you may experience 1) vertigo (dizziness) or even 2) an urge to jump, usually experienced as some external force drawing you to the edge.

**Elevator phobia.** This phobia may involve a fear that the cables will break and the elevator will crash *or* a fear that the elevator will get stuck and you will be trapped inside. You may have panic reactions, but you have no history of panic disorder or agoraphobia.

**Airplane phobia.** This most often involves a fear that the plane will crash. Alternatively, it can involve a fear that the cabin will depressurize, causing you to asphyxiate. Phobias about planes being hijacked or bombed are relatively common. It is quite common for people to fear the confinement of being on a plane, without any ability to exit, for a fixed period of time. When flying, you might also have a fear of having a panic attack. Otherwise, you likely have no history of panic disorder or agoraphobia. Fear of flying is a very common phobia. Approximately 10 percent of the population will not fly at all, while an additional 20 percent experience considerable anxiety while flying.

**Doctor or dentist phobias.** This can begin as a fear of painful procedures (injections, having teeth filled) conducted in a doctor's or dentist's office. Later it can generalize to anything having to do with doctors or dentists. The danger is that you may avoid needed medical treatment.

**Phobias of thunder and/or lightning.** Almost invariably, phobias of thunder and lightning begin in childhood. When they persist beyond adolescence, they are classified as specific phobias.

**Blood-injury phobia.** This is a unique phobia in that you have a tendency to faint (rather than panic) if exposed to blood or your own pain through injections or inadvertent injury. In response to the phobic situation, your heart rate and blood pressure will initially rise and then subsequently fall, in what is called a *vasovagal response*. People with blood-injury phobia tend to be both physically and psychologically healthy in other regards.

**Disease phobia (hypochondria).** Usually, this phobia involves a fear of contracting and/or ultimately succumbing to a specific illness, such as a heart attack or cancer. With disease phobias, you tend to seek constant reassurance from doctors and will avoid any situation that reminds you of the dreaded disease.

Specific phobias are common and affect approximately 10 percent of the population (rates go as high as 16 percent among adolescents). However, since they do not always result in severe impairment, only a minority of people with specific phobias actually seek treatment. Most types of phobias occur in men and women about equally. Animal phobias tend to be more common in women, while disease phobias are more common in men. In general, women are twice as likely to report specific phobias as men, but this may reflect a difference in who seeks treatment. Among adults over sixty, the prevalence of specific phobias tends to drop.

As previously mentioned, specific phobias are often childhood fears that were never outgrown. In other instances, they may develop after a traumatic event, such as an accident, a natural disaster, an illness, or a visit to the dentist—in other words, as a result of conditioning. A final cause is childhood *modeling*. Repeated observation of a parent with a specific phobia can lead a child to develop it as well.

## Current Treatment

Since specific phobias generally do not involve spontaneous panic attacks, some of the treatments for panic, such as panic control therapy, interoceptive exposure, and medication, are usually not included.

*Relaxation training.* Abdominal breathing and deep muscle relaxation are practiced on a regular basis to reduce symptoms of anxiety that occur both when facing the specific phobia and when experiencing worry (anticipatory anxiety) about having to deal with the phobic situation. (See chapter 4.)

*Cognitive therapy.* Fearful thoughts that tend to perpetuate the specific phobia are challenged and replaced. For example, "What if I panic because I feel trapped aboard an airplane?" would be replaced with more realistic and supportive thoughts, such as "While I may not be able to leave the airplane for two hours, I *can* move around, such as leaving my seat to go to the bathroom several times if needed. If I start to feel panicky, I have many strategies for coping that I can use, including abdominal breathing, talking to my companion, listening to a relaxing tape, or taking medication, if necessary." Coping statements, such as "I've handled this before and I can handle it again" or "This is just a thought; it has no validity," are also useful. These supportive coping statements are rehearsed until they are internalized. (See chapter 8.)

*Exposure.* This involves gradually facing the phobic situation through a series of incremental steps. For example, fear of flying would be faced first in imagination only (imagery exposure), then by watching planes land and take off, then by boarding a grounded plane, then by taking a short flight, and, finally, by taking a longer flight. A support person might accompany you first through all the steps, then you'd try them on your own. For some phobias, it's difficult to do real-life exposure—for example, if you're afraid of earthquakes. Treatment would then emphasize cognitive therapy and then exposure to imagined scenes of earthquakes (or watching movies about earthquakes). Imagery and real-life exposure are described in chapter 7.

*Virtual reality exposure therapy.* In a small number of settings with appropriate technology, specific phobias have been treated with *virtual reality exposure therapy*. Virtual reality exposure therapy (VRT) uses specifically programmed equipment with large screens to simulate phobic situations such as spiders, heights, flying, speaking in public, and even closed-in spaces. As with real-life exposure, the client is exposed to a highly detailed hierarchy of phobic scenes that utilize visual, auditory, and even tactile cues to enhance a sense of presence and immersion in the situation. The clinician can adjust the intensity of each situation as well as identify triggers that are uniquely associated with the client's specific phobia. The client is also given controls, such as a joystick, to allow movement and interaction within the simulated environment. The client's progress through a succession of scenes can be closely monitored. Difficult scenes can be repeated until the client learns that the situation is not truly harmful. Early research with VRT conducted in the 1990s found marked reduction of fears of heights, comparable to real-life exposure for acrophobia. Since that time, the range of applications has been extended to treat veterans for post-traumatic stress disorder (where combat scenes are re-created with the opportunity to achieve mastery over adverse conditions of combat). More recently, VRT has been used to treat depression in adolescents. The client enters the role of a character that travels through a fantasy world, combatting their virtual negative thoughts. As with any form of specialized therapy, clinicians who administer VRT need to be properly trained. There has been a problem with untrained therapists who simply purchase the equipment and proceed to use it without specialty training. Research indicates that virtual exposure can be effective and transfer well to the real-life phobic situation. A detailed summary of research on the efficacy of VRT with respect to heights, fear of flying, and PTSD can be found in Rothbaum (2006). For the reference, see the section on specific phobia under "Further Reading" at the end of this chapter.

To sum up, specific phobia is usually a benign disorder, particularly if it begins as a common childhood fear. Though it may last for years, it rarely gets worse and it often diminishes over time. Typically, it is not associated with other psychiatric disturbances. People with specific phobias are usually functioning at a high level in all other respects.

# Generalized Anxiety Disorder

Generalized anxiety disorder (GAD) is characterized by chronic anxiety that persists for at least six months *but is unaccompanied by panic attacks, phobias, or obsessions.* You simply experience persistent anxiety and worry without the complicating features of other anxiety disorders. To be given a diagnosis of generalized anxiety disorder, your anxiety and worry must focus on two or more stressful life circumstances (such as finances, relationships, health, work problems, or school performance) for a majority of days during a six-month period. It's common, if you're dealing with generalized anxiety disorder, to have a large number of worries and to spend a lot of your time worrying, yet you find it difficult to exercise much control over your worrying. Moreover, the intensity and frequency of the worry are always out of proportion to the actual likelihood of the feared events happening.

In addition to frequent, hard-to-control worry, generalized anxiety disorder involves having at least three of the following six symptoms (with some symptoms present more days than not over the past six months):

- Tension—feeling keyed up

- Being easily fatigued

- Difficulty concentrating

- Restlessness

- Irritability

- Muscle tightness

- Difficulties with sleep

- Difficulty controlling worrying

Generalized anxiety disorder is frequently associated with physical symptoms such as tension headaches, irritable bowel syndrome, high blood pressure, insomnia, and even osteoporosis. However, the presence of any or all of these physical problems does not necessarily imply a diagnosis of generalized anxiety disorder, which is based primarily on the presence of ongoing worry.

You are likely to receive a diagnosis of generalized anxiety disorder if your worry and associated symptoms cause you significant distress and/or interfere with your ability to function occupationally, socially, or in other important areas.

If a doctor tells you that you suffer from generalized anxiety disorder, he or she has probably ruled out possible medical causes of chronic anxiety, such as hyperventilation, thyroid problems, or drug-induced anxiety (alcohol or benzodiazepine withdrawal). Generalized anxiety disorder often occurs together with depression, a condition sometimes referred to as "mixed anxiety-depressive disorder." In such instances, a careful history will usually reveal which disorder—the generalized anxiety or the depression—came first.

Generalized anxiety disorder can develop at any age. In children and adolescents, the focus of worry often tends to be on performance in school or sports events. In adults, the focus can vary but is usually a common theme like finances, personal relationships, health, or job responsibilities. At any given time, about 4 percent of adults experience generalized anxiety disorder; a total of 9 percent experience it over their entire life span. Women are approximately twice as likely to experience the disorder as men (3.4 percent versus 1.9 percent). Incidence is highest for persons aged thirty to sixty and tends to decline later in life. People of European descent are more likely to develop GAD than those of non-European descent.

Although there are no specific phobias associated with generalized anxiety disorder, one view propounded by Aaron Beck and Gary Emery (2005) suggests that the disorder is sustained by "basic fears" of a broader nature than specific phobias, such as:

- Fear of losing control

- Fear of not being able to cope

- Fear of failure

- Fear of rejection or abandonment

- Fear of death and disease

Generalized anxiety disorder can be aggravated by any stressful situation that elicits these fears, such as increased demands for performance, intensified marital conflict, physical illness, or *any situation that heightens your perception of danger or threat.*

The underlying causes of generalized anxiety disorder are unknown. It is likely to involve a combination of heredity, neurobiology, and predisposing childhood experiences, such as excessive parental expectations, parental abandonment and rejection, or parents modeling worry behavior. Cumulative stress in adolescence or adulthood triggers the onset of GAD based on these predisposing causes. A more complete discussion of generalized anxiety disorder and its treatment may be found in chapter 10, Overcoming Worry.

## Current Treatment

*Relaxation training.* Abdominal breathing and deep relaxation techniques are practiced on a regular basis to directly reduce anxiety. A physical exercise program may also be included in the treatment. (See chapters 4 and 5.)

*Cognitive therapy.* Fearful self-talk underlying specific worry themes is identified, challenged, and replaced with more realistic thinking. When you worry, you overestimate the odds of something negative happening and underestimate your ability to cope if something bad does, in fact, happen. Cognitive therapy aims to correct both types of distorted thinking. You would also work on changing negative beliefs, or "metabeliefs," about worry itself. These include both beliefs that worry will help you avoid something negative, such as "If I worry about it, it won't happen," and fearful beliefs about worry itself, such as "My worries are uncontrollable" or "I'll go crazy from worrying." Realistic self-statements and constructive beliefs are consistently practiced and internalized over time.

*Worry exposure.* In worry exposure, you do repeated and prolonged exposure to fearful images (your worst-case scenarios) of what you're worried about. In these images, you include strategies you would use to reduce anxiety and cope with the situation.

*Reducing worry behaviors.* You identify overly cautious "safety behaviors" that tend to reinforce worrying. For example, if you tend to call your spouse or child several times a day to check on them, you would reduce the frequency of this behavior.

*Problem solving.* This means taking systematic action to solve the problem you're worried about. In short, you focus on solutions to the problem that worries you instead of the worry itself. If there is no practical solution, you work on changing your attitude toward the situation—that is, learning to accept what you can't change.

*Disruption.* A variety of disruption techniques can be helpful for worries that do not lend themselves easily to cognitive therapy or problem solving. Common disruptive activities include talking to a friend, journaling, gardening, exercise, puzzle solving, arts and crafts, or cooking. Note that these activities are practiced with the attitude of proactively *disrupting* the worry, rather than fleeing or escaping it through distraction.

*Medication.* For moderate to severe cases of generalized anxiety disorder, SSRI medications such as Zoloft, Luvox, Lexapro, or Celexa may be used. The serotonin-norepinephrine reuptake inhibitor (SNRI) medications such as Effexor and Pristiq have also been found to be effective in treating generalized anxiety disorder. Another medication, Buspar, has been used for many years to treat worry and generalized anxiety. It is still occasionally used as a first-line medication treatment for GAD. Buspar may sometimes be combined with an SSRI medication to enhance the SSRI's effectiveness. Benzodiazepines such as Xanax, Ativan, and Klonopin are often used to treat GAD, though some psychiatrists are wary because of their potential for tolerance, dependence, and abuse. Neurontin (gabapentin), a mood stabilizer that has an anxiety-reducing effect, has also been used to treat GAD. (More information about medications can be found in chapter 18.)

*Mindfulness practice.* Mindfulness is an attitude of simply witnessing the ongoing stream of your thoughts and feelings in the present moment without judgment. It originated in Buddhist meditation practice but is now being used as a common treatment for stress, depression, and generalized anxiety. (For further information about mindfulness practice, see chapter 19.)

*Lifestyle and personality changes.* Such changes are basically similar to the methods described for panic disorder: stress management, increased downtime, regular exercise, eliminating stimulants and sweets from your diet, resolving interpersonal conflicts, and changing attitudes toward perfectionism, an excessive need to please others, or the excessive need to control.

Please note that a detailed discussion of strategies and techniques for overcoming worry may be found in chapter 10, Overcoming Worry.

## Obsessive-Compulsive Disorder

In the *DSM-5* formulation of psychiatric disorders, obsessive-compulsive disorder (OCD) is described in a separate chapter of its own apart from other anxiety disorders. It is listed with other *OC spectrum disorders* such as body dysmorphic disorder (distorted perception of one's body), trichotillomania (hair-pulling disorder), hoarding disorder, excoriation (skin-picking disorder), and substance/medication-induced obsessive-compulsive disorder. More will be said about these disorders in the next section. The placement of obsessive-compulsive disorder (as well as OCD spectrum disorders) in a chapter of its own is based on certain neurobiological differences in the causes of OCD from other anxiety disorders.

Some people naturally tend to be more neat, tidy, and orderly than others. These traits can be useful in many situations, both at work and at home. In obsessive-compulsive disorder, however, they are carried to an extreme and disruptive degree. Obsessive-compulsive people can spend many hours cleaning, tidying, checking, or ordering, to the point that these activities interfere with the rest of the business of their lives.

*Obsessions* are recurring ideas, thoughts, images, or impulses that seem senseless but nonetheless continue to intrude into your mind. Common examples include recurring images of violence, thoughts of doing violence to someone else, fears of leaving on lights or your stove or perhaps leaving your door unlocked, or fears of contamination by germs from touching doorknobs, light switches, toilets, and many other things. You recognize that these thoughts or fears are irrational and you try to suppress them, but they continue to intrude into your mind for hours, days, weeks, or longer. These thoughts or images are not excessive worries about real-life problems and are usually unrelated to any real-life problems.

*Compulsions* are behaviors or rituals that you perform to dispel the anxiety brought up by obsessions. For example, you may wash your hands numerous times to dispel a fear of being contaminated, check the stove again and again to see if it is turned off, order and arrange things in a set way, or look continually in your rearview mirror while driving to assuage anxiety about having hit somebody. You realize that these rituals are unreasonable, yet you feel compelled to perform them to ward off the anxiety associated with your particular obsession. The conflict between your wish to be free of the compulsive ritual and the irresistible desire to perform it is a source of anxiety, shame, and even despair. Eventually, you may cease struggling with your compulsions and give over to them entirely.

Obsessions may occur by themselves, without necessarily being accompanied by compulsions. In fact, about 20 percent of the people who suffer from obsessive-compulsive disorder only have obsessions, and these often center around fears of causing harm to a loved one or having disquieting sexual thoughts.

The most common compulsions include washing, checking, and counting. If you are a washer, you are constantly concerned about avoiding contamination. You avoid touching doorknobs, shaking hands, or coming into contact with any object you associate with germs, filth, or a toxic substance. You can spend literally hours washing hands or showering to reduce anxiety about being contaminated. Women more often have this compulsion than men. Men outnumber women as checkers, however. Doors have to be repeatedly checked to dispel obsessions about being robbed; stoves are repeatedly checked to dispel obsessions about starting a fire; or roads are repeatedly checked to dispel obsessions about having hit someone. In the counting compulsion, you must count up to a certain number or repeat a word a certain number of times to dispel anxiety about harm befalling you or someone else.

Obsessive-compulsive disorder is often accompanied by depression. Preoccupation with obsessions, in fact, tends to wax and wane with depression. This disorder is also typically accompanied by phobic avoidance—such as when a person with an obsession about dirt or germs avoids public restrooms or touching doorknobs. Sometimes avoidance interferes with the person's social or occupational functioning. The World Health Organization ranks OCD among the ten most handicapping conditions across all disorders.

It is very important to realize that as bizarre as obsessive-compulsive behavior may sound, it has nothing to do with "being crazy." You usually recognize the irrationality and senselessness of your thoughts and behavior, and you are very frustrated (as well as depressed) about your inability to control them.

Obsessive-compulsive disorder is different from compulsive behavior disorders such as gambling and overeating. People with compulsive behavior disorders derive some pleasure from their compulsive activities, whereas people with OCD neither want to perform their compulsions (except to reduce fear) nor derive any pleasure from doing so. In the *DSM-5*, there are diagnostic specifiers to indicate the few people who have little or no insight into their OCD beliefs as being illogical.

Obsessive-compulsive disorder used to be considered a rare behavior disturbance. However, recent studies have shown that about *2 to 3 percent of the general population* may suffer, to varying degrees, from obsessive-compulsive disorder. About 1.5 percent actually seek treatment. The reason prevalence rates have been underestimated up to now is that most sufferers have been very reluctant to tell anyone about their problem. Women seem to be affected slightly more than men, but boys are more commonly affected in childhood than girls. The average age of onset of OCD is 19.5 years. Onset of symptoms is typically gradual. Without treatment, remission of OCD in adulthood is low, typically less than 20 percent. With effective treatment, partial to full recovery is possible in up to 60 percent of cases.

The causes of obsessive-compulsive disorder are unclear. There is some evidence that a deficiency of a neurotransmitter substance in the brain known as serotonin, or a disturbance in serotonin metabolism, is associated with the disorder. This is borne out by the fact that many sufferers improve when they take medications that increase brain serotonin levels, such as clomipramine (Anafranil), or specific serotonin-enhancing antidepressants, such as fluoxetine (Prozac), fluvoxamine (Luvox), sertraline (Zoloft), or escitalopram (Lexapro). It also appears that people with OCD have excessive activity in certain parts of the brain, such as the prefrontal cortex and the caudate nucleus. See chapter 2 for a more detailed description of the latest research on the neurobiology of obsessive-compulsive disorder. OCD has a high degree of heritability, with 57 percent of identical twins both showing symptoms of the disorder versus 22 percent of fraternal twins.

## Current Treatment

*Relaxation training.* As with all of the anxiety disorders, abdominal breathing and deep relaxation skills are practiced on a daily basis to help reduce anxiety symptoms. (See chapter 4.)

*Cognitive therapy.* Fearful, superstitious, or guilty thoughts associated with obsessions are identified, challenged, and replaced. For example, the idea "If I have a thought of doing harm to my child, I might act on it" is replaced with "The thought of doing harm is just random noise caused by the OCD. It has no significance. Just having the thought doesn't mean I'll do it." (See chapter 8.)

*Exposure and response prevention (ERP).* This technique consists of exposure to situations that aggravate obsessions, followed by enforced prevention from performing rituals or compulsions. For example, if you've been washing your hands every time you touch a doorknob, you'd be instructed to touch doorknobs and either reduce the number of times you wash your hands or refrain from washing at all. Similarly, if you check the door five times whenever you leave your house, you would be required to gradually reduce the number of checks to one. You and your therapist devise a variety of situations, preferably in your home setting. Then you continually practice exposing yourself to these situations and desist from performing the compulsions (response prevention). Usually, your therapist or a support person accompanies you to monitor your compliance in not performing compulsions. When your problem involves obsessions only, without compulsions, any neutralizing thoughts or covert rituals you use to reduce anxiety caused by your obsessions need to be stopped. You would also work on accepting your obsessions without trying to make them go away. (For further information on exposure and response prevention in treating OCD, see the book *Stop Obsessing: How to Overcome Your Obsessions and Compulsions* by Edna Foa and Reid Wilson, or *The OCD Workbook* by Bruce Hyman and Cherry Pedrick.)

*Medication.* Medications such as Anafranil and the SSRI medications, including Prozac, Luvox, Lexapro, Celexa, and Zoloft, help about 60 to 70 percent of those with OCD. SNRIs such as Effexor and Cymbalta may also be used. Long-term use of medication is fairly common with OCD, although in some cases the cognitive and exposure/response prevention strategies described above may suffice. Effective doses of SSRI or SNRI medications are usually higher for OCD than for other anxiety disorders, and benefits from these medications tend to appear only after two to three months at higher doses. Low doses of antipsychotic medications such as Zyprexa and Risperdal have been found to be useful adjuncts in the treatment of OCD for some people, which indicates that part of the brain mechanisms underlying OCD involve the role of dopamine receptors. The use of SSRI or SNRI medications is often part of the normal treatment protocol for OCD. It is necessary to take the medication long term, as discontinuation often results in a return of the original OCD symptoms.

*Lifestyle and personality changes.* Essentially, the same lifestyle and personality changes described for panic disorder and generalized anxiety disorder apply to OCD.

The strategies presented in this workbook will be helpful if you are affected by obsessive-compulsive disorder. Because OCD is often a severe and debilitating problem, it is highly recommended that you consult a professional who is well versed in the use of behavioral methods, such as exposure and response prevention, as well as in the use of appropriate medications. This workbook can complement behavioral and pharmacological treatment approaches.

## Obsessive-Compulsive Spectrum Disorders

OC spectrum disorders share commonalities in their neurobiological basis with OCD. (See chapter 2 for details on the neurobiology of OCD.) The OC spectrum disorders vary in their manifestation. These are the most common OC spectrum disorders:

**Body dysmorphic disorder:** a preoccupation with perceived flaws or defects in physical appearance

**Excoriation:** recurrent skin picking (resulting in lesions) with repeated attempts to stop

**Hoarding disorder:** a difficulty with discarding possessions that results in significant clutter in one's personal living area

**Trichotillomania:** a recurrent pulling out of one's hair (resulting in noticeable hair loss) with repeated attempts to decrease or stop pulling

**Hypochondriasis:** a preoccupation about having a serious illness with excessive attention to bodily symptoms that are taken as evidence of that illness

OC spectrum disorders have become a specialty area of their own and are typically treated by therapists who specialize in OCD, and who adopt exposure and response prevention techniques to the specific OC spectrum disorder involved.

Several other OCD-related disorders are mentioned in the full *DSM-5* chapter on OCD. These include instances where OCD or OC spectrum disorders can be directly attributed to a medical condition, or appear to be manifestations of substance-induced intoxication or withdrawal symptoms.

# Trauma- and Stressor-Related Disorders

As is the case with obsessive-compulsive disorder, *DSM-5* presents post-traumatic stress disorder (PTSD) in a chapter of its own. The chapter, entitled "Trauma- and Stressor-Related Disorders," includes several other stress-related problems. This new chapter unifies all psychiatric disorders thought to arise in response to a traumatic or highly stressful event (or events). In addition to post-traumatic stress disorder, *acute stress disorder* refers to the same constellation of symptoms as PTSD (including intrusive memories of the trauma, distressing dreams or nightmares, flashbacks, and dissociative symptoms such as depersonalization), except that these symptoms are apparent *three days to one month* following the initial stressor. When these symptoms persist *past one month*, a diagnosis of post-traumatic stress disorder is deemed appropriate.

The *DSM-5* chapter also includes the diagnostic category of *adjustment disorders*. The distinguishing characteristic of adjustment disorders is that they consist of a group of maladaptive symptoms following within three months of a significant life stressor. However, the symptoms are not in the same range or severity as PTSD symptoms, yet they do include marked distress out of proportion to the severity of the instigating stressor and impairment of social or occupational functioning. Adjustment disorders do not include dissociative symptoms such as depersonalization and derealization (see below), but they are specified in *DSM-5* according to whether they include anxiety, depression, or mixed anxiety and depression.

Two other disorders affecting children under five years of age are mentioned in the chapter. *Reactive attachment disorder* constitutes a pattern showing severe social withdrawal, and the child's apparent lack of capacity to seek or respond to comfort when distressed. In contrast, *disinhibited social engagement disorder* reflects a pattern of behavior where the child approaches unfamiliar adults and fails to show normal social inhibition or reticence in doing so.

## *Post-Traumatic Stress Disorder*

The essential feature of post-traumatic stress disorder (PTSD) is the development of disabling psychological symptoms following a traumatic event. It was first identified during World War I, when soldiers were observed to suffer chronic anxiety, nightmares, and flashbacks for weeks, months, or even years following combat. This condition came to be known as "shell shock."

Post-traumatic stress disorder can occur in anyone in the wake of a severe trauma outside the normal range of human experience. These are traumas that would produce intense fear, terror, and feelings of helplessness in anyone and include natural disasters, such as fires, earthquakes or tornadoes; serious accidents like car, train, or plane crashes; and rape, assault, or other violent crimes against you or your immediate family. It appears that the symptoms are more intense and longer lasting when the trauma is personal, as in rape or other violent crimes. *Observation* of someone else suffering a severe trauma can be sufficient to induce post-traumatic stress disorder. Even learning that a traumatic event has occurred to a close family member or significant other can be a source of trauma.

Among the variety of symptoms that can occur with post-traumatic stress disorder, the following nine are particularly common:

- Repetitive, distressing thoughts about the event, often intrusive and unwanted

- Nightmares related to the event

- Flashbacks so intense that you feel or act as though the trauma were occurring all over again

- An attempt to avoid thoughts or feelings associated with the trauma

- An attempt to avoid activities or external situations associated with the trauma—such as developing a phobia about driving after you have been in an auto accident

- Emotional numbness—being out of touch with your feelings

- Losing interest in activities that used to give you pleasure

- Persistent symptoms of increased anxiety, such as difficulty falling or staying asleep, difficulty concentrating, startling easily, or irritability and outbursts of anger

- Exaggerated negative beliefs such as "I'm ruined" or "Nobody can be trusted"

For you to receive a diagnosis of post-traumatic stress disorder, these symptoms need to have persisted for at least one month (with less than one month's duration, the appropriate diagnosis is acute stress disorder). In addition, the disturbance must be causing you significant distress, interfering with social, vocational, or other important areas of your life. In *DSM-5*, PTSD can be diagnosed on the basis of the above symptom profile, or with the addition of *dissociative symptoms* such as depersonalization or derealization. *Depersonalization* is a sense of detachment from yourself, as though you are an outside observer of your own mental processes or body. *Derealization* is the perception of unreality, with your entire surroundings appearing unreal, dreamlike, or distant.

If you suffer from post-traumatic stress disorder, you tend to be anxious and depressed. Sometimes you will find yourself acting impulsively, suddenly changing residence or going on a trip with hardly any plans. If you have been through a trauma where others around you died, you may suffer from guilt about having survived.

Post-traumatic stress disorder can occur at any age and affects about 9 percent of the population at some time in their life. Children with the disorder tend not to relive the trauma consciously but continually reenact it in their play or in distressing dreams. The highest rates of PTSD are found among survivors of rape, military combat, or ethnically motivated confinement and/or persecution. The onset of full-spectrum PTSD can be delayed by months or even years; however, at least some symptoms are typically evident one week to three months following the traumatic event.

There is good evidence that susceptibility to post-traumatic stress disorder has a hereditary component. A recent study bringing together more than twenty thousand people participating in eleven multiethnic studies around the world builds a strong case for the role of genetics in PTSD (Duncan, Ratanatharathorn, et al. 2017). Also, for identical twins exposed to combat in Vietnam, if one identical twin developed the disorder, the odds were higher that the other identical twin would, as compared with fraternal twins.

## Current Treatment

Treatment for post-traumatic stress disorder is complex and multifaceted. Many of the strategies described above for other anxiety disorders are helpful, but additional techniques may be used as well.

*Relaxation training.* Abdominal breathing and progressive muscle relaxation techniques are practiced to better control anxiety symptoms. (See chapter 4.)

*Cognitive therapy.* Fearful or depressed thinking is identified, challenged, and replaced with more productive thinking. For example, guilt about having been responsible for the trauma—or having survived when someone you loved did not—would be challenged. You would reinforce yourself with supportive, constructive thoughts, such as "What happened was horrible, and I accept that there is nothing I could have done to prevent it. I'm learning now that I can go on." (See chapters 8 and 9.)

*Exposure therapy.* A therapist or support person helps you confront fearful situations that you want to avoid because they trigger strong anxiety. In imaginal exposure, you would repeatedly go back over fearful memories of events, objects, and persons associated with the original trauma. In real-life exposure, you would return to the actual situation where the trauma occurred. For example, if you were assaulted in an elevator, you would return to the elevator several times. Repeated exposure helps you understand that the fearful situation is no longer dangerous. (See chapter 7.)

*Imagery rescripting.* In imagery rescripting, a therapist asks you to revisualize a situation that was traumatic as a child or adolescent but from the standpoint of being an empowered, strong adult, capable of handling the situation. For example, if you were physically abused as a child, you would imagine going back to the original situation as your adult self rather than as a child, and then confronting the abuser and dealing with the abuser in a strong, empowered way. An additional phase might include going back to the situation as a strong adult accompanied by your child self, with the adult confronting the abuser on behalf of the child. Imagery rescripting is a common technique used with PTSD and has also been used successfully with social phobias that are based on childhood and adolescent traumatic social experiences (Wild and Clark 2011).

*Medication.* SSRI medications, such as Zoloft, Luvox, Prozac, or Celexa, are often helpful in alleviating PTSD symptoms. Especially when these symptoms are severe and long lasting, a course of medication lasting one or two years might be utilized. Tranquilizers such as Xanax or Klonopin might be used on a more short-term basis. (See chapter 18.)

*Support groups.* Support groups are particularly helpful in enabling PTSD victims to realize that they are not alone. Support groups for rape or crime survivors are often available in larger metropolitan areas. Considerable research indicates that social support offers protective effects in both avoiding and recovering from the disorder.

*EMDR.* Eye movement desensitization and reprocessing (EMDR) is often helpful in enabling PTSD victims to retrieve and work through memories of the original traumatic incident. The technique may be used to accelerate the course of therapy and/or overcome resistance to exposure. Studies show EMDR to be equally effective as cognitive behavioral therapy and exposure with various anxiety disorders and a first-line treatment for PTSD. Please go to the website for the EMDR Institute at emdr.com for further information.

For a comprehensive summary of treatment for PTSD, see *The PTSD Workbook,* 3rd ed., by Mary Beth Williams and Soili Poijula.

It's important to add that the treatment for any anxiety disorder may include marital or family therapy. Interpersonal problems with spouses and/or family may serve to perpetuate anxiety and undermine the success of treatment until these issues are addressed. Family therapy is also useful in educating family members about how to understand, support, and, in some cases, set limits with the family member suffering with the anxiety disorder.

# Additional Anxiety Disorders in the *DSM-5*

Two additional anxiety disorders, which were originally added to *DSM-IV,* were retained in *DSM-5.*

### Anxiety Disorder Due to Another Medical Condition

This diagnostic category is reserved for situations in which significant anxiety (in the form of either panic attacks or generalized anxiety) is a direct physiological effect of a specific medical condition. Numerous types of medical conditions can cause anxiety, including endocrine conditions (hyper- and hypothyroidism, pheochromocytoma, hypoglycemia), cardiovascular conditions (congestive heart failure, pulmonary embolism), metabolic conditions (vitamin $B_{12}$ deficiency, porphyria), and neurological conditions (vestibular problems, encephalitis). For a more complete listing, see the section in chapter 2 entitled "Medical Conditions That Can Cause Panic Attacks or Anxiety."

### Substance-Induced Anxiety Disorder

This category is used when generalized anxiety or panic attacks are determined to be the direct physiological effect of a substance, whether a drug of abuse, a medication, or a toxin exposure. The anxiety may be a result either of exposure to the substance or of withdrawal from it. For example, if you had no previous history of an anxiety disorder, then suddenly developed panic attacks as a result of withdrawing too quickly from a medication, you would receive this diagnosis.

## Self-Diagnosis Questionnaire

The following questionnaire is designed to help you identify which particular anxiety disorder you may be dealing with. It is based on the official classification of anxiety disorders used by mental health professionals and known as the *DSM-5* (*Diagnostic and Statistical Manual of Mental Disorders*, Fifth Edition).

1.  Do you have spontaneous anxiety attacks that come out of the blue? (Only answer "yes" if you do *not* have any phobias.)   Yes _____ No _____

2.  Have you had at least one such attack in the last month?   Yes _____ No _____

3.  If you had an anxiety attack in the last month, did you worry about having another one? Or did you worry about the implications of your attack for your physical or mental health? Yes _____ No _____

4.  In your worst experience with anxiety, did you have four or more of the following symptoms?

    ☐  Shortness of breath or a smothering sensation

    ☐  Dizziness, a light-headed or unsteady feeling

    ☐  Heart palpitations or rapid heartbeat

    ☐  Trembling or shaking

    ☐  Sweating

    ☐  Choking

    ☐  Nausea or abdominal distress

    ☐  Feelings of being detached or out of touch with your body

    ☐  Numbness or tingling sensations

    ☐  Flushes or chills

    ☐  Chest pain or discomfort

    ☐  Fear of dying

    ☐  Fear of going crazy or doing something out of control

    If your answers to 1, 2, 3, and 4 were yes, stop. You've met the conditions for **panic disorder**.

    If your answer to 1 was yes, but your anxiety reaction involved three or fewer of the symptoms listed under 4, you're experiencing what are called *limited-symptom attacks*, but do not have full-blown panic disorder.

    If you have panic attacks *and* phobias, go on.

5. Does fear of having panic attacks cause you to avoid going into certain situations? Yes _____ No _____

> If your answer to 5 was yes, stop. It is likely that you are dealing with **agoraphobia**. See question 6 to determine the extent of your agoraphobia.

6. Which of the following situations do you avoid because you are afraid of panicking?

   ☐ Going far away from home

   ☐ Shopping in a grocery store

   ☐ Standing in a grocery store line

   ☐ Going to department stores

   ☐ Going to shopping malls

   ☐ Driving on freeways

   ☐ Driving on surface streets far from home

   ☐ Driving anywhere by yourself

   ☐ Using public transportation (buses, trains, etc.)

   ☐ Going over bridges (whether you're the driver or the passenger)

   ☐ Going through tunnels (as driver or passenger)

   ☐ Flying in planes

   ☐ Riding in elevators

   ☐ Being in high places

   ☐ Going to a dentist's or doctor's office

   ☐ Sitting in a barber's or beautician's chair

   ☐ Eating in restaurants

   ☐ Going to work

   ☐ Being too far from a safe person or safe place

   ☐ Being alone

   ☐ Going outside your house

   ☐ Other

   > The number of situations you checked above indicates the extent of your agoraphobia and the degree to which it limits your activity.
   >
   > If your answer to 5 was no, but you do have phobias, go on.

7. Do you avoid certain situations *not* primarily because you are afraid of panicking but because you're afraid of being embarrassed or negatively evaluated by other people (which could subsequently lead you to panic)?   Yes _____ No _____

    If your answer to 7 was yes, stop. It's likely that you are dealing with **social phobia**. See question 8 to determine the extent of your social phobia.

8. Which of the following situations do you avoid because of a fear of embarrassing or humiliating yourself?

    □ Sitting in any kind of group (for example, at work, in school classrooms, in social organizations, or in self-help groups)

    □ Giving a talk or presentation before a small group of people

    □ Giving a talk or presentation before a large group of people

    □ Parties and social functions

    □ Using public restrooms

    □ Eating in front of others

    □ Writing or signing your name in the presence of others

    □ Dating

    □ Any situation in which you might say something foolish

    □ Other

    The number of situations you checked indicates the extent to which social phobia limits your activities.

    If your answers to questions 5 and 7 were no, but you have other phobias, continue.

9. Do you fear and avoid any one (or more than one) of the following?

    □ Insects or animals, such as spiders, bees, snakes, rats, bats, or dogs

    □ Heights (high floors in buildings, tops of hills or mountains, high-level bridges)

    □ Driving

    □ Tunnels

    □ Bridges

    □ Elevators

    □ Airplanes (flying)

    □ Doctors or dentists

    □ Thunder or lightning

☐   Water

☐   Blood

☐   Injections or medical procedures

☐   Illness such as heart attacks or cancer

☐   Darkness

☐   Other

10. Do you have high degrees of anxiety usually *only* when you have to face one of these situations?   Yes _____ No _____

   If you checked one or more items in 9 and answered yes to 10, stop. It's likely that you're dealing with a **specific phobia**. If not, proceed.

11. Do you feel quite anxious much of the time but do *not* have distinct panic attacks, do *not* have phobias, and do *not* have specific obsessions or compulsions?   Yes _____ No _____

12. Have you been prone to excessive worry for at least the last six months?   Yes _____ No _____

13. Has your anxiety and worry been associated with at least three of the following six symptoms?

   ☐   Tense—feeling keyed up

   ☐   Being easily fatigued

   ☐   Difficulty concentrating or mind going blank

   ☐   Irritability

   ☐   Muscle tension

   ☐   Sleep disturbance (difficulty falling or staying asleep, or restless and unsatisfying sleep)

   If your answers to 11, 12, and 13 were yes, stop. It's likely that you're dealing with **generalized anxiety disorder**. If you answered yes to 11 but no to 12 or 13, you're dealing with an anxiety condition that is not severe enough to qualify as generalized anxiety disorder.

14. Do you have recurring intrusive thoughts such as about hurting or harming a close relative, being contaminated with dirt or a toxic substance, fearing you forgot to lock your door or turn off an appliance, or an unpleasant fantasy of catastrophe? (You recognize that these thoughts are irrational, but you can't keep them from coming into your mind.)   Yes _____ No _____

15. Do you perform ritualistic actions such as washing your hands, checking, or counting to relieve anxiety over irrational fears that enter your mind?   Yes _____ No _____

   If you answered yes to 14 but no to 15, you are probably dealing with **obsessive-compulsive disorder**, but have obsessions only.

   If you answered yes to 14 and 15, you're probably dealing with **obsessive-compulsive disorder**, with both obsessions and compulsions.

If you answered no to 14 and 15 and most or all of the preceding questions, but you still have anxiety or anxiety-related symptoms, you may be dealing with post-traumatic stress disorder or a nonspecific anxiety condition. Use the section in this chapter on post-traumatic stress disorder to determine whether your symptoms fit this category.

## Co-Occurrence of Anxiety Disorders

In the years that have passed since the first edition of *The Anxiety & Phobia Workbook* was published, it has become increasingly apparent that many people are dealing with more than one anxiety disorder. For example, one survey of people with panic disorder found that 15 to 30 percent also have social phobia, 10 to 20 percent have a specific phobia, 25 percent have generalized anxiety disorder, and 8 to 10 percent have obsessive-compulsive disorder. People with agoraphobia quite often have social phobias and/or obsessive-compulsive difficulties. If you find that your particular condition fits the description for more than one anxiety disorder, you are not alone.

## Further Reading

### *Panic Disorder*

Barlow, David, and Michelle Craske. *Mastery of Your Anxiety and Panic: Workbook.* 4th ed. New York: Oxford University Press, 2006.

Beckfield, Denise F. *Master Your Panic and Take Back Your Life.* 3rd ed. Atascadero, CA: Impact Publishers, 2004.

Isensee, B., H. U. Wittchen, M. Stein, M. Hofler, and R. Leib. 2003. "Smoking Increases the Risk of Panic: Findings from a Prospective Community Study." *Archives of General Psychiatry* 60(7): 692–700.

Weekes, Claire. *Hope and Help for Your Nerves.* New York: Signet, 1990.

Wilson, Reid. *Don't Panic: Taking Control of Anxiety Attacks.* 3rd ed. New York: Collins Living/ HarperCollins, 2009.

Zuercher-White, Elke. *An End to Panic.* 2nd ed. Oakland, CA: New Harbinger Publications, 1998.

### *Agoraphobia*

Beckfield, Denise F. *Master Your Panic and Take Back Your Life.* 3rd ed. Atascadero, CA: Impact Publishers, 2004.

Feninger, Mani. *Journey from Anxiety to Freedom.* New York: Three Rivers Press, 1997.

Pollard, C. Alec, and Elke Zuercher-White. *The Agoraphobia Workbook.* Oakland, CA: New Harbinger Publications, 2003.

## Social Phobia

Antony, Martin, and Richard Swinson. *The Shyness & Social Anxiety Workbook*. 3rd ed. Oakland, CA: New Harbinger Publications, 2017.

Butler, Gillian. *Overcoming Social Anxiety and Shyness: A Self-Help Guide Using Cognitive Behavioral Techniques*. New York: Basic Books, 2008.

Kendler, K., L. Karkowski, and C. Prescott. 1999. "Fears and Phobias: Reliability and Heritability." *Psychological Medicine* 29(3): 539–53.

Rapee, Ronald. *Overcoming Shyness and Social Phobia*. Lanham, MD: Rowan & Littlefield Publishers, 1998.

Schneier, Franklin, and Lawrence Welkowitz. *The Hidden Face of Shyness: Understanding and Overcoming Social Anxiety*. New York: Avon Books, 1997.

## Specific Phobia

Bourne, Edmund J. *Overcoming Specific Phobia: Therapist Protocol and Client Manual* (two-book set). Oakland, CA: New Harbinger Publications, 1998.

Brown, Duane. *Flying Without Fear*. 2nd ed. Oakland, CA: New Harbinger Publications, 2009.

Rothbaum, Barbara Olson. "Virtual Reality Exposure Therapy," 227–44. In *Pathological Anxiety*, edited by Barbara Olson Rothbaum. New York: Guilford Press, 2006.

## Generalized Anxiety Disorder

Beck, Aaron, and Gary Emery et al. *Anxiety Disorders and Phobias: A Cognitive Perspective*. New York: Basic Books, 2005.

Copeland, Mary Ellen. *The Worry Control Workbook*. Oakland, CA: New Harbinger Publications, 1998.

Orsillo, Susan M., and Lizabeth Roemer. *The Mindful Way Through Anxiety: Break Free from Chronic Worry and Reclaim Your Life*. New York: Guilford Press, 2011.

White, John. *Overcoming Generalized Anxiety Disorder: Therapist Protocol and Client Manual*. Oakland, CA: New Harbinger Publications, 1999.

## Obsessive-Compulsive Disorder

Foa, Edna, and Reid Wilson. *Stop Obsessing: How to Overcome Your Obsessions and Compulsions*. Rev. ed. New York: Bantam Books, 2001.

Frost, Randy, and Gail Steketee. *Stuff: Compulsive Hoarding and the Meaning of Things.* New York: Mariner Books/Houghton Mifflin Harcourt, 2011.

Hyman, Bruce, and Troy Dufrene. *Coping with OCD: Practical Strategies for Living Well with Obsessive-Compulsive Disorder.* Oakland, CA: New Harbinger Publications, 2008.

———, and Cherry Pedrick. *The OCD Workbook.* 3rd ed. Oakland, CA: New Harbinger Publications, 2010.

Schwartz, Jeffrey M. *Brain Lock: Free Yourself from Obsessive-Compulsive Behavior.* New York: ReganBooks, 1996.

## Post-Traumatic Stress Disorder

Allen, Jon G. *Coping with Trauma: Hope Through Understanding.* 2nd ed. Washington, DC: American Psychiatric Association Publishing, 2005.

Duncan, Laramie E., Andrew Ratanatharathorn, et al. April 2017. "Largest GWAS (N=20,070) Yields Genetic Overlap with Schizophrenia and Sex Differences in Heritability." *Molecular Psychiatry,* 23: 666–73.

England, Diane. *The Post-Traumatic Stress Disorder Relationship.* Avon, MA: Adams Media, 2009.

Matsakis, Aphrodite. *Trust After Trauma: A Guide to Relationships for Survivors and Those Who Love Them.* Oakland, CA: New Harbinger Publications, 1998.

Schiraldi, Glenn. *The Post-Traumatic Stress Disorder Sourcebook: A Guide to Healing, Recovery, and Growth.* Revised and expanded 2nd ed. New York: McGraw-Hill, 2016.

Seidler, G. H., and F. E. Wagner. 2006. "Comparing the Efficacy of EMDR and Trauma-Focused Cognitive Behavioral Therapy in the Treatment of PTSD: A Meta-analytic Study." *Psychological Medicine* 36(11): 1515–22.

Wild, Jennifer, and David M. Clark. 2011. "Imagery Rescripting of Early Traumatic Memories in Social Phobia." *Cognitive Behavioral Practice* 18(4): 433–43.

Williams, Mary Beth, and Soili Poijula. *The PTSD Workbook: Simple, Effective Techniques for Overcoming Traumatic Stress Symptoms.* 3rd ed. Oakland, CA: New Harbinger Publications, 2016.

## Children's Anxiety Disorders

Spencer, Elizabeth D., Robert Dupont, and Caroline Dupont. *The Anxiety Cure for Kids: A Guide for Parents and Children.* Hoboken, NJ: Wiley, 2003.

Wood, Jeffrey J., and Bryce McLeod. *Child Anxiety Disorders: A Family-Based Treatment Manual for Practitioners.* New York: Norton, 2008.

# 2

# Major Causes of Anxiety Disorders

If you are dealing with one of the anxiety disorders, you are likely to be concerned with the causes of your problem. You probably ask yourself, "Why do I have panic attacks? Is it something hereditary, or is it the way I was brought up? What causes phobias to develop? Why am I afraid of something I know isn't dangerous? What causes obsessions and compulsions?"

The symptoms of anxiety disorders often seem irrational and inexplicable: it is only natural to raise the question "Why?" But before considering in detail the various causes of anxiety disorders, there are two general points you should bear in mind. First, although learning about the causes of anxiety disorders can give you insight into how these problems develop, such knowledge is not necessary to overcome your particular difficulty. The various strategies for overcoming anxiety disorders presented in this workbook—such as relaxation, exercise, exposure, changing self-talk and mistaken beliefs, or dealing with feelings—do not depend on a knowledge of underlying causes to be effective. However interesting the information in this chapter may be, it is not necessarily what "cures." Second, be wary of the notion that there is one primary cause, or type of cause, for any of the anxiety disorders. Whether you are dealing with panic attacks, social phobia, generalized anxiety, or obsessive-compulsive disorder, recognize that there is no one cause that, if removed, would eliminate the problem. Anxiety problems are brought about by a variety of causes operating on numerous different levels: heredity, biology, family background and upbringing, conditioning, recent stressors, your self-talk and personal belief system, your ability to express feelings, and so on. The range of chapters in this book indicates the many different levels on which you can understand the causes of and the means of recovering from anxiety disorders.

Some experts in the field of anxiety disorders propose "single-cause" theories. Such theories tend to greatly oversimplify anxiety disorders and are susceptible to one of two mistaken lines of reasoning: the *biological fallacy* and the *psychological fallacy*. The biological fallacy assumes that a particular type of anxiety disorder is caused *solely* by some biological or physiological imbalance in the brain or body. For example, there has recently been a tendency to reduce the causation of panic disorder, as well as obsessive-compulsive disorder, to a strictly biological level. Panic disorder is viewed as arising from a dysfunction in parts of the brain, such as the *amygdala* and the *locus coeruleus*. Obsessive-compulsive disorder is thought to be caused by a deficiency in a particular neurotransmitter substance in the brain called *serotonin*—or a dysregulation in the serotonin system of neurons in the brain. (A *neurotransmitter* is a chemical substance that allows nerve impulses to be transmitted from one nerve cell to another.)

It is helpful to know that there may be physiological dysfunctions involved in panic disorder and obsessive-compulsive disorder. This certainly has implications for treatment of these problems. But this does not mean that panic attacks and obsessive-compulsive disorder are physiological disturbances only. The question remains: *What caused the physiological disturbance itself?*

Perhaps chronic stress due to psychological conflict causes the amygdala and locus coeruleus to malfunction in panic disorder. Or perhaps chronically suppressed anger sets up a disturbance in brain serotonin levels that is a contributing cause of obsessive-compulsive disorder. Psychological conflicts and repressed anger may, in turn, have been caused by a person's upbringing. Because any particular physiological disturbance may have originally been set up by stress or other psychological factors, it is a fallacy to assume that anxiety disorders are solely (or even primarily) caused by physiological imbalances.

The psychological fallacy makes the same kind of mistake in the opposite direction. It assumes that, say, social phobia or generalized anxiety disorder is caused by having grown up with parents who neglected, abandoned, or abused you, resulting in a deep-seated sense of insecurity or shame that causes your current phobic avoidance and anxiety as an adult. While it may be true that your family background *contributed* in an important way to your current problems, is it reasonable to assume that this is the *only* cause? Again, not really. To do so overlooks the possible contributions of hereditary and biological factors. After all, not all children who grow up in dysfunctional families develop anxiety disorders. It is more plausible to assume that your problem is a result of *both* 1) a hereditary predisposition toward anxiety (and possibly phobia) *and* 2) early childhood conditions that fostered a sense of shame and/or insecurity.

In sum, the idea that your particular difficulties are *just* a physiological disturbance or *just* a psychological disturbance neglects the fact that nature and nurture are interactive. Biological disturbances may be "set up" by stress or psychological factors; psychological problems, in turn, may be influenced by inborn biological disturbances. There is simply no way to say which came first or which is the so-called "ultimate" cause. By the same token, a comprehensive approach to recovery from panic, phobias, or anxiety cannot restrict itself to treating physiological or psychological causes in isolation. A variety of strategies dealing with several different levels, including biological, behavioral, emotional, mental, interpersonal, and even spiritual factors, is necessary for a full and lasting recovery. This multidimensional approach to recovery is discussed in the next chapter and assumed throughout this book.

The causes of anxiety disorders vary not only according to the level at which they occur but also according to the time period over which they operate. Some are *predisposing causes*, which set you up from birth or childhood to develop panic or anxiety later on. Some are *recent* or *short-term* causes—circumstances that *trigger* the onset of, say, panic attacks or agoraphobia. Others are *maintaining* causes—factors in your current lifestyle, attitudes, and behavior that serve to keep anxiety disorders going once they have developed. The remainder of this chapter examines each of these types of causes in more detail. A section on biological causes is included to acquaint you with some of the better-known hypotheses about the role of the brain in causing panic attacks and anxiety.

An outline of the causes of anxiety disorders follows.

## Causes of Anxiety Disorders

### Long-Term Predisposing Causes

1. Heredity

2. Childhood circumstances

- Your parents communicate an overly cautious view of the world.

- Your parents are overly critical and set excessively high standards.

- Emotional insecurity and dependence.

- Your parents suppress your expression of feelings and self-assertiveness.

3. Cumulative stress over time

## Biological Causes

1. The physiology of panic

2. Panic attacks

3. Generalized anxiety

4. Obsessive-compulsive disorder

5. Further details about how antidepressant medications work

6. Medical conditions that can cause panic attacks or anxiety

## Short-Term, Triggering Causes

1. Stressors that precipitate panic attacks

- Significant personal loss

- Significant life change

- Stimulants and recreational drugs

2. Conditioning and the origin of phobias

3. Trauma, simple phobias, and post-traumatic stress disorder

## Maintaining Causes

1. Avoidance of phobic situations

2. Reliance on safety behaviors

3. Anxious self-talk

4. Mistaken beliefs

5. Withheld feelings

6. Lack of assertiveness

7. Lack of self-nurturing skills

8. Muscle tension

9. Stimulants and other dietary factors

10. High-stress lifestyle

11. Low self-esteem

12. Lack of meaning or sense of purpose

# Long-Term, Predisposing Causes

## Heredity

Are anxiety disorders inherited? The limited evidence that exists to date would argue that they are—at least in part. For example, it is estimated that 15 to 25 percent of children growing up with at least one agoraphobic parent become agoraphobic themselves, while the rate of agoraphobia in the general population is only 5 percent. This fact in itself doesn't prove that agoraphobia is inherited, however, because it could be argued that children *learn* from their parents to be agoraphobic.

More compelling evidence comes from studies of identical twins who, of course, have exactly the same genetic makeup. If one identical twin has an anxiety disorder, the probability of the other identical twin having an anxiety disorder ranges from 31 to 88 percent, depending on the study you're looking at. By comparison, when fraternal twins (whose genes are no more similar than those of siblings born at different times) are studied, the probability is much lower. If one fraternal twin has an anxiety disorder, the odds of the other having an anxiety disorder range from about 0 to 38 percent—again, depending on the study. Having the same genetic makeup as someone else with phobias or anxiety makes it *more than twice as likely* that you will have a similar problem. Interestingly, the percentages of anxiety disorders for fraternal twins are generally higher than the incidence in the population (about 8 to 10 percent). This would argue that growing up in the same family—having the same parenting—contributes at least something to the development of anxiety disorders. Both nature and nurture seem to have an impact.

What is it that is inherited? Based on what is known at this time, it seems that you don't inherit agoraphobia, social phobia, or even panic attacks specifically from your parents. What is inherited seems to be a *general personality type* that predisposes you to be overly anxious. This is a volatile, excitable, reactive personality that is more easily set off by any slightly threatening stimulus than is the personality of individuals without anxiety disorders. Once you are born with this highly reactive personality, you might develop one or another anxiety disorder, depending on your particular environment and upbringing. For example, whether you develop agoraphobia or social phobia might depend on how much you learned to feel ashamed in situations where you were expected to perform. Whether you develop panic attacks might depend on the nature and degree of stress you're exposed to during adolescence and early adulthood. In short, while heredity might cause you to be born with a more reactive, excitable nervous system, childhood experiences, conditioning, and stress all serve to shape the particular type of anxiety disorder you subsequently develop.

Recent research in the field of behavior genetics has begun to hone in on specific genes associated with anxiety disorders. For example, the seventeenth chromosome (we all have twenty-three) contains a gene known as SERT (serotonin transfer gene), which functions in the manufacture of the brain neurotransmitter serotonin. People with the "short" form of the gene tend to be more predisposed to develop anxiety disorders (as well as mood disorders such as depression), while people with the "long" form of the gene have a degree of protection, in spite of childhood and adult stress, from developing problems with anxiety.

## Childhood Circumstances

What childhood experiences or family environments might predispose you to develop a particular anxiety disorder? Unfortunately, very little research on this topic has been done. Researchers have found that panic attacks and agoraphobia in adulthood are often preceded by separation anxiety disorder in childhood. This is a condition in which children experience anxiety, panic, or somatic symptoms when separated from their parents, as when going to school or even before going to sleep. Later on as adults, these same people experience anxiety when separated from a "safe" person or place. The conditions that might lead to separation anxiety disorder in the first place are matters for speculation.

What follows is a list of childhood circumstances that might predispose you to develop anxiety disorders. The list is based on my own experience with clients over several years. These factors are especially relevant if you are dealing with agoraphobia or social phobia, but may be applicable to other anxiety disorders as well.

- *Your parents communicate an overly cautious view of the world.* Parents of people with phobias either tend to have phobias themselves or are more fearful and anxious than average. Often they are overly concerned about potential dangers to their child. They are likely to say things like "Don't go out in the rain—you'll catch a cold," "Don't watch TV so much. You'll ruin your eyes," or "Be very careful," again and again. The more they communicate a fearful, overcautious attitude toward their child, the more that child comes to view the world as a "dangerous" place. When you learn that the outside world is threatening, you automatically restrict your exploration and risk taking. You grow up with a tendency to worry excessively and be overly concerned with safety.

- *Your parents are overly critical and set excessively high standards.* Children growing up with critical, perfectionist parents are never quite sure of their own acceptability. There is always some doubt about whether you are "good enough," or sufficiently worthy. As a result, you are constantly striving to please your parents and maintain their approval. As an adult, you may be overly eager to please, "look good," and "be nice" at the expense of your true feelings and capacity for assertiveness. Having grown up always feeling insecure, you may become very dependent on a safe person or safe place, and may restrict yourself from entering public or social situations where there is a risk of "losing face." You often come to internalize your parents' values, becoming exceptionally perfectionist and self-critical (as well as critical of others).

- *Emotional insecurity and dependence.* Up to the age of four or five, children are utterly dependent on their parents, especially their primary parent. Any conditions that create insecurity during this time can lead to excessive dependency and clinging later on. Excessive criticism and perfectionist standards on the part of parents seem to be a common source of insecurity for people who later develop anxiety disorders. *However, experiences of neglect, rejection, abandonment through divorce or death, and physical or sexual abuse can also produce the kind of basic insecurity (as well as emotional dependency) that forms a background for anxiety disorders.*

  Growing up in a family in which one or both parents are alcoholic is also a common contributing factor in 20 to 25 percent of the clients I've seen. As described in a number of popular books on the subject, adult children of alcoholics grow up with characteristics such as 1) obsession with control, 2) avoidance of feelings, 3) difficulty trusting others, 4) overresponsibility, 5) all-or-nothing thinking, and 6) excessive eagerness to please, at the expense of their own needs. Although not all adult children of alcoholics develop anxiety disorders, the above characteristics are commonly seen in many people who have problems with panic and/or phobias.

  A common denominator in the background of adult children of alcoholics, adult survivors of other forms of abuse, and most people who develop anxiety disorders is a deep-seated sense of insecurity. Perhaps the degree of insecurity and the way children respond to it will determine whether they later develop a specific type of anxiety disorder—as opposed to, say, an addictive personality or some other behavior disturbance. When children respond to insecurity with *excessive dependency*, the stage is set for overreliance on a safe person or safe place later in life. This is a common background for agoraphobia.

- *Your parents suppress your expression of feelings and self-assertiveness.* Parents not only may foster dependency but may also suppress your innate capacity to express your feelings and assert yourself. For example, as a child you may have been continually reprimanded or punished for speaking out, acting impulsively, or getting angry. Subsequently, you grew up exerting a restrictive, even punitive, attitude toward your own expression of impulses and feelings. If these impulses and feelings are suppressed over a long period of time, their sudden recurrence under stress may produce anxiety or even panic. Frequently, people who learned to bottle up their feelings and self-expression as children are tense, more prone to be anxious, and unable to express themselves as adults. Of course, this form of suppression in childhood can also lead to depression and passivity later on. In both cases, learning to express your feelings and becoming more assertive can have a very beneficial effect.

Reading about the four factors just discussed may have stimulated you to think about what happened in your own childhood. Use the *Family Background Questionnaire* on the next page to further explore what circumstances in your family may have contributed to your own problems with anxiety.

# *Family Background Questionnaire*

Use the following questionnaire to reflect on your childhood. Can you identify what conditions might have contributed to your current problem with anxiety?

1. Did either of your parents suffer from panic attacks or phobias?

2. Did you have a brother, sister, grandparent, or other relative who had panic attacks or phobias?

3. Did either of your parents seem excessively prone to worry?

4. Did either of your parents seem overly concerned about potential dangers that could befall you or other family members?

5. Did your parents encourage exploration of the outside world, or did they cultivate an attitude of caution, suspicion, or distrust?

6. Do you feel that your parents were overly critical or demanding of you? If so, how did you feel in response to this criticism?

   ☐ Put down or diminished      ☐ Ashamed or guilty

   ☐ Hurt or rejected            ☐ Angry or rebellious

7. As a child, did you feel free to express your feelings and impulses? How were feelings dealt with in your family?

   ☐ Openly expressed            ☐ Punished

   ☐ Denied

8. Was it okay for you to cry? How did your parents respond when you cried?

9. Was it okay to express anger? How did your parents respond when you got angry?

10. What was your role in the family? How were you perceived relative to other children in the family?

11. Do you feel that you grew up feeling insecure? Which of the following might have contributed to your insecurity?

    ☐ Excessive criticism by your parents

    ☐ Excessive punishment

    ☐ Your parents made you feel ashamed

    ☐ Your parents made you feel guilty

    ☐ Your parents neglected you

    ☐ One or both parents abandoned you through death or divorce

☐ Physical abuse

☐ Sexual abuse

☐ Parental alcoholism

12. If you grew up insecure, how did you respond to your feelings of insecurity?

☐ By becoming very dependent on your family (Did you have difficulty leaving home?)

☐ By becoming very independent of your family (Did you leave home early?)

☐ By becoming angry or rebellious

## Cumulative Stress over Time

A third contributing factor in the development of anxiety disorders is the influence of *cumulative* stress over time. When stress persists without letup over a period of time, such as several months or years, it tends to accumulate. This sort of stress is more enduring than the normal, temporary stresses of moving, the holiday season, or a short-term financial setback. Cumulative stress can arise from unresolved psychological conflicts lasting over many years. Or it can be due to difficulties in one area of your life—such as problems with your marriage or physical health—that persist over a long period of time. Finally, it may be due to the accretion of a large number of *life events*. Life events include changes in the course of your life that require an adjustment and reordering of your priorities, such as going off to college, changing jobs, getting married or leaving an intimate relationship, moving to a new location, having a baby, or having your children leave home. While one or two life events every year is a common and manageable experience, a series of many of them stretching over one or two years' time can lead to a state of chronic stress and exhaustion.

The concept of life events arose from the work of Dr. Richard Holmes and Dr. Thomas Rahe, who developed an instrument called the *Life Events Survey* (also known as *The Social Readjustment Scale*) to assess the number and severity of life events that occur in a two-year period. They used the survey specifically to predict a person's risk of developing physical disease. However, the survey can also be used as a general measure of cumulative stress. You can get an estimate of your own level of cumulative stress by completing the *Life Events Survey* on the next page.

For many years, it has been known that stress can increase your risk of developing psychosomatic disorders, such as high blood pressure, headaches, or ulcers. Only recently has it been recognized that *psychological disorders* may also be an outcome of cumulative stress. Over time, stress can affect the neuroendocrine regulatory systems of the brain, which play an important role in mood disorders, such as depression and anxiety disorders. Stress is nonspecific in its action; it simply has the greatest impact on the weakest point in your system. If this happens to be your cardiovascular system, you may develop high blood pressure or migraine headaches. If it is the neuroendocrine and neurotransmitter systems of your brain, you will be more subject to developing a behavior disorder such as mood swings, generalized anxiety, or panic disorder. In short, cumulative stress might produce headaches, fatigue, or panic attacks, depending on your particular point of greatest vulnerability. That point of vulnerability may, in turn, be influenced

# Life Events Survey

| Life Event | Average Stress Score |
|---|---|

Death of spouse  100
Divorce 73
Marital separation     65
Jail term     63
Death of close family member     63
Personal injury or illness  53
Marriage     50
Being fired from work     47
Marital problems     45
Retirement  45
Change in health of family member     44
Pregnancy     40
Sexual difficulties     39
Gain of new family member  39
Business readjustment     39
Change in finances     38
Death of close friend 37
Change to different line of work     36
Change in number of arguments with spouse     35
Mortgage or loan for major purchase (such as a home)     31
Foreclosure of mortgage or loan     30
Change in responsibilities at work 29
Son or daughter leaving home     29
Trouble with in-laws  29
Outstanding personal achievement     28
Spouse begins or stops work  26
Beginning or finishing school  26
Change in living conditions     25
Revision of personal habits     24
Trouble with boss     23
Change in work hours or conditions     20
Change in residence  20
Change in school     20
Change in recreation  19
Change in church activities     19
Change in social activities     18
Mortgage or loan for lesser purchase (such as a car or TV)     17
Change in sleeping habits     16
Change in number of family get-togethers  15
Change in eating habits     15
Vacation     13
Holiday season  12
Minor violations of the law     11

Determine which life events have occurred in your life over the past two years and add up your total stress score. For example, if you got married, changed to a different line of work, changed residence, and took two vacations, your total stress score would be 50 + 36 + 20 + 13 + 13 = 132. If your total stress score is near 150, you are less likely to be suffering the effects of cumulative stress. If it is between 150 and 300, you may be suffering from chronic stress, depending on how you perceived and coped with the particular life events that occurred. If your score is over 300, it is likely you are experiencing some detrimental effects of cumulative stress. Please note that the stress scores on the above survey are averaged over many people. The degree to which any particular event is stressful to you will depend on how you perceive it.

by heredity. It is likely, then, that genes, cumulative stress, and childhood circumstances all contribute to the genesis of a particular anxiety disorder, as suggested in this diagram:

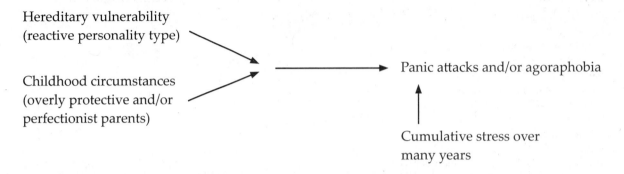

When you examine long-term causes, it turns out that no *one* of them may be sufficient, by itself, to produce a particular anxiety disorder. You may live twenty years with a hereditary vulnerability to panic attacks and yet never have one. Then life events in your twenties might produce enough cumulative stress to activate what had been only a potential—and you have your first panic attack. If you grew up feeling insecure and were taught that the outside world is dangerous, you may go on to develop agoraphobia. If you grew up feeling ashamed when you performed, perhaps your particular type of phobic avoidance will be less territorial and more social (in other words, a social phobia).

## Biological Causes

*Biological causes* refer to physiological imbalances in the body or brain that are associated with anxiety disorders. It is important to recognize that such imbalances are not necessarily the *ultimate causes* of anxiety disorders and may *themselves* be caused by

- A specific hereditary vulnerability

- Cumulative stress over time

- A hereditary vulnerability that is brought out by cumulative stress

Once again, it is likely that genes, life history, and stress all work together to bring about the disturbances underlying anxiety disorders.

Recent research has pointed to different types of biological explanations for different types of anxiety disorders. The type of malfunction associated with spontaneous panic attacks is probably different from the type associated with generalized anxiety disorder. And both of these, in turn, are different from physiological imbalances associated with obsessive-compulsive disorder. Each of these is discussed separately below.

Our state of knowledge about biological causes underlying anxiety disorders is still very tentative and incomplete. The brain mechanisms considered in this chapter, which are discussed after an initial section on the physiology of panic, should be viewed as hypothetical—not proven facts.

Finally, it is important to realize that even though there may be a physiological imbalance in the brain underlying your particular anxiety disorder, there is no reason to assume you can't correct it. *If you are willing to make lifestyle changes to reduce stress and upgrade your level of physical wellness, any physiological imbalances associated with panic, phobias, anxiety, or obsessions will tend to diminish and perhaps disappear altogether.* These lifestyle changes include making time for daily relaxation, an exercise program, good nutrition, social support, and self-nurturing activities. (See the relevant chapters in this workbook.) An alternative way to correct a biological imbalance is to rely on prescription medications that specifically alter the functioning of your brain. Medications work well in overcoming the physiological causes of anxiety disorders—though, in my opinion, they should be viewed as a last line of defense. It is often possible to correct physical imbalances *simply* by upgrading your level of health and wellness.

Later in this section you will read about mechanisms in the brain that are thought, based on recent research, to underlie panic attacks, generalized anxiety, and obsessive-compulsive disorder. First, however, is a description of the basic physiology of a panic attack—something that is much better understood.

## The Physiology of Panic

What happens to your body during a panic attack? Panic is an extreme version of an alarm reaction your body *naturally* goes through in response to any type of threat. Years ago, Walter Cannon described this as the *fight-or-flight response.* It is a built-in mechanism that enables all higher animals to mobilize a great deal of energy quickly in order to cope with predators or other immediate threats to their survival. This alarm reaction serves us well in situations that are realistically dangerous. Unfortunately, most of us also experience the fight-or-flight reaction in response to any situation that is viewed as *psychologically* dangerous, threatening, or overwhelming. An argument with your spouse or having to get up and go to work after a bad night's sleep can cause a pronounced stress response because *you perceive* it as threatening or overwhelming, even though it poses no direct risk to your survival.

In the case of a panic attack, there may be no perceived threat at all—the reaction may come on "out of the blue," without any noticeable provocation. Somehow the natural fight-or-flight response has gotten out of control. That it occurs out of context and without apparent reason suggests that the brain mechanisms that control the response aren't functioning properly. The current hypothesis about the nature of this dysfunction is described in the next section. The physiology of panic itself, however, is better known.

Your nervous system has two separate actions: *voluntary* and *involuntary.* There is a voluntary nervous system that moves your muscles and obeys your direct command. Your involuntary nervous system, on the other hand, regulates automatic functions that are ordinarily outside voluntary control, such as your heartbeat, respiration, and digestion. This involuntary system is itself divided into two branches: the *sympathetic* and *parasympathetic* nervous systems. The sympathetic nervous system is responsible for mobilizing a number of reactions throughout your body whenever you're emotional or excited. The parasympathetic nervous system has an opposite function. It maintains normal, smooth functioning of your various internal organs during times when you are calm and at rest.

In a panic attack, your sympathetic nervous system sets off several different bodily reactions rapidly and intensely. First, it causes your adrenal glands to release large amounts of adrenaline. What you feel is a sudden "jolt," often accompanied by a feeling of dread or terror. Within seconds, the excess adrenaline can cause 1) your heart to race, 2) your respiration to become rapid and shallow, 3) profuse sweating, 4) trembling and shaking, and 5) cold hands and feet. Your sympathetic nervous system also produces muscle contractions (the most extreme case of this is when animals "freeze" in fear), possibly leading you to experience strong contractions in your chest or throat along with a fear of not being able to breathe. Other reactions caused by the sympathetic nervous system include excess release of stomach acid, inhibition of digestion, release of red blood cells by the spleen, release of stored-up sugar by the liver, an increase in metabolic rate, and dilation of the pupils.

All of these reactions occur to a lesser degree when you are emotional or excited. The problem in panic is that they peak to such an extreme level that you feel overwhelmed and terrified, and have a strong urge to run. It is important to realize that the adrenaline released during panic tends to be reabsorbed by the liver and kidneys within a few minutes. If you can "ride out" the bodily symptoms of panic without fighting them or telling yourself how horrible they are, they will tend to subside within a short time. Chapter 6 will describe strategies for learning to observe rather than react to the bodily symptoms of panic. By breathing properly and making supportive, calming statements to yourself, you can learn to manage panic instead of scaring yourself into a much more intense reaction.

While the physiology of panic is well understood, the mechanisms in the brain that initiate these physiological reactions are less well understood. The following section presents two recent hypotheses about particular imbalances in the brain thought to be responsible for panic attacks.

## Panic Attacks

Your brain is by far the most complex system in your body, consisting of over one hundred billion brain cells or neurons. At any given moment in time, millions of nerve impulses are being transmitted along multiple pathways that interconnect various regions of your brain. Every time a single nerve impulse moves from one nerve cell to the next, it must cross a space. Individual nerve cells are not connected but are separated by tiny spaces called *synapses*. It has been known for some time that the process by which a nerve impulse moves across a synapse is chemical in nature. Microscopic amounts of chemicals secreted into the synapse allow transmission of a nerve impulse from one neuron to the next. These chemicals are called *neurotransmitters*; there are over twenty different types of them in the brain.

It appears that there are different systems in the brain that are especially sensitive to particular neurotransmitters. Each system consists of a vast network of nerve cells (*neurons*) that are sensitive to a particular neurotransmitter. One system, called the *noradrenergic system*, seems to be especially sensitive to a neurotransmitter substance called *norepinephrine*. Another system, the *serotonergic system*, contains neurons especially sensitive to a neurotransmitter substance called *serotonin*. Yet another system, the *glutamatergic system*, is especially sensitive to the stimulating neurotransmitter *glutamate*. These three systems have a large number of receptor sites (sites on nerve cells that respond to neurotransmitters) in some of the major structures of the brain that are activated during a panic attack. Specifically, the *amygdala*—a structure in your brain—is thought to play a key role in instigating panic. Research has found that the amygdala does not act alone but works in concert with a variety of other structures that all contribute to stimulating panic. These structures include "higher" brain centers such as the prefrontal cortex and insula, which serve to modulate sensory information, interpreting it as "dangerous" or "safe." Such information is stored in memory in a part of the brain called the *hippocampus*. The higher brain centers and the hippocampus interface directly with the amygdala. The amygdala, in turn, instigates panic by stimulating a variety of other brain structures, including 1) the *locus coeruleus*, which contributes to general behavioral and physiological arousal, 2) the *hypothalamus*, which regulates the release of adrenaline (via the pituitary gland, stimulating your adrenal glands) and also stimulates your sympathetic nervous system (see the previous section), 3) the *periaqueductal gray region*, which stimulates defensive and avoidance behavior, and, finally, 4) the *parabrachial nucleus*, which stimulates increased respiration.

Within your brain, panic attacks are more likely to occur when this entire system is *overly sensitized*, perhaps from having been previously activated too frequently, too intensely, or both. Thus, the neurological basis for panic is not exactly a "chemical imbalance," as your doctor may have told you, but an overly sensitized "fear system," including all of the above brain structures. Researchers believe that deficiencies of the neurotransmitters serotonin and norepinephrine may contribute to *insufficient inhibition* of the amygdala, locus coeruleus, and associated structures that make up this fear system. That is why SSRI antidepressants and SNRI antidepressants that affect the metabolism of serotonin and/or norepinephrine available throughout your brain can diminish panic attacks (as well as other anxiety disorders). An older class of antidepressants, the tricyclic antidepressants, can also be effective in reducing the symptoms of anxiety disorders. (See chapter 18 for further information on these various types of antidepressant medications.) Over a period of two to four weeks, these medications seem to be able to *stabilize* and *desensitize* an overly sensitized amygdala, locus coeruleus, and associated fear system.

What *causes* the original oversensitization of the fear system remains unclear at this time. One hypothesis is that changes in this system can take place as a result of acute stress or as the long-term result of multiple stressors over time. Although this hypothesis remains unproven, it seems likely that *cumulative stress contributes in an important way to the onset of panic attacks* (as discussed earlier in this chapter). If this hypothesis about stress altering the amygdala and the fear system turns out to be true, an important implication follows: *the most effective long-term treatment for brain dysfunctions associated with panic disorder is a consistent and comprehensive program for reducing stress in your life*. Medications can certainly help restabilize structures in your brain that contribute to panic and anxiety in the short run. Yet without changes in your lifestyle, such as regular relaxation and exercise, good time management, proper nutrition, personal support, and constructive attitudes—changes that allow you to live more simply and peacefully—panic and anxiety will tend to return after the medications are withdrawn.

An additional hypothesis for the causation of panic attacks has to do with the prefrontal cortex. This is a "higher" cortical brain center that comes into play *after* the amygdala surges with sudden fear in response to a potential threat. The prefrontal cortex helps you evaluate your environment to see whether a legitimate threat really exists or not. If no threat appears to exist, the prefrontal cortex exerts a "top down" influence on the amygdala so that you can dismiss the potential threat and not continue further into panic. It is believed that this link between the prefrontal cortex and the amygdala may be impaired in people prone to panic disorder. That is, the prefrontal cortex fails to adequately tone down the amygdala, allowing fear to continue to gain momentum until a full-blown panic attack occurs.

## Generalized Anxiety

Benzodiazepine tranquilizers, such as Xanax, Ativan, or Klonopin, can effectively reduce anxiety in generalized anxiety disorder (GAD) as well as other anxiety disorders (including anticipatory anxiety in phobias). It has been discovered that a specific receptor system in the brain, the GABA system, is uniquely sensitive to benzodiazepine drugs. This system consists of neurons that are sensitive to the neurotransmitter gamma-aminobutyric acid (GABA for short). GABA functions naturally in the brain as an *inhibitory* neurotransmitter—it tends to inhibit, or "tone down," brain activity, particularly in the limbic system, which is the brain's center for emotions. Thus GABA is associated with the brain's own natural calming response. When you give people GABA directly, or give them drugs that increase the activity of the GABA system, their anxiety decreases.

It appears that benzodiazepine tranquilizers like Xanax stimulate the GABA system to be more active, just as the neurotransmitter GABA itself does. That is why these tranquilizers tone down anxiety, as well as any other form of emotional arousal.

What is going on with the GABA system in people who are chronically anxious? Several hypotheses have been proposed. There may be a deficiency of GABA itself, resulting in less inhibitory activity of the GABA system. Or there may be a deficiency of some naturally occurring benzodiazepine substance in the brain (yet to be identified), which leads to reduced activity of the GABA system. Perhaps there are too many GABA receptors relative to the amount of GABA available. The situation is quite complicated because brain activation (hence anxiety) is controlled not only by the GABA system but also by the serotonin and norepinephrine systems (and even other neurotransmitter systems as well). Moreover, brain research has found that these systems all interact and modulate each other. Suffice it to say that all of these systems play a role in the neurobiological basis of generalized anxiety disorder.

## Obsessive-Compulsive Disorder

The same reasoning that applied to generalized anxiety disorder also applies to obsessive-compulsive disorder (OCD). The effectiveness of specific drugs, such as clomipramine (Anafranil) and SSRI antidepressants (selective serotonin reuptake inhibitors)—fluoxetine (Prozac), sertraline (Zoloft), paroxetine (Paxil), and fluvoxamine (Luvox)—in reducing obsessive-compulsive symptoms tells us something about the possible biological mechanisms for obsessive-compulsive disorder. These drugs are known to increase the amount of a specific neurotransmitter substance, serotonin, in the brain. They do so more effectively than other classes of antidepressant medications. So we know that serotonin (and the serotonin system of the brain) plays an important role in the neurobiological basis of OCD.

Research has identified an OCD "neurocircuit" in the brain involving three brain structures: the *orbitofrontal cortex*, *thalamus*, and *caudate nucleus*. These structures define a circuit, or "loop," that brain imaging studies have found to be overly active in persons with OCD. When you worry, the orbitofrontal cortex sends a worry signal to the thalamus, which in turn sends the signal back (via the caudate nucleus) to the orbitofrontal cortex for interpretation. In normal people, this cycle happens only once or a few times. In people with OCD, however, because of a problem in the caudate nucleus, the signal goes back and forth and "loops" many, many times. It appears that SSRIs work by toning down excess activity of this OCD circuit. Many serotonin neurons in the brain are inhibitory in function, and there appears to be an abundance of these inhibitory neurons in the structures that make up the OCD loop, especially the caudate. Thus, increasing serotonin in the brain increases the activity of the inhibitory serotonin neurons, which in turn "brakes" excess activity in the OCD circuit.

Another brain structure involved in OCD is the *anterior cingulate gyrus*. One function of the cingulate is to enable you to flexibly shift attention from one topic to another. When the cingulate isn't functioning properly, you can more easily get "stuck" or get locked in to a particular theme, as is the case when you are obsessing on something. It appears that SSRI medications help the cingulate function better. Brain imaging research has also found that cognitive behavioral therapy, specifically exposure and response prevention, can normalize brain function in the structures associated with OCD. It's exciting to see that a strictly psychological intervention can result in lasting changes in brain function similar to what drugs can accomplish.

## Further Details About How Antidepressant Medications Work

The following section provides a more technical explanation of how antidepressant medications work. It may be of particular interest to those who hope to study medicine or have an interest in brain physiology. If this is not you, feel free to move ahead to the next section, "Medical Conditions That Can Cause Panic Attacks or Anxiety."

Scientific understanding of how antidepressant medications work to reduce anxiety and depression has evolved over the past two decades. Selective serotonin reuptake inhibitor medications (SSRIs) work by blocking the reuptake of serotonin, a major brain neurotransmitter, at the *synapse*, a tiny space between every nerve connection in the brain. More serotonin remains in the synapse because it is blocked from being reabsorbed by the nerve cell leading up to a given synapse (reabsorption at the presynaptic nerve cell normally happens in the absence of the medication).

Nerve transmission in the brain involves propagation of nerve impulses (electrical signals produced by ion exchanges) along the distance of nerve cells or neurons. Among the many billions of neurons in your brain, there are literally trillions of tiny spaces among them—the synapses—which serve to separate *incoming neurons* (specifically their elongated *axons*) from numerous *outgoing neurons* (whose receiving terminals are called *dendrites*).

Antidepressant medications (both SSRIs and SNRIs—see chapter 18, Medications for Anxiety, for more information) *block the reuptake of serotonin* at the synapse. They do this by actually blocking the reabsorption of serotonin at the sites of the presynaptic axons. The result is that these medications increase the amount of free serotonin in the synapse.

With more serotonin (as well as norepinephrine with the SNRIs) in the synapse, why don't antidepressant medications have an *immediate* effect in diminishing anxiety or depression? Neurobiological research has determined that the efficacy of these medications is not caused *directly by increasing amounts of serotonin* they produce in the brain's synapses. What actually happens is that the added serotonin *downregulates the* number *of postsynaptic (dendritic) receptor sites.* In plain English, the increased serotonin at the synapse reduces the number of postsynaptic receptor sites. Why? Because not as many receptor sites are needed to process the increased amount of synaptic serotonin. This process of downregulation and reduction of postsynaptic sites *takes time,* usually two or three weeks at the very least. *The fact that downregulation takes time is the reason why antidepressant medications don't work immediately but take two or three weeks to begin to show therapeutic effects.* In fact, SSRIs and SNRIs can take up to a full twelve weeks to demonstrate their maximum therapeutic effects. The full downregulation effect may just take that long.

A brief summary of the downregulation process may also be found in the section "SSRI Antidepressant Medications" in chapter 18, Medications for Anxiety.

More recently, evidence has also shown that depression is accompanied by decreased levels of *brain-derived neurotrophic factor* (BDNF), most specifically in the hippocampus region of the brain (a section associated with formation of new memories and learning). This is sometimes referred to as the "neurotrophic hypothesis" of depression (and commonly anxiety as well). The neurotrophic hypothesis proposes that increased depression/anxiety is associated with *reduced* levels of BDNF in the hippocampus. So SSRI medications also alleviate depressive or anxiety symptoms by increasing BDNF levels. Further discussion of the neurotrophic hypothesis is beyond the scope of this chapter.

One final idea being explored recently is that antidepressant medications, both as a result of postsynaptic downregulation as well as increased BDNF activity, result in increased *neuronal plasticity* of the brain, especially in key areas such as the amygdala, hippocampus, and caudate. Several studies have found very impaired neuronal plasticity in depression, and, even more critical, in people with suicidal behavior. We've known for some time that various agents can increase brain plasticity (or the ability of undamaged areas to take over for impaired or damaged brain areas). The ability of antidepressant treatments to promote increased neuronal plasticity is yet another promising indication of their ability to reduce both depression as well as suicide.

## Medical Conditions That Can Cause Panic Attacks or Anxiety

The physiology of panic described at the beginning of this section is well established. But the various proposed explanations of the biological mechanisms involving different neurotransmitter systems of the brain are, at present, still under investigation. It is important to keep in mind that these biological hypotheses apply to a majority *but not all cases* of panic attacks and generalized anxiety. Sometimes panic reactions or anxiety can arise from medical conditions that are quite separate from recognized anxiety disorders. Hyperthyroidism and hypoglycemia, for example, can cause panic attacks that are by all appearances identical to those seen in panic disorder. A calcium or magnesium deficiency or an allergy to certain food additives can also produce panic or anxiety. So can excessive caffeine intake. When these conditions are corrected, the anxiety disappears.

Any of the following conditions might be a cause of panic attacks or generalized anxiety. The first six are the ones most frequently seen.

- *Hyperventilation syndrome.*

Rapid, shallow breathing at the level of your chest can sometimes lead to excessive lowering of carbon dioxide in your bloodstream. This results in symptoms very similar to those of a panic attack, including light-headedness, dizziness, feelings of unreality, shortness of breath, trembling, and/or tingling in your hands, feet, or lips. These symptoms, in turn, may be perceived as dangerous and may stimulate a bona fide panic attack. (See the section on abdominal breathing in chapter 4 for further discussion of hyperventilation.)

- *Hypoglycemia.*

For a large number of people, blood sugar levels can fall too low as a result of improper diet or simply stress. When this happens, such people experience a variety of symptoms similar to a panic reaction, including anxiety, shakiness, dizziness, weakness, and disorientation. Hypoglycemia can cause panic attacks, or, more often, can aggravate panic reactions that are caused by other factors. (See chapter 16 for a detailed discussion.)

- *Hyperthyroidism.*

Excessive secretion of thyroid hormone can lead to heart palpitations (rapid heartbeat), sweating, and generalized anxiety. Other symptoms of hyperthyroidism include weight loss, elevated body temperature, insomnia, and bulging eyes. If you have several of the above symptoms, you might want to have your doctor do a thyroid panel to see if this condition is contributing to your anxiety or panic symptoms. (See chapter 17 for more information about how thyroid conditions can affect anxiety.)

- *Mitral valve prolapse.*

Mitral valve prolapse is a harmless condition that causes heart palpitations. It is caused by a slight defect in the valve separating the upper and lower chambers on the left side of your heart. Blood moves through the mitral valve as it passes from the upper to the lower chamber. With mitral valve prolapse, the valve doesn't close completely and some of the blood can flow back from the lower to the upper chamber, causing the heart to beat out of rhythm. The resulting rhythm disturbance can be disconcerting enough to cause some people to panic—but it is *not* dangerous. Mitral valve prolapse is *not* a cause of heart attacks.

For reasons that are unclear, mitral valve prolapse occurs more frequently in people with panic disorder than in the population at large. In severe cases, it can be treated through the use of beta-blocking drugs such as Inderal.

- *Premenstrual syndrome (PMS).*

If you are a woman, it is important to observe whether your panic reactions (or generalized anxiety) worsen around the time just before your period. If so, treating your PMS may be enough to alleviate your problem with panic or anxiety. Treatment usually involves improvements in diet and exercise, taking supplements such as vitamin $B_6$, and in some cases taking natural progesterone. (See chapter 17 for a more detailed discussion.)

- *Inner ear disturbances.*

For a small proportion of the population, panic attacks seem to be associated with a disturbance in balance caused by swelling of the inner ear (due to infection, allergy, Ménière's disease, or other problems). If dizziness, light-headedness, and/or unsteadiness are a *prominent* part of your problem with anxiety or panic, you may want to consult an otolaryngologist to check the labyrinth system of your inner ear.

Other medical conditions that can cause panic or anxiety include the following:

- Acute reaction to cocaine, amphetamines, caffeine, aspartame, appetite suppressants, asthma medications, steroids, or other stimulants

- Withdrawal from alcohol, sedatives, or tranquilizers

- Thyrotoxicosis

- Cushing's syndrome

- Adrenal tumor

- Parathyroid disease

- Partial complex seizures (temporal lobe epilepsy)

- Post-concussion syndrome

- Deficiencies of calcium, magnesium, potassium, niacin, vitamin $B_{12}$

- Emphysema

- Pulmonary embolism

- Cardiac arrhythmias

- Congestive heart failure

- Essential hypertension

- Environmental toxins such as mercury, carbon dioxide, hydrocarbons, food additives, pesticides

To adequately rule out any medical conditions that could be causing or aggravating your particular problem, have your doctor give you a thorough physical examination, including a blood panel, before adopting behavioral and psychological strategies for recovery. Keep in mind, though, that the above medical conditions (with the exception of hyperventilation and hypoglycemia) contribute to panic or anxiety in only a minority of cases.

## Short-Term, Triggering Causes

Long-term causes such as heredity, childhood environment, and cumulative stress create a *predisposition* to anxiety disorders. Yet it takes more specific conditions, operating over a short period of time, to actually trigger panic attacks or cause a phobia to develop. In this section we will briefly consider:

- Specific stressors that often precede a first panic attack

- Conditioning processes that produce phobias

- The role of trauma in certain simple phobias and post-traumatic stress disorder

## Stressors That Precipitate Panic Attacks

A first panic attack is often preceded by a stressful event or situation. In my experience with people already vulnerable to panic disorder as a result of the predisposing factors previously described, the following three types of stressors often preceded their first panic attack:

- *Significant personal loss.*

Loss of a significant person through death, divorce, or separation seems very frequently to be a trigger of a first panic attack. Other major losses, such as loss of employment, loss of health through illness, or a major financial reversal, can also precipitate a first panic attack.

- *Significant life change.*

A major life event causing a period of adjustment lasting several months can sometimes precipitate a first panic attack. Examples of such an event might include getting married, having a baby, going off to college, changing jobs, going into the military, making a geographical move, or developing a protracted physical illness.

It may be that *any major stressor*, whether it is a significant loss or a major life change, can trigger a first panic attack in an individual who is already vulnerable for other reasons.

- *Stimulants and recreational drugs.*

It is not uncommon for a first panic attack to occur after excessive intake of caffeine. Often people are unaware that their use of caffeine is excessive until a full-blown panic attack brings it to their attention.

Even more common is the incidence of panic attacks in people using cocaine or amphetamine-related drugs. Cocaine is such a strong stimulant that it may cause panic attacks even in people who are *not* predisposed to panic disorder by the long-term factors previously described. Amphetamines, especially recreational methamphetamine, frequently trigger panic attacks. In addition, high doses of marijuana as well as withdrawal from narcotics, barbiturates, or tranquilizers can also jolt a person into a first panic attack.

## Conditioning and the Origin of Phobias

A phobia is a persistent and unreasonable fear of a specific object, activity, or situation that results in a compelling desire to avoid that dreaded object, activity, or situation. There are three characteristics that distinguish a phobia from ordinary, everyday fears. First, you are *persistently* afraid of the object or situation over a long period of time. Second, you know that your fear is *unreasonable*, even though this recognition does not help to dispel it. Finally, what is most characteristic of a phobia is your *avoidance* of the feared situation. Being unreasonably afraid of something is not yet a phobia; the phobia begins when you actually start avoiding what you fear.

What is avoided tends to vary among the different types of phobias. If you are agoraphobic, you tend to avoid situations where you're afraid you can't easily escape if you have a panic attack—examples include checkout lines in grocery stores, freeways, elevators, and bridges. If you have a social phobia, you tend to avoid situations where you fear you might humiliate or embarrass yourself in front of others—examples include public speaking, parties, public restrooms, and job interviews. Simple phobias lead you to fear potential death or injury from causes such as natural disasters or certain animals. Or you may have an enormous fear of being trapped.

How do these phobias develop? There are two types of processes that are most commonly responsible: *conditioning* and *trauma*. Trauma isn't always involved in the creation of a phobia, but conditioning processes are always present. There are two types of conditioning that contribute to the formation of a phobia: 1) *conditioning by association* and 2) *conditioning by avoidance*.

In *conditioning by association*, a situation that was originally neutral begins to elicit strong anxiety because on one particular day you panicked or had a strong anxiety reaction in that same situation. For example, you're driving on the freeway and spontaneously have a panic attack. The panic is made worse by fearful thoughts, such as "How do I get out of here?" or "What if I get into an accident?" Your mind forms a strong association between being on the freeway and experiencing anxiety, so that later, being on, being near, or even thinking about freeways elicits anxiety. In short, you have *learned* an association between freeways and anxiety. By the same token, experiencing strong anxiety the first time you try public speaking may lead to an association between the two. Subsequently, every time you attempt to speak before others, or even think about doing so, strong anxiety is automatically triggered.

Conditioning by association may cause you to develop a fear toward a particular situation or object, but it does not by itself create a phobia. Only when you start to *avoid* that situation or object do you "learn" to be phobic. A time-honored principle in behavioral psychology is that any behavior that is rewarded tends to be repeated. Avoiding a situation you're anxious about is obviously rewarded—the reward being the reduction of anxiety. Each time you avoid the situation, the reward of being relieved of anxiety follows, and so your avoidance behavior gets strengthened and tends to be repeated. Your avoidance works very well in saving you from anxiety.

Learning to stay away from a fearful situation because it is rewarding to do so is what constitutes *conditioning by avoidance*. Avoidance conditioning is the most critical process in the formation of any phobia. It is directly reversed and overcome by the processes of imagery and real-life exposure described in chapter 7.

## Trauma, Simple Phobias, and Post-Traumatic Stress Disorder

Agoraphobia and social phobia tend to develop primarily as a result of the conditioning processes just described. Certain simple phobias, on the other hand, can develop in the wake of specific traumatic experiences. As a child, you might develop a phobia about bees as a result of unknowingly picking up a bee and getting stung. This is really an example of conditioning by association. The fear you feel at the time of getting stung causes you to develop an automatic association between bees and fear. Avoidance conditioning can then come into play if you subsequently start to avoid or run away from bees whenever you see them.

By the same token, being in an auto accident can cause a person to subsequently fear driving or even being in a car. Or nearly drowning may lead to a subsequent phobia about water. Many simple phobias can be traced back to some kind of traumatic incident in childhood. Others—especially those we have from a very early age, like the fear of darkness or fears of insects—may be part of our evolutionary heritage. Such fears may have been biologically programmed into the nervous systems of all mammals to promote survival of the species. These inborn fears people often grow up with cannot be considered phobias unless 1) they lead to persistent avoidance and 2) they persist into adulthood.

A different outcome of trauma is the occurrence of post-traumatic stress disorder, which was described in chapter 1. No specific phobias develop; instead, you tend to develop an array of symptoms that "re-create" the original trauma. Distressing recollections and dreams about what happened are the mind's attempt to gain control of the original event and neutralize the emotional charge it carries.

## Maintaining Causes

The maintaining causes of anxiety disorders are what tend to keep them going. They involve ways of thinking, feeling, and coping that serve to perpetuate anxiety, panic, or phobias. Much of this workbook is devoted to helping you deal with these maintaining causes. Of the four types of causes we are considering, only the maintaining ones operate in the here and now and are thus the easiest to deal with. The following list of maintaining causes isn't exhaustive and includes only those that are most obvious. Maintaining causes will be considered in greater detail throughout the rest of this workbook.

### *Avoidance of Phobic Situations*

Phobias develop because it is very rewarding to avoid facing situations that cause you anxiety. As long as you continue to avoid dealing with a phobic situation, activity, or object, the phobia will remain securely in place. Trying to think or reason your way out of a phobia simply won't work if you continue to avoid confronting it directly. As long as you avoid a situation, you will be prone to worry about whether you can ever handle it.

Overcoming a phobia means that you unlearn certain responses while relearning others. When you finally begin to face the situation, you *unlearn* both 1) the "fear-in-advance," or the anticipatory anxiety about possibly panicking in the situation, and 2) the avoidance of the situation itself. At the same time, you give yourself the opportunity to *learn* that you can enter—and remain in—a phobic situation without undue anxiety. You can learn to tolerate and eventually be comfortable in any phobic situation if you approach it in sufficiently small steps. The imagery and real-life exposure processes discussed in chapter 7 are intended to foster this type of learning.

## Reliance on Safety Behaviors

Safety behaviors are self-protective maneuvers you undertake to avoid fear. Usually they tend to backfire and aggravate your fear. Fleeing fear begets fear. Relinquishing safety behaviors means taking a stance where you accept and endure fear. The payoff is that you ultimately learn you can handle your fear, often more easily than you had anticipated.

Some common types of safety behaviors follow.

*Procrastination.* For example, you have an upcoming music recital or speech before a group of people. Instead of giving yourself ample time to prepare, you wait until the last minute and then stress yourself out trying to adequately prepare in much too short a time, leading to much more anxiety.

*Overpreparation.* You have a demanding task coming up such as a final exam or, as in the previous example, a live musical performance. You spend excessive time overpreparing for it, leading to "anticipatory anxiety" (anxiety ahead of a somewhat demanding situation) that makes you miserable for several days before the actual event. By the time you get to the actual performance, you may feel exhausted or have lost sleep because of excessive preparation and attendant anxiety.

*Reassurance seeking.* For example, your heart is beating unusually hard or fast because you've been under excessive stress for the past day or two. This is a normal occurrence for many people. You fear you might have some serious heart affliction or even be susceptible to a heart attack. For reassurance, you make an appointment with your primary care doctor or even a cardiologist and run tests such as a stress test and an echocardiogram. Even if the tests come out fine, you may still harbor doubt and ask the doctors to perform additional tests. Had you waited three or four days, the heart symptoms might have naturally subsided as your stress passed. The impulse to seek reassurance only adds to your fear.

*Overchecking.* Let's say you have occasional episodes of rapid heartbeat (not even technical tachycardia, which is a sustained period of greater than 100 beats per minute). As above, your condition may be due to excessive stress, rushing around too much and at too fast a pace for a few days, or simply drinking too much coffee. Even though your heart is designed to beat at up to 100 beats a minute for days at a time with no real danger, you resort to constantly checking your pulse to check your heart rate. Perhaps you check up to twenty or thirty times per day, a few times each hour. Eventually, if you aren't satisfied that your heart rate has settled down, you call your primary care physician or even a cardiologist to check if something is truly wrong. Even if half or more of your pulse rate checks are in the entirely normal range (70 to 99 beats per minute), you keep checking to make sure you are okay. The constant checking of your heart rate only serves to aggravate your anxiety.

Or your husband is late in getting home (perhaps due to an extended work schedule or excessive traffic), and you become worried and keep calling him, despite the fact that he provides a reasonable explanation for being late. A single phone call is not enough. Of course, the situation can get much worse if your husband decides to turn off his phone in order to stop receiving repeated calls.

*Perfectionism.* Striving for perfection can create not only potential anxiety but also increased disillusionment and even depression. Perfectionism often rears its head in advance of demanding tasks, such as going to a college admissions or job interview, taking a final exam or a job certification exam, or perhaps doing a live musical performance. Striving for complete perfection prior to or during such a situation tends to backfire. Your overwrought expectations lead you to feel overly anxious, or even ashamed, up to and during the actual task itself, sometimes interfering with your best performance. For more information about perfectionism and how to deal with it, see the section on perfectionism in chapter 11, Personality Styles That Perpetuate Anxiety.

*Overreliance on a support person.* In working on facing a long-standing phobia, it often helps at the outset to have a support person go with you. For example, if you're making your first flight after many years of avoiding flying, having someone accompany you can provide both distraction and reassurance to help mitigate your anxiety. Or perhaps you have a phobia of going to the doctor for a routine exam, and you've let yourself stay away from medical practitioners for a few years. It may be quite helpful to have someone accompany your when you make your first visit to the doctor in a long time. Just having the support person sit in the waiting room while you're having the checkup may be sufficient.

Support people are a kind of "crutch" that can help you when you *first* face a phobic situation you've avoided for years. However, if you keep taking your support person with you in every case of facing the fear, you will never learn that you can become capable of handling the fear on your own. In order to *complete* exposure to most phobias, it's necessary to relinquish the safety behavior of having a support person along. Then you can learn to be fully confident about your ability to overcome the fear. This is especially important in situations where you *really need to be able to confront a situation without always needing someone to be with you,* such as staying home alone or driving far away from home.

*Rituals.* Before you face a demanding situation, such as flying or going to the dentist, you may try to assuage your anxiety with a ritual, such as saying a prayer four times or taking along a special security object such as teddy bear or certain piece of jewelry. The ritual serves to foster the false belief that you can *only* handle the situation by performing the ritual. Ultimately, though, you can only gain confidence in your ability to *fully* handle the situation by relinquishing the ritual and learning that nothing terrible happens by entering the situation without the ritual. You may want to do this in degrees (such as entering the situation by saying a fewer number of prayers or taking just a stuffed ball instead of a stuffed teddy bear) before you attempt to finally enter the situation free of any ritual.

**To reduce reliance on safety behaviors, utilize the following three guidelines.**

1. **Notice** you are engaging in safety behavior(s) in order to protect yourself from anxiety.

2. **Expose rather than oppose.** Desist from fighting or fleeing an uncomfortable exposure situation (facing what you fear). The key to overcoming safety behaviors is *full acceptance* of the situation and your ability to *tolerate discomfort* (as long as discomfort doesn't soar to an overwhelming degree, which is usually unlikely).

3. **Cope.** Rely on your most helpful *coping strategies* to move through exposure to an uncomfortable situation and tolerate the discomfort. Quite a number of coping strategies are available, so pick the ones that you personally find most helpful.

In chapter 6, Coping with Panic Attacks, you will find a list of coping strategies in the section "Coping Strategies to Counteract Panic at an Early Stage," such as abdominal breathing, utilizing coping statements, speaking with a support person nearby or on the phone, or engaging in physical activity, to name a few. All of these strategies can help reduce and eventually eliminate anxiety that interferes with your goals. When you use coping strategies, make sure you use them *proactively to disrupt your tendency to avoid facing your fear*. This is critical. You don't want to use a coping strategy as if it were just another safety signal: a maneuver you use to flee your fear. Coping strategies are helpful at the beginning of facing a difficult situation, but they are not intended to last forever.

The *ultimate* accomplishment in proactively dealing with fear, whether it's fear of an external situation, fear of internal bodily sensations, or simply excessive worry, is to *dispense even with coping strategies and just face the fear full on*, without any aids or assists. See chapter 7, Exposure for Phobias, for further explanation of the distinction between what might be called "coping exposure" versus "mastery exposure."

Whether you learn to face your fears with the help of a coping strategy such as abdominal breathing, or whether you face your fear without the assistance of any strategy whatsoever, you learn two very important lessons: 1) you are able to handle the fear well without all the anticipatory anxiety you might have previously had about the fear, and 2) even if fully facing your fear isn't entirely comfortable, you discover that you overestimated how bad it might be, and that it isn't as bad as you anticipated.

## Anxious Self-Talk

Self-talk is what you say to yourself in your own mind. It is the internal monologue that you engage in much of the time, although it may be so automatic and subtle that you don't notice it unless you step back and pay attention. Much of your anxiety is created by statements you make to yourself beginning with the words "what if"—for example, "What if I have another panic attack?" "What if I lose control of myself while driving?" "What will people think if I get anxious while standing in line?" This type of self-talk *anticipates* the worst before it even happens. The more common term for it is simply *worry*.

Self-talk can also contribute to creating a full-blown panic attack. Such an attack may start off with bodily symptoms such as tightness in the chest and heart palpitations. If you can accept and "flow with" these symptoms without letting them scare you, they will soon peak and then subside. However, all too often you tell yourself such things as "Oh no—I'm going to panic!" "What if I have a heart attack?" "I've got to get out of here, but I can't!" "People will think I'm weird if I have to rest or lean on something for a minute because my legs feel weak." This scare-talk only aggravates the physical symptoms, which in turn produce even more extreme scare-talk, leading to a vicious circle that produces a full-blown panic attack.

The good news is that you can learn to recognize anxiety-provoking self-talk, stop it, and replace it with more supportive and calming statements to yourself. The subject of self-talk is dealt with in detail in chapter 8.

## Mistaken Beliefs

Your negative self-talk comes from underlying mistaken beliefs about yourself, others, and "the way the world is." For example, if you believe that you can't be safely alone, you will talk yourself and everyone else into assuming that there must always be someone with you. If you truly believe that life is always a struggle, then you will tell yourself that something is wrong when you start to feel better or when others offer you help. A belief that the outside world is dangerous does not promote an attitude of trust or a willingness to take risks necessary to overcome a condition like agoraphobia.

Revamping your basic beliefs about yourself and your life takes more time and work than simply reversing anxious self-talk. Yet to do so will have far-reaching effects on your self-esteem, your willingness to accept imperfections in yourself and others, and your long-term peace of mind. The subject of mistaken beliefs is considered in detail in chapter 9.

## Withheld Feelings

Denying feelings of anger, frustration, sadness, or even excitement can contribute to a state of *free-floating anxiety*. Free-floating anxiety is when you feel vaguely anxious without knowing why. You may have noticed that after you let out your angry feelings or have a good cry you feel calmer and more at ease. Expressing feelings can have a distinct physiological effect that results in a reduced level of anxiety.

As mentioned earlier, anxiety-prone people are often born with a predisposition to be more emotionally reactive or volatile. Yet they often grow up in families where obtaining parental approval takes precedence over expressing their needs and feelings. As adults, they still feel it is more important to attain perfection or always be pleasing than to express strong feelings. This tendency to deny deep emotions can lead to a chronic state of tension and anxiety. It is believed by some that the *external* danger avoided by the phobic is actually a stand-in for a deeper-lying *internal* danger: the fear of long-repressed feelings resurfacing. Panic may occur when such feelings "threaten" to break through. For example, if you have a phobia about water, this might be viewed as a stand-in for a deeper-lying fear of denied feelings. Or a fear of ferocious animals might symbolize a deeper-lying fear of experiencing your own anger and the unmet needs from which it flows. In my view, this emotion-based theory of phobias may be at least partially right.

Fortunately, it is possible to *learn* to recognize and express your feelings more easily and frequently. Excessive ventilation of feelings, especially anger, may not always be productive, yet it is important to at least know *what* you are feeling and then allow your feelings some form of expression. Doing so will substantially lower your level of anxiety and reduce your tendency to panic. This topic is dealt with in chapter 13.

## Lack of Assertiveness

In order to express feelings to other people, it is important that you develop an assertive style of communicating that allows you to express yourself in a direct, forthright manner. Assertive communication strikes the right balance between submissiveness, where you are afraid to ask for what you want at all, and aggressiveness, where you demand what you want through coercion or threat. If you are prone to anxiety and phobias, you will tend to act submissively. You avoid asking directly for what you want and are afraid to express strong feelings, especially anger. Often you are afraid of imposing on others; you don't want to compromise your self-image as someone who is pleasing and nice. Or you are afraid that assertive communication will alienate the one person you feel dependent on for your basic sense of security. The problem with a lack of assertiveness is that it breeds feelings within you of resentment and confinement. And resentment and a sense of confinement are notorious for aggravating anxiety and phobias.

It's possible to *learn* to be assertive and directly express your wants and feelings. An introduction to this type of communication is presented in chapter 14.

## Lack of Self-Nurturing Skills

Common to the background of many people with anxiety disorders is a pervasive sense of insecurity. This is especially apparent in agoraphobia, where the need to stay close to a safe place or safe person can be so strong. Such insecurity arises from a variety of conditions in childhood, including parental neglect, abandonment, abuse, overprotection, or overcriticism, as well as alcoholism or chemical dependency in the family. Since they never received consistent or reliable nurturing as children, adult survivors of these various forms of deprivation often lack the capacity to properly take care of their own needs. Unaware of how to love and nurture themselves, they suffer low self-esteem and may feel anxious or overwhelmed in the face of adult demands and responsibilities. This lack of self-nurturing skills only serves to perpetuate anxiety.

The most lasting solution to parental abuse and deprivation is to become a good parent to yourself.

## Muscle Tension

When your muscles are tense, you feel "uptight." Muscle tension tends to restrict your breathing. And when your breathing is shallow and restricted, you are more likely to experience anxiety. Tense muscles also help keep your feelings suppressed, which, as discussed above, can increase anxiety. You may have noticed that when your body is tense, your mind has a greater tendency to race. As you relax the muscles throughout your body, your mind will begin to slow down and become calmer. A founder of systematic methods of relaxation, Edmund Jacobson, once said, "An anxious mind cannot exist in a relaxed body." Body and mind are inextricably related in anxiety.

You can reduce your level of muscle tension on a consistent basis by maintaining daily programs of deep relaxation as well as vigorous exercise. Either one of these alone can reduce muscle tension, but the combination has an even more profound effect. Detailed guidelines for incorporating relaxation and exercise into your lifestyle are presented in chapters 4 and 5.

## Stimulants and Other Dietary Factors

Stimulants such as caffeine and nicotine can aggravate anxiety and leave you more vulnerable to panic attacks. You may not even be aware of their impact until you reduce or eliminate them from your life. For some people, panic attacks go away completely when they eliminate caffeine from their diets (this is caffeine from not only coffee but also tea, cola beverages, and over-the-counter medications). For other people, additional dietary factors, such as sugar and food additives, can aggravate or occasionally even cause panic reactions.

The nutrition-anxiety connection has hardly been explored in either popular or technical books on anxiety disorders. Chapter 16 of this book takes a detailed look at this connection.

## High-Stress Lifestyle

The role of stress both as a predisposing agent and as a short-term cause of anxiety disorders has been described earlier. It is not surprising that a stressful lifestyle perpetuates problems with anxiety. The frequency of panic attacks and the severity of phobias tends to wax and wane depending on how well you cope with the daily stresses of living. Getting a handle on all of the maintaining causes of anxiety discussed in this section—self-talk, mistaken beliefs, withheld feelings, lack of assertiveness, lack of support, muscle tension, and diet—will go a long way toward reducing stress in your life. Other factors associated with stress that are not dealt with in this workbook include time management, Type A personality, and communication. These have been discussed in many excellent popular books on stress management—for example, *Guide to Stress Reduction*, revised edition, by John Mason and *The Relaxation & Stress Reduction Workbook*, 7th edition, by Martha Davis, Elizabeth Eshelman, and Matthew McKay. (See the reading list at the end of this chapter.)

## Lack of Meaning or Sense of Purpose

It has been my repeated experience that clients experience relief from anxiety as well as phobias when they come to feel that their life has meaning, purpose, and a sense of direction. Until you discover something larger than self-gratification—something that gives your life a sense of purpose—you may be prone to feelings of boredom and a vague sense of confinement because you are not realizing all of your potential. This sense of confinement can be a potent breeding ground for anxiety, phobias, and even panic attacks.

Issues of meaninglessness and purposelessness, and their relationship to psychological well-being, have been dealt with in depth by existential psychologists such as Victor Frankl and Rollo May. Several ways of confronting and working on these issues in your own life are presented in chapter 21.

## Investigating the Causes of Your Anxiety

1. Which of the following factors do you feel might be helping to maintain your particular difficulty?

    ☐ Avoidance of phobic situations

    ☐ Reliance on safety behaviors

    ☐ Anxious self-talk

    ☐ Mistaken beliefs

    ☐ Withheld feelings

    ☐ Lack of assertiveness

    ☐ Lack of self-nurturing skills

    ☐ Muscle tension

    ☐ Stimulants and other dietary factors

    ☐ High-stress lifestyle

    ☐ Low self=esteem

    ☐ Lack of meaning or sense of purpose

2. Can you rank these maintaining causes according to how much you feel they influence your condition? Which ones do you feel are most important for you to work on?

3. Specify three maintaining causes that you would seriously be willing to work on in the next month.

# Further Reading

Davis, Martha, Elizabeth Robbins Eshelman, and Matthew McKay. *The Relaxation & Stress Reduction Workbook.* 7th ed. Oakland, CA: New Harbinger Publications, 2019.

Holmes, Thomas, and Richard Rahe. 1967. "Social Readjustment Rating Scale." *Journal of Psychosomatic Research* 11: 213–18.

Mason, John. *Guide to Stress Reduction.* Rev. ed. Berkeley, CA: Celestial Arts, 2001.

McKay, Matthew, Michelle Skeen, and Patrick Fanning. *The CBT Anxiety Solution Workbook: A Breakthrough Treatment for Overcoming Fear, Worry, and Panic.* Oakland, CA: New Harbinger Publications, 2017.

Preston, John, John O'Neal, and Mary C. Talaga. *Handbook of Clinical Psychopharmacology for Therapists.* 8th ed. Oakland, CA: New Harbinger Publications, 2017.

True, W. R., J. Rice, and S. A. Eisen. 1993. "A Twin Study of Genetic and Environmental Contributions to Liability for Post-Traumatic Stress Symptoms." *Archives of General Psychiatry* 50(4): 257–64.

# 3

# Recovery: A Comprehensive Approach

Chapter 2 demonstrated how many different types of factors are contributing causes of anxiety disorders. Heredity, physiological imbalances in the brain, childhood deprivation and faulty parenting, and the cumulative effect of stress over time can all work to bring about the onset of panic attacks, agoraphobia, or any of the other anxiety disorders. The maintaining causes of these disorders—what keeps them going—are many and varied as well. Such factors can operate at the level of your body (for example, shallow breathing, muscle tension, or poor nutrition), emotions (such as withheld feelings), behavior (avoidance of phobic situations), mind (anxious self-talk and mistaken beliefs), and "whole self" (such as low self-esteem or a lack of self-nurturing skills).

If the causes of anxiety disorders are so varied, then an adequate approach to recovery needs to be, too. It is the basic philosophy of this workbook that the most effective approach for treating panic, phobias, or any other problem with anxiety is one that addresses the *full range* of factors contributing to these conditions. This type of approach can be called "comprehensive." It assumes that you can't just give someone the "right" medication and expect panic or generalized anxiety to go away. Nor can you just deal with childhood deprivation, having someone work through the emotional consequences of bad parenting, and expect the problems to disappear. By the same token, you can't just teach people new behaviors and new ways of talking to themselves and expect these things alone to resolve their problems. Some therapists still treat anxiety disorders solely as psychiatric conditions that can be "cured" by medication, or solely as childhood developmental problems, or solely as behavior problems, but the trend in recent years has been away from such single-gauged approaches. Many practitioners have discovered that problems with anxiety go away only temporarily when merely one or two contributing causes are dealt with. Lasting recovery is achieved when you are willing to make basic and comprehensive changes in habit, attitude, and lifestyle.

This chapter outlines and illustrates a comprehensive approach to recovery that has evolved over the past twenty years. What makes this approach truly comprehensive is that it offers interventions addressing seven different levels of contributing causes. These levels are as follows:

- Physical

- Emotional

- Behavioral

- Mental

- Interpersonal

- Whole self

- Existential and spiritual

Some brief descriptions of these levels, and a preview of the rest of the chapters in this workbook, follow.

## Physical Level

Physical-level causes include possible physiological imbalances in the brain and body (see the section on biological causes in chapter 2). Such causes also include 1) shallow breathing, 2) muscle tension, 3) bodily effects of cumulative stress, and 4) nutritional and dietary factors (such as excess caffeine or sugar in your diet). Strategies for dealing with physical-level causes can be found in five different chapters in this workbook. Chapter 4 offers breathing techniques to help modify your breathing pattern from the shallow, chest-level breathing that contributes to anxiety. That chapter also provides two deep relaxation techniques designed to reduce muscle tension and the effects of stress—progressive muscle relaxation and passive muscle relaxation. When practiced on a regular basis, either of these techniques can help you feel calmer in general, often making it unnecessary to rely on tranquilizers.

Chapter 5 on exercise makes a strong case for getting involved in a program of regular aerobic exercise. Many of my clients have found regular exercise to be the *single most effective* strategy for reducing muscle tension, stress, and hence anxiety (both chronic and acute). Chapter 16 discusses a variety of dietary changes that can help reduce anxiety. These include eliminating stimulants and substances that stress the body and relying more on foods and supplements that promote a calmer disposition. Chapter 17 examines a variety of health issues that can aggravate anxiety—conditions such as adrenal exhaustion, PMS, seasonal affective disorder, and insomnia. All need to be dealt with in a comprehensive program for overcoming anxiety. Finally, chapter 18 discusses situations where it is *appropriate* for you to take medication, along with the risks and benefits of each of the major types of medications used to treat anxiety disorders.

## Emotional Level

Suppressed feelings—especially withheld anger—can be a very important contributing cause to both chronic anxiety and panic attacks. Often feelings of panic are merely a front for buried feelings of anger, frustration, grief, or desperation. Many people with anxiety disorders grew up in families that discouraged the expression of feelings. As an adult, you may have difficulty just identifying what you *are* feeling, let alone expressing those feelings. Chapter 13 provides specific guidelines and strategies for:

- Recognizing symptoms of suppressed feelings

- Identifying what you are feeling

- Learning to express your feelings

- Communicating your feelings to someone else

# Behavioral Level

Phobias persist because of a single behavior: avoidance. As long as you avoid driving on freeways, crossing bridges, speaking in public, or being in your home alone, your fear about these situations will persist. Your phobia is maintained because your avoidance behavior is so well rewarded: you don't have to reckon with the anxiety you'd experience if you confronted what you fear. Chapter 7 describes strategies that have been found to be very effective in dealing with phobias. Exposure through imagery allows you to first confront your fear mentally, imagining over and over that you can handle it well. Real-life exposure involves confronting your phobia in actuality—but with the help of a support person and in small increments. Perhaps the most important feature of both types of exposure is that they break down into small steps the process of confronting what you fear.

Certain behaviors tend to encourage panic attacks. Trying to fight or resist panic will usually only aggravate it. Most of the time it is impossible to will your way out of panic. Chapter 6 suggests strategies you can use to minimize panic when it first develops. Learning to observe and "go with it" instead of reacting to the bodily symptoms of panic is perhaps the most important behavioral shift you can make. Specific techniques such as talking to another person, distracting your mind, becoming physically active, expressing needs and feelings, doing abdominal breathing, and repeating coping statements can all foster an increased capacity to *actively disrupt panic symptoms* rather than passively react to them.

# Mental Level

What you say to yourself internally—what is called *self-talk*—has a major effect on your state of anxiety. People with all types of anxiety disorders tend to engage in excessive "what-if" thinking, imagining the worst possible outcome in advance of facing what they fear. Scaring yourself through what-if scenarios is what has traditionally been called "worry." Self-critical thinking and perfectionist self-talk (statements to yourself that start with "I should," "I have to," or "I must") also promote anxiety.

Chapter 8 presents specific strategies for recognizing and *countering* destructive thinking patterns. By reconstructing negative self-talk into more supportive, confidence-building statements, you can begin to undo the long-standing habits of worry, self-criticism, and perfectionism that perpetuate anxiety.

Beneath anxiety-provoking self-talk are *mistaken beliefs* about yourself, others, and the world that produce anxiety in very basic ways. For example, if you see yourself as inadequate compared to others—or view the outside world as a dangerous place—you'll tend to remain anxious until you revise these basic attitudes. Chapter 9 offers strategies for both identifying and countering mistaken beliefs that contribute to anxiety.

# Interpersonal Level

Much of the anxiety people experience arises from difficulties in interpersonal relationships. When you have difficulty communicating your real feelings and needs to others, you may find yourself swallowing frustration to the point where you're chronically tense and anxious. The same is true when you're unable to set limits or say no to unwanted demands or requests from others. Chapter 14 offers a variety of strategies for learning to stand up for your rights and express your true wants and feelings. Assertive communication provides ways to express what you want or don't want in a manner that preserves respect for other people. Learning to be assertive is a very important part of the recovery process, especially if you're dealing with agoraphobia or social phobia.

Being able to talk about your condition with others is also an important step in the recovery process. Ways to do this are discussed at the end of chapter 6.

# "Whole Self" Level (Self-Esteem)

Of all the contributing causes to anxiety disorders, low self-esteem is among the deepest. You may have grown up in a dysfunctional family, which, through various forms of deprivation, abuse, or neglect, fostered your low sense of self-worth. As a result, you may carry into adulthood deep-seated feelings of insecurity, shame, and inadequacy, which tend to show up, on a more noticeable level, as panic attacks, fear of confronting the outside world (agoraphobia), fear of humiliation (social phobia), or generalized anxiety. Frequently, low self-esteem is tied in with all of the various contributing causes described above—in particular, lack of assertiveness, self-critical or perfectionist self-talk, and difficulty expressing feelings.

There are many ways to build self-esteem. Developing a positive body image, working toward and achieving concrete goals, and countering negative self-talk with validating affirmations can all help. Chapter 15 provides specific strategies and exercises for strengthening your feelings of self-worth.

# Existential and Spiritual Level

Sometimes people can improve on all of the levels previously described and yet remain anxious and unsettled. They seem to have a vague sense of dissatisfaction, emptiness, or boredom about life, which can lead to panic or to chronic, generalized anxiety. Certain of my clients have found that the ultimate "solution" to their problem with anxiety was to find a broad purpose or direction that gave their life greater meaning. Frequently, this involved taking up a vocation that fulfilled their true talents and interests. In one case, it involved developing an artistic talent that provided a creative outlet. Anxiety symptoms (as well as depression) can be the psyche's way of pushing you to explore and actualize an unrealized potential in your life, whether this involves intellectual development, emotional development, or even getting more in touch with your body. Instead of regarding your panic or phobias *merely* as a reaction to negative physical, emotional, or mental factors, you may be surprised to discover that they represent a call to realize your full potential.

For many individuals, a deep spiritual commitment and involvement provides a significant pathway to recovery from anxiety problems. Twelve-step programs have demonstrated the potency of spiritual awakening in the area of addictions—and the same is true for recovery from anxiety disorders. Developing a connection with a Higher Power (call it God, Spirit, or whatever you like) can provide a profound means for achieving inner security, strength, peace of mind, and an attitude that the outer world is a benevolent place. An existential-spiritual level of recovery is considered in chapter 21.

# Four Examples of a Comprehensive Recovery Program

The preceding section may have helped broaden your understanding of the various levels that come into play in a comprehensive approach to recovery from anxiety disorders. To make this more concrete, I want you to consider what such an approach would look like in four specific cases. These four examples are the same ones that were presented at the beginning of chapter 1 and reflect the four most common types of anxiety disorders seen by therapists: panic attacks, agoraphobia, social phobia, and obsessive-compulsive disorder. As you read through each of the examples, you may begin to formulate what strategies you want to include in your own recovery program. The *Problem Effectiveness Chart* and *Weekly Practice Record* that follow these examples will enable you to work out your own unique program in greater detail.

## Susan: Panic Disorder

You may remember from chapter 1 that Susan was awakened every night by panic attacks marked by heart palpitations, dizziness, and a fear that she was going to die. She would get up and try to make these symptoms go away, becoming more and more anxious when they didn't, to the point where she might spend an hour or more walking about her house. Terrified and confused, she worried about whether she was going to have a heart attack. After a week of recurring panic episodes, she made an appointment with a cardiologist.

Let's suppose that her cardiologist was enlightened about anxiety disorders. After ruling out any heart problems, the cardiologist diagnosed her panic disorder and sent her to a therapist who specialized in the treatment of phobias and panic. This therapist utilized a comprehensive treatment approach with a number of components designed to diminish Susan's problem on a physical, emotional, and mental level.

First, the therapist sent her back to a medical doctor, an internist, to rule out any other possible physical bases for her problem, such as hyperthyroidism, hypoglycemia, mitral valve prolapse, or a calcium-magnesium deficiency. Once these possible medical conditions were ruled out, Susan began her recovery program by learning abdominal breathing techniques (see chapter 4) that helped her slow down the physiological arousal response that accompanies a panic attack. She was also asked to practice progressive muscle relaxation on a daily basis (chapter 4) to train her body to enter into a relaxed state easily. Regular practice of progressive muscle relaxation had a cumulative effect (and the same would be true for regular practice of any other deep relaxation technique, such as visualization or meditation). After several weeks, Susan noticed that she was feeling more relaxed *all the time*. In addition to breathing and deep relaxation techniques, she was asked to maintain a program of regular, vigorous exercise (see chapter 5). She had discretion in choosing the type of exercise to do, but preferably it was to be aerobic exercise lasting for a half hour four to five times per week. Regular exercise worked together with the breathing techniques and deep relaxation to help relieve excess muscle tension, metabolize excess adrenaline, reduce vulnerability to sudden surges of anxiety, and increase Susan's overall sense of well-being. This combination of relaxation and exercise alone went a long way to significantly reduce the intensity and frequency of her panic attacks.

Susan's therapist also discovered that she was drinking three to four cups of coffee per day. Although for some people this might be a manageable amount, most individuals dealing with panic disorder find that their condition is aggravated by even small amounts of caffeine. Susan was asked to gradually taper off her caffeine consumption and replace regular with decaffeinated coffee. Her therapist also recommended a balanced diet, consisting largely of whole, unprocessed foods with minimal sugar and salt. She was also advised to take high-potency vitamin B-complex, vitamin C, and calcium-magnesium supplements (see chapter 16).

Susan was then taught specific techniques for interrupting the onset of panic when she first began to notice the approach of symptoms (see chapter 6). These techniques included calling a friend, physically exerting herself by doing housework, or writing out her feelings in a journal if she was feeling angry or frustrated. Special emphasis was given to her self-talk—what she said to herself at the very onset of feeling panic symptoms. Her therapist found that Susan had a tendency to scare herself into a high state of panic by internally saying such things as "What if I have a heart attack?" "I can't stand this!" or "I've got to get out of here!" She was taught to replace this "scare-talk" with more positive, self-supportive statements, such as "I can handle these sensations," "I can flow with this and wait for my anxiety to diminish," or "I can let my body do its thing and this will pass." After practicing these "coping statements" repeatedly (see the section "Coping Statements" in chapter 6, Coping with Panic Attacks), Susan found that she could more easily manage early body symptoms of panic rather than react to them. After a while she was able to minimize severe panic reactions altogether. Her therapist also helped Susan identify some of the fundamental mistaken beliefs underlying much of her behavior (see chapter 9). She began to let go of such basic assumptions about herself, such as "I have to be completely successful at everything I do," "Life is a struggle," and "Everything must be totally predictable and in control." She was able to take life a little more easily and view its inevitable challenges with more perspective. The net result was a significant reduction in her overall level of anxiety.

A final issue associated with Susan's panic reactions was her tendency to completely suppress her anger and frustration. Early on, her therapist noticed that Susan was most vulnerable to panic on days when she had encountered numerous frustrating situations at work. She had grown up in a family where everyone was supposed to always do their best without ever complaining. Direct expression of feelings and needs was discouraged—she had learned to keep up a pleasant front both to strangers and friends, no matter how she was feeling inside. Although Susan couldn't believe it at first, she eventually concluded that her panic reactions were sometimes nothing more than intense feelings of frustration and anger in disguise. Her exercise program helped her discharge some of these feelings. She also found it helpful to write her feelings down in a journal whenever she noticed herself beginning to feel on-edge (see chapter 13).

Susan's recovery program consisted of a variety of interventions on a physical, behavioral, emotional, and mental level, as summarized below.

*Physical*     Breathing exercises
Regular practice of deep relaxation
Regular aerobic exercise
Elimination of caffeine
Nutritional improvements, including vitamin supplements

*Behavioral*     Coping techniques to abort panic reactions at their onset—such as abdominal breathing and distraction techniques

*Emotional*     Identifying some panic reactions as anger in disguise
Learning to express frustrations verbally and in writing

*Mental*     Changing scare-talk at the onset of panic to supportive, calming self-talk
Practicing coping affirmations
Reevaluating underlying mistaken beliefs and adopting a more relaxed, easygoing perspective on life

It was through a combination of all these interventions that Susan was able to find lasting relief from her panic attacks. Six months from the time she began her program, she was still occasionally anxious but only rarely experienced symptoms of panic. On the occasions when she did, she had a variety of tools that allowed her to dissipate the reaction before it gained momentum.

For Susan, it was possible to achieve a lasting recovery from panic without the use of prescription medications. This is not always the case. When panic is so frequent or severe that it interferes with your work, relationships, or general ability to function (or when it does not yield to approaches like those discussed above), it may be appropriate to take medication. An antidepressant medication such as Zoloft (sertraline), taken over a period of six months to one year, can often be quite helpful in these instances (see chapter 18).

## Cindy: Agoraphobia

You may recall Cindy's case from the example in the first chapter. She not only had panic attacks but was also beginning to avoid situations such as grocery stores, restaurants, and movie theaters, where she was afraid she might have an attack. She was also very concerned that she might have to stop going to work. This avoidance of situations out of fear of panic is the hallmark of agoraphobia. What would a comprehensive recovery program for Cindy look like?

Just about all the interventions described in the example of Susan were also used in Cindy's case, because she, too, was experiencing panic attacks. Breathing techniques, regular practice of progressive muscle relaxation, regular (if possible, aerobic) exercise, and nutritional improvements were all necessary to help her reduce the physiological component of panic (see the corresponding chapters in this workbook). She also learned the same coping techniques for panic so that she was able to *act* rather than *react* when she felt the first bodily symptoms of panic coming on (see chapter 6). Cindy also worked on changing counterproductive self-talk (see chapter 8). In her case, this was especially important—not only for coping with panic itself but also for curbing her excessive tendency to worry about panicking when she went to work. Finally, Cindy, just like Susan, needed to reexamine some of her basic mistaken beliefs about herself, such as "I can't make mistakes," "I must always be pleasing to everybody," and "Success is everything." She developed affirmations to counter these beliefs and made an audio recording of them that she listened to every night as she went to sleep (see chapter 9).

It was important for Cindy to work not only on her panic reactions but on her avoidance behavior as well. At the outset, she was avoiding crowded public situations, such as grocery stores, restaurants, and movie theaters, and had nearly reached the point where she was afraid to go to work. In only a few weeks, she had severely limited where she would go. It was through the processes of imagery and real-life exposure that she learned to reenter all these situations and be comfortable with them (see chapter 7). There were three phases in this process. First, she broke down the goal of reentering each specific situation into a series of steps. For example, in the case of the grocery store, she had eight steps:

1. Spending one minute near the entrance of the store

2. Spending one minute inside the door of the store

3. Going halfway to the back of the store, spending one minute there, and then leaving

4. Going to the back of the store, spending one minute there, and then leaving

5. Spending three minutes in the store without buying anything

6. Buying one item and going through the express checkout line

7. Buying three items and going through the express checkout line

8. Buying three items and going through a regular checkout line

The second phase involved practicing imagery exposure—going through each of these steps in her *imagination* until she could visualize the final step in detail without feeling any anxiety.

Third, Cindy practiced real-life exposure, going through each of the eight steps in real life. She practiced each step several times at first with the help of a support person—usually her boyfriend—and then tried it out alone. For example, after she had mastered step 3 by herself, she started practicing step 4 with her support person. She found that the process worked best if she temporarily stopped, attempting not to exit the situation, any time she felt anxiety coming on so strongly that she felt it might get out of control. Yet it was easier to advance from one step to the next if she didn't "overexpose" or resensitize herself by pushing herself to the point of feeling intense anxiety. If her anxiety did start to feel as though it was becoming out of control, Cindy would temporarily step out of the situation and then return to it as soon as possible.

Cindy undertook this three-phase process—1) breaking the goal down into steps, 2) imagery exposure, and 3) real-life exposure—with each of her specific phobias. By practicing exposure on a regular basis, she was able after three months to reenter all the situations she had previously avoided and to feel comfortable with them.

Cindy had a high degree of self-motivation. The consistent encouragement and reinforcement she got from her boyfriend, who always accompanied her on her first run of entering a phobic situation, sped up her progress considerably.

The most direct and efficient way to overcome any fear is simply to face it. If you are agoraphobic, however, the prospect of confronting long-standing fears can seem overwhelming at first. Cindy learned that this confrontation process can be made manageable if it is broken down into sufficiently small steps that are first negotiated in the imagination.

Apart from overcoming her phobias, another important part of Cindy's recovery was learning to be assertive (see chapter 14). A major part of the stress that contributed to her first panic attack came from her inability to say no to unreasonable demands placed on her by her boss. Cindy's friends also noted that she couldn't stand up for her rights or say no to her boyfriend for fear of his leaving her. She had grown up in a family where her father had left when she was eight. In addition, her mother was very demanding and critical. Consequently, Cindy was never quite sure that she was loved, and she had a deep-seated insecurity about being abandoned. As a child she feared that standing up for herself would jeopardize the tenuous and conditional love she received from her mother. Cindy carried this pattern of dependency and fear of abandonment into adulthood and replayed it in her relationship with her boyfriend. In subtle ways, it actually served to reinforce her agoraphobia. On an unconscious level, she felt that if she were dependent on her boyfriend to take care of her, he would never leave her.

During her recovery, Cindy realized that she wanted to rework her "life script." She was feeling increasingly frustrated about always accommodating everyone else, and she began to recognize the need to develop a stronger sense of herself and her own rights. Through learning to be assertive, she discovered that she could ask for what she wanted, say no to what she didn't want, and still obtain the love and support she needed from her boyfriend and others. In fact, she was surprised to find that everyone, including her boyfriend, respected her more for being able to stand up for herself. The independence Cindy gained from learning to confront situations she had previously avoided went hand in hand with the independence she gained from developing a more assertive interpersonal style. There was no longer any need for her agoraphobia because there was no longer any need for the dependency that maintained it.

Because of the insecurity and fear of abandonment left over from her childhood, it was also critical for Cindy to work on her self-esteem (see chapter 15). She discovered that the only remedy for the inadequate parenting she had received was to become a good parent to herself. She did this in part by improving her body image and countering her *inner critic* (self-critical inner dialogue) with affirmations of self-acceptance and self-worth.

In sum, Cindy's recovery program for agoraphobia contained all of the elements of Susan's program for panic attacks *plus* imagery and real-life exposure to overcome her specific avoidances. It was also necessary for Cindy to address assertiveness and self-esteem issues. She needed to overcome feelings of insecurity and a fear of abandonment that she had carried over from childhood—an insecurity and fear that tended to reinforce her agoraphobia. Her total program involved interventions on six different levels:

| | |
|---|---|
| *Physical* | Breathing exercises |
| | Regular practice of deep relaxation |

|  | Regular aerobic exercise |
|  | Nutritional improvements, including vitamin supplements |
| *Behavioral* | Coping techniques to abort panic reactions at their onset |
|  | Imagery and real-life exposure to overcome specific phobias |
| *Emotional* | Learning to identify and express feelings |
| *Mental* | Countering negative self-talk that contributed to panic attacks as well as worry about panicking |
|  | Countering underlying mistaken beliefs with self-supporting affirmations |
| *Interpersonal* | Developing a more assertive interpersonal style |
| *Whole Self* | Developing self-esteem through |

*Whole Self*  Developing self-esteem through

- Working on her body image

- Overcoming her inner critic

It took Cindy about a year to fully implement these interventions. At the end of one year, she was close to being free of her agoraphobia as well as panic attacks. She decided to go back to school part-time to train to become a registered nurse while continuing her job as a medical secretary.

## Steve: Social Phobia

You may recall from chapter 1 that Steve had difficulty attending meetings at work. He would clam up in group sessions and feared that his coworkers would look upon him critically for not contributing. His very worst fear was of being asked to give a presentation before a group. When this finally happened, he was so terrified that he felt he might have to quit his job.

Steve's problem fits the picture of a social phobia very well—he feared embarrassment and humiliation as a result of being unable to perform in a group situation. His recovery program depended heavily on the processes of imagery and real-life exposure.

Like Susan and Cindy, Steve required a comprehensive treatment approach. Because he tended generally to be anxious much of the time, the same strategies were needed that were used to reduce the physical component of anxiety for Susan and Cindy. Steve first learned abdominal breathing techniques to reduce anxiety on a short-term basis. He found these to be very helpful in reducing the apprehension that came up when he was asked to attend meetings at work. He also practiced a deep relaxation technique twice a day. In Steve's case, meditation seemed to work better than progressive muscle relaxation for soothing his active mind (see chapter 19). He also found that jogging four times a week made a substantial improvement in his level of tension and anxiety (see chapter 5). Finally, he learned that when he reduced his consumption of refined sugar, his mood swings diminished and he was less prone to bouts of depression (see chapter 16). By upgrading his overall health and wellness, Steve became more confident about tackling his social phobia.

The phobia of being in meetings at work was dealt with first through visualizing attending meetings in imagery. As in Cindy's case, Steve broke down the goal of being able to handle meetings into steps:

1. Sitting in a small group (fewer than five people) for fifteen minutes

2. Sitting in a small group for forty-five minutes to one hour

3. Sitting in a larger group for fifteen minutes

4. Sitting in a larger group for forty-five minutes to one hour

5. Repeating steps 1 to 4, but making at least one comment during the course of the meeting

6. Repeating steps 1 to 4, but making at least two comments during the meeting

7. Giving a one-minute presentation before a small group

8. Giving a three-minute presentation before a small group

9. Giving a five- to ten-minute presentation before a small group

10. Repeating steps 7 to 9 with a larger group

After he had successfully practiced exposure in his imagination, Steve undertook the mission to conquer his fear of groups in real life (see chapter 7). First, he sat down with his boss and discussed his problem. He explained that he wanted to be able to participate in meetings and was working through a specific step-by-step program to overcome his phobia. He made an arrangement with his boss to attend only small, short meetings; he had permission to temporarily leave if his anxiety level became too high. After mastering small, brief meetings, he would be able to progress to larger and longer ones. Knowing he would always be free to retreat if he needed to, he felt more willing to undertake real-life exposure. After working up to a point where he could verbally participate in large meetings, he began to work on his fear of making a presentation. Instead of starting out trying to do this at work, Steve decided to take a course in public speaking at a local junior college. The demands for performance in a classroom setting, where everyone was learning, seemed less intense than the expectations at work. After completing the public speaking class, he arranged to make a brief presentation at work before a small group of coworkers he knew well. From there, he progressed to larger groups, to longer presentations, and finally to speaking before groups of strangers.

Steve continued to feel anxious when he got up before a group, but he was now able to *handle* his anxiety through a combination of abdominal breathing techniques and coping statements: "I can ride through this anxiety and be fine"; "As soon as I get started, I'll be fine"; "What I have to say is worthwhile—everyone will be interested." With time and practice, he got to the point where he no longer feared making presentations and, in fact, looked forward to them as an opportunity to contribute his own insights and ideas.

Besides practicing exposure, Steve, like Cindy, worked on assertiveness and self-esteem (see chapters 14 and 15). He had grown up in a family where he was the youngest of three brothers.

Always being bossed around by his older brothers, he had learned to suppress his own feelings and ideas. Throughout his life, he had been afraid to stand up for himself. This fear played no small role in his difficulty with speaking up or making presentations before a group. Through practicing assertiveness skills, he learned how to express his feelings and wants to others directly. He was pleasantly surprised to find that others usually appreciated and were interested in what he had to say.

As the youngest child in his family, Steve had also been "babied" during childhood. He grew up with an underlying fear of standing up as his own person and assuming full responsibility as an adult. He had to work on self-esteem to realize that he was just as valuable, important, and able to contribute as anyone else. Steve's program for recovery from social phobia contained many of the same components as Cindy's program for recovery from agoraphobia. The only significant difference was that Steve didn't have to deal with panic; his phobia centered around fears of embarrassment and humiliation rather than fears of losing control during a panic attack. All of the following strategies contributed to his recovery, with real-life exposure perhaps being the most crucial:

| | |
|---|---|
| *Physical* | Breathing exercises |
| | Regular practice of deep relaxation |
| | Regular aerobic exercise |
| | Nutritional improvements (specifically, reducing sugar intake and thus hypoglycemic mood swings) |
| *Behavioral* | Imagery exposure |
| | Real-life exposure, including taking a public speaking class prior to making presentations at work |
| *Emotional* | Learning to identify and express feelings |
| *Mental* | Countering negative self-talk |
| | Countering mistaken beliefs |
| *Interpersonal* | Developing an assertive interpersonal style |
| *Whole Self* | Working on reducing his worry about how he might appear to others in group situations |
| | Overcoming listening to the voice of his inner critic |

## Mike: Obsessive-Compulsive Disorder

Mike, you may recall, was a successful businessman who had a recurring, irrational fear while driving that he had run over a person or an animal. So strong and insistent was this fear that he continually had to retrace the route he'd just driven to assure himself that no one was lying in the street. By the time he sought treatment, his compulsion to check was so strong that he needed to retrace his route three or four times before he could go on. Because he felt both ashamed and powerless to control his behavior, he was also significantly depressed—a common complaint of people with obsessive-compulsive disorder. Mike's problem was an example of the "checking" type of obsessive-compulsive disorder. But the comprehensive recovery program he undertook could apply equally well to other forms of obsessive-compulsive disorder, including washing, counting, or other compulsions.

In many respects, Mike's road to recovery was similar to that of Susan, Cindy, and Steve in the preceding examples. His therapist asked him to practice breathing exercises, progressive muscle relaxation, and aerobic exercise on a daily basis to reduce the physiological component of his anxiety. Mike also reduced the amount of caffeine and sugar in his diet and started taking high-potency B-complex and vitamin C supplements with breakfast and dinner. Mike felt so much better from these practices alone that there were certain days that he didn't need to retrace his driving route at all. However, his problem didn't disappear altogether.

Mike worked on changing his inner dialogue, or self-talk, while driving. Instead of always asking himself, "What if I hit someone?" he learned to counter with the statement, "If I hit anything, I certainly would hear it or feel it. But this hasn't happened, so I'm okay." Repeating this reassuring statement over and over helped him reduce the number of times he needed to retrace his route from three or four to one or two, though it didn't dispel his obsession completely.

Another helpful intervention was learning to identify and express his angry feelings. Mike found that by getting angry with his compulsion to check and shouting "No!" very loudly in his car, he could sometimes dissipate his anxiety enough so that he didn't have to check. Getting in touch with and acknowledging his frustrations also helped him reduce stress in other areas of his life apart from his specific problem with checking. Yet expressing needs and feelings was not enough, any more than the physical and mental strategies he had tried, to completely resolve his obsessive-compulsive problem.

From his reading on the subject, Mike learned that obsessive-compulsive disorder responds best to the combination of two specific interventions:

- Exposure and response prevention, a behavioral intervention

- Medication—specifically, antidepressant medications such as clomipramine (Anafranil) and fluoxetine (Prozac)

Under the supervision of his therapist, Mike practiced exposure and response prevention in two steps. First, he was instructed to reduce to one the number of times he retraced his route. He had already brought the frequency down from four or five repetitions to two or three, and over the course of a month he was able to reduce the number further, to one. At this point, his therapist rode with him in the car and instructed Mike, whenever he felt the urge to retrace, to pull the car over to the side of the road and stop. Mike then waited several minutes for the anxiety he felt about not retracing his route to subside. Then he resumed his driving. After two weeks of practicing response prevention with his therapist, Mike was finally able to do it on his own. It was very liberating to Mike not to have to spend so much time and energy on retracing his driving route.

A problem that remained, though, was that he couldn't get the obsession about having run over someone out of his mind completely—even though positive self-talk had helped somewhat.

He continued to be vigilant while driving and was depressed that he had so little control over his thoughts.

Mike's therapist referred him to a psychiatrist who instructed him about the medication fluvoxamine (see the section "SSRI Antidepressant Medications" in chapter 18), a drug that has been effective in eliminating or reducing the symptoms of obsessive-compulsive disorder in about 50 percent of the cases in which it has been used. Within three weeks of starting the medication, Mike found that his obsessions had diminished and that his depression had lifted significantly. He began to relax and enjoy driving again, free of any concern about having hit someone. Mike's doctor told him that he would need to stay on the medication for one year, at which point he would reduce the dose to a maintenance dose that he would continue long-term.

Although Mike's obsessive-compulsive disorder responded quite well to the combination of interventions described above, he continued to feel depressed from time to time. It became apparent to his therapist that Mike was feeling somewhat bored with his line of work and with his life in general. The final phase of his recovery program involved making two major adjustments that added meaning and direction to his life. First, he decided to make a career change. Over the course of a year, he moved from a corporate position in marketing to starting a small retail business of his own. All his life, Mike had had a strong interest in music but had never done anything to fulfill it. So, as a second step, he began taking piano lessons. After a year, he took this pursuit a step further, bought a synthesizer, and began to compose his own original piano pieces. This creative outlet added a new dimension to Mike's life and enabled him to express a previously unrealized potential. It was after this that his depression fully lifted.

The most critical component of Mike's recovery from obsessive-compulsive disorder was the combination of response prevention and medication. The crux of his recovery from depression was the combination of overcoming his obsessive-compulsive disorder *and* developing a creative outlet that gave his life a new dimension of meaning. His total program for recovery can be summarized as follows:

| | |
|---|---|
| *Physical* | Breathing exercises |
| | Regular practice of deep relaxation |
| | Regular aerobic exercise |
| | Nutritional improvements plus vitamin supplements |
| *Behavioral* | Exposure and response prevention to eliminate checking |
| *Emotional* | Learning to identify and express anger and frustration |
| *Mental* | Self-talk to counter fears about having run over someone |
| *Medication* | Taking fluvoxamine for one year at a higher dose, then continuing after a year at a maintenance dose |
| *Existential/ Spiritual* | Pursuing a creative interest in playing the piano and musical composition |

# Developing Your Own Recovery Program

By this point, you've likely gained a better idea about three things: 1) the wide range of strategies used in a comprehensive recovery program, 2) the specific types of strategies employed, and 3) how such strategies are actually implemented in specific cases.

You can now begin to develop your own recovery program. The following two charts are designed to assist you with this. The first is the *Problem Effectiveness Chart*. It correlates different types of anxiety disorders with specific chapters in this workbook. Chapters that are particularly relevant for *everyone* with the disorder are marked with an "X." Those chapters that are often relevant are marked with a lowercase "x." Your choice of strategies will, of course, depend on the nature and causes of your particular difficulty. After reading the first three chapters of this workbook, you should have some idea of which strategies to emphasize.

## Problem Effectiveness Chart

| "Ordinary" Anxiety | Post-Traumatic Stress Disorder | Obsessive-Compulsive Disorder | Generalized Anxiety Disorder | Specific Phobia | Social Phobia | Agoraphobia | Panic Attacks | |
|---|---|---|---|---|---|---|---|---|
| X | X | X | X | X | X | X | X | Relaxation |
| X | X | X | X | X | X | X | X | Exercise |
|   |   |   |   |   | x | X | X | Coping Techniques for Panic |
|   |   |   |   | X | X | X | X | Exposure |
| X | X | X | X | X | X | X | X | Self-Talk |
| X | X | X | X | X | X | X | X | Mistaken Beliefs |
| X | X | X | X |   | X | X | X | Expressing Feelings |
| x | x | x | x |   | X | X |   | Assertiveness |
| X | X | X | X | X | X | X | X | Self-Esteem |
| X | X | X | X | X | X | X | X | Nutrition |
|   | X | X | x |   | x | x | X | Medication |
| x | x | x | x |   | x | x | x | Meaning/Spirituality |

The second chart, called the *Weekly Practice Record*, enables you to outline in detail your own personal program for recovery. The chart lists all the specific strategies and skills offered in this workbook. Following each skill, in parentheses, is the recommended frequency for practice in a one-week time period. This chart enables you to check off, for each day of the week, which exercises you have practiced.

Since this is a weekly chart, you may want to *make fifty-two copies* of it to take you through at least a one-year time period. (Of course, your actual recovery may turn out to take significantly less than one year.) A downloadable version of the form is available online; see the very back of this book for more information.

At the top of the chart, be sure to specify the dates of the particular week as well as your goals for that week. At the bottom of the chart, you can estimate, on a scale of 0 to 100 percent, how much you believe you have recovered up to the time of that particular week. (Note: Be prepared for your level of recovery to be marked by progressions and regressions from week to week.) It is obvious that you will not implement *all* of the strategies recommended in this workbook *every* week. As you go through each chapter, you'll likely emphasize the skills taught in that chapter. There are four particular skills, though, worth practicing *five to seven times a week* for fifty-two weeks a year, regardless of the type of anxiety disorder you happen to be dealing with:

1.  A deep relaxation technique such as muscle relaxation, visualization, or meditation

2.  One half-hour of vigorous exercise

3.  Good nutritional habits

4.  Countering negative self-talk or using affirmations to counter mistaken beliefs

If you happen to have phobias, there is one additional strategy recommended for practice three to five times a week until you are phobia-free:

5.  Incremental real-life exposure

Beyond these guidelines, you will be working out for yourself how much time you need to spend with the various other strategies that constitute your particular recovery program.

A *consistent commitment over time* to practicing strategies that are helpful to you is what will make the difference between a partial and a complete recovery. The *Weekly Practice Record* is designed to help keep you on track with your personal program for recovery over the long haul.

## *Weekly Practice Record*

Goals for Week                                                Date:

1.

2.

3.

| | Mon | Tues | Wed | Thurs | Fri | Sat | Sun |
|---|---|---|---|---|---|---|---|
| Used deep breathing technique (6–7) | | | | | | | |
| Used deep relaxation technique* (5–7) | | | | | | | |
| Did one half-hour vigorous exercise (5–7) | | | | | | | |
| Used coping techniques to manage panic** | | | | | | | |
| Practiced countering negative self-talk (5–7) | | | | | | | |
| Used affirmations to counter mistaken beliefs (5–7) | | | | | | | |
| Practiced imagery exposure (3–5) | | | | | | | |
| Practiced real-life exposure (3–5) | | | | | | | |
| Identified/expressed feelings** | | | | | | | |
| Practiced assertive communication with significant other** | | | | | | | |
| Practiced assertive communication to avoid manipulation** | | | | | | | |
| Self-esteem: worked on improving body image** | | | | | | | |
| Self-esteem: took steps toward achieving goals** | | | | | | | |
| Self-esteem: worked on countering inner critic** | | | | | | | |
| Nutrition: eliminated caffeine/sugar/stimulants (7) | | | | | | | |
| Nutrition: ate only whole, unprocessed foods (5–7) | | | | | | | |
| Nutrition: used antistress supplements (5–7) | | | | | | | |
| Medication: used appropriate medications as prescribed by doctor (7) | | | | | | | |
| Meaning: worked on discovering/realizing life purpose** | | | | | | | |
| Spirituality: utilized spiritual beliefs and practices to reduce anxiety** | | | | | | | |

Estimated percent recovery (0 percent to 100 percent): _____     * e.g., progressive muscle relaxation, visualization, or meditation
** Recommended frequency varies depending on focus

# Necessary Ingredients for Undertaking Your Own Recovery Program

By now, you may have some idea of the strategies you want to utilize for your own recovery. The *Weekly Practice Record* will enable you to specify, on a weekly basis, the particular strategies and skills you incorporate in your personal program. You may have already guessed, though, that recovery entails much more than just a series of strategies. Your ability to *implement* the strategies recommended in this workbook depends entirely on your attitude, commitment, and motivation to really *do* something about your problem. Your recovery depends on the extent to which you can adopt and incorporate the five necessary ingredients described below.

## 1. Taking Responsibility—In a Context of Support

Do you feel responsible for your problem? Or do you attribute it to some quirk of heredity, abusive parents, or the stressful people in your life? Even if you feel you aren't solely responsible for having created your disorder, you are the one who is ultimately responsible either for holding on to it or for doing something about it. It may be difficult initially to accept the idea that the decision is yours whether to maintain or whether to overcome your problem. Yet accepting full responsibility is the most empowering step you can take. If you are the one who keeps your condition going, you are also the one with the power to change and outgrow it.

Taking responsibility means you don't blame anyone else for your difficulties. It also means that you don't blame *yourself*. Is there truly any justification for blaming yourself that you have panic attacks, phobias, or obsessions and compulsions? Is it truly your fault that you developed these problems? Is it not more accurate to say that you've done the best you could in your life up to now with the knowledge and resources at your disposal? While it's up to you to change your condition, there is simply no basis for judging or blaming yourself for having it.

Taking responsibility for overcoming your condition does *not* mean that you have to do it all alone. In fact, the opposite is true: you are more likely to be willing to change and to take risks when you feel adequately supported. A most important prerequisite for undertaking your own program for recovery is to have an adequate support system. This can include your spouse or partner, one or two close friends, and/or a support group or class specifically set up to assist people with anxiety disorders.

## 2. Motivation—Overcoming Secondary Gains

Once you've decided to acknowledge your share of the responsibility for your problem, your ability to actually do something about it will depend on your motivation. Do you feel truly motivated to change? Enough so that you'll be willing to learn and incorporate several new habits of thought and behavior into your daily routine? Enough so that you'll be willing to make some basic changes in your lifestyle?

Psychologist David Bakan once made the observation that "suffering is the great motivator of growth." If you are experiencing considerable distress from your particular problem, you're likely to be strongly motivated to do something about it. A basic belief in your self-worth can also be a strong motivation for change. If you love yourself enough to feel that you sincerely deserve to have a fulfilling and productive life, you simply won't settle for being impeded by panic, phobias, or other anxiety symptoms. You will demand more of life than that.

This brings up the issue of what interferes with motivation. Any person, situation, or factor that consciously or unconsciously *rewards you for holding on to your condition* will tend to undermine your motivation. For example, you may want to overcome your problem with being housebound. However, if consciously or unconsciously you don't want to deal with facing the outside world, getting a job, and earning an income, you will tend to keep yourself confined. Consciously, you want to overcome agoraphobia, yet your motivation is not strong enough to overcome the unconscious "payoffs" for not recovering.

Many years ago, Sigmund Freud referred to the idea of unconscious payoffs as "secondary gains." Wherever there is strong resistance to recovering from any chronic, disabling condition—whether it is an anxiety disorder, depression, addiction, or obesity—secondary gains are often operative. If you find that you have difficulty developing or *sustaining* motivation to do something about your condition, it's important to ask yourself, "What payoffs am I getting for staying this way?" The list below enumerates some of the more common secondary gains that can keep you stuck:

- A deep-seated belief that you "don't deserve" to recover and lead a normal life—that you're unworthy of being reasonably happy. When self-punishment is a secondary gain, it is often the case that you're punishing yourself to get back at someone else. Self-punishment also can occur because you feel guilty about your condition. The way out of guilt and the tendency to hold yourself back is to work on your self-esteem (see chapter 15).

- A deep-seated belief that "it's too much work" to truly change. After all, you may already be feeling stressed out and overwhelmed. Now you are being asked to take on considerably more responsibility and work in order to recover. Unconsciously, it may just seem like too much work, leaving you discouraged about ever breaking out of your condition. The solution to this dilemma is to replace your assumption of "too much work" with more positive beliefs, such as "I don't have to be completely well tomorrow—I can take small steps toward recovering at my own pace" or "Any goal can be achieved if broken down into sufficiently small steps." (The 12-step recovery programs have abbreviated these constructive attitudes with the slogan "One day at a time.")

- If you're agoraphobic and relatively housebound, you may be attached to the payoffs you get from your spouse or partner. These include attention, being taken care of, and being financially supported, or, in general, not having to deal with adult responsibilities.

- Your spouse or partner may be getting payoffs from your being dependent on him or her, the reverse of the last situation. These can include the opportunity to take care of, control, and even take responsibility for your life (this is a case of *codependency*—see chapter 15). The payoff can also be assurance that you will never leave. That is, your partner may fear that if you fully recover and become more independent, you'll leave. You need to realize that you won't be held back by your partner's secondary gains unless you are unconsciously colluding with him or her to maintain them.

The above is only a partial list of secondary gains. They may or may not apply in your case. If you feel that you're having difficulties with motivation at any point in your recovery, it's important to raise the question "What is the payoff for avoiding change?"

## 3. Making a Commitment to Yourself to Follow Through

The initial motivation and enthusiasm you have when you first decide to do something about your problem is usually sufficient to get you started. The real test is in following through. Are you willing to make a commitment to *consistently* practice skills and strategies that work for you over the many months and sometimes years that it takes to achieve a full and lasting recovery? In my experience, it is difficult to sustain a high level of motivation over such periods of time unless you have a deep and sincere *commitment* to persist with your recovery program until you're fully satisfied with the results. On a practical level, this means going out and exercising, practicing exposure, or working on your self-esteem even on those days when you don't feel like it. It means that you get up and keep going even after you've had a setback that makes you wonder whether you'll *ever* feel better. While your motivation may wax and wane, a personal commitment to follow through with your program is what is going to make the difference between a partial and a complete recovery.

## 4. Willingness to Take Risks

It is simply not possible to change or grow in any area of your life unless you are willing to take some risks. To recover means being willing to experiment with new ways of thinking, feeling, and acting that may be unfamiliar to you at first. It also means giving up some of the payoffs for not changing, as were described in the section on motivation. If you are dealing with phobias, the way to overcome them is simply to face the situations you've been avoiding—gradually and in your imagination at first. If you are dealing with panic attacks, it may be necessary to risk relinquishing some control and learning to flow with unpleasant bodily sensations instead of resisting and fighting them. If you're dealing with obsessions and compulsions, it may be necessary to risk experiencing anxiety when you resist engaging in compulsive behavior. Or it may be necessary to risk taking a prescription medication.

An effective program for recovery is predicated upon your willingness to risk trying out new behaviors that may cause you *more* anxiety at first yet, which in the long run, can be quite helpful. As in the case of taking responsibility, having support from others who believe in you and back you up will make taking risks considerably easier.

## 5. Defining and Visualizing Your Goals for Recovery

It's difficult to tackle and then overcome a problem unless you have a clear, concrete idea of the goal you're aiming for. Before embarking on your own program for recovery, it is important that you answer the following questions:

- "What are the most important positive changes I want to make in my life?"

- "What would a complete recovery from my present condition look like?"

- "Specifically, how will I think, feel, and act in my work, my relationships with others, and my relationship with myself once I've fully recovered?"

- "What new opportunities will I take advantage of once I've fully recovered?"

Once you've defined what your own recovery might be like, it can be very helpful to practice *visualizing* it. During the time you allocate for practicing deep relaxation, take a few minutes to imagine what your life would look like if you were entirely free of your problems. Visualize in detail any changes in your work, recreational activities, and relationships, and the body image and appearance you would like to achieve. To assist you in developing this positive scenario, use the space below or preferably a separate sheet of paper to write out a "script" of how your life would *ideally* look when you have fully recovered. Be sure to cover as many different areas of your life as possible.

### Ideal Scenario for My Life After I've Recovered

Practicing visualizing your goals for recovery on a daily basis (preferably in a relaxed state) will increase your confidence about succeeding. This practice will actually make a full recovery more likely. There is abundant philosophical evidence—both ancient and modern—that what you believe in with your whole heart and see with your whole mind has a strong tendency to come true.

## Summary of Things to Do

1.  Review the case histories in this chapter and examine the *Problem Effectiveness Chart* to determine which chapters of this workbook are relevant to your particular problem.

2.  Decide in what order you're going to work with the various chapters that are relevant to you. The most critical chapters of the book, which you might consider reading first, are chapters 4 through 8.

3.  Make fifty-two copies of the *Weekly Practice Record* to monitor your personal recovery program for one year. (Your recovery, of course, may take less than one year, or perhaps more.)

4.  Reread the final section, "Necessary Ingredients for Undertaking Your Own Recovery Program," to reinforce in your mind the five keys to a successful and complete recovery: *taking responsibility, motivation* (including overcoming secondary gains), *commitment, a willingness to take risks,* and *defining and visualizing goals.*

# 4

# Relaxation

The capacity to relax is at the very foundation of any program undertaken to overcome anxiety, phobias, or panic attacks. Many of the other skills described in this book, such as exposure, changing negative self-talk, or becoming assertive, build on a capacity to achieve deep relaxation.

Relaxation is more than unwinding in front of the TV set or in the bathtub at the end of the day—though, without doubt, these practices can be relaxing. The type of relaxation that really makes a difference in dealing with anxiety is the *regular, daily* practice of some form of *deep relaxation*. Deep relaxation refers to a distinct physiological state that is the exact opposite of the way your body reacts under stress or during a panic attack. This state was originally described by Herbert Benson in 1975 as the *relaxation response*. It involves a series of physiological changes, including:

- Decrease in heart rate

- Decrease in respiration rate

- Decrease in blood pressure

- Decrease in skeletal muscle tension

- Decrease in metabolic rate and oxygen consumption

- Decrease in analytical thinking

- Increase in skin resistance

- Increase in alpha wave activity in the brain

Regular practice of deep relaxation for twenty to thirty minutes on a daily basis can produce, over time, a generalization of relaxation to the rest of your life. That is, after several weeks of practicing deep relaxation once per day, you will tend to feel more relaxed all the time.

Numerous other benefits of deep relaxation have been documented over the past forty years. These include:

- Reduction of generalized anxiety. Many people have found that regular practice also reduces the frequency and severity of panic attacks.

- Preventing stress from becoming cumulative. Unabated stress tends to build up over time. Entering into a state of physiological quiescence once a day gives your body the opportunity to recover from the effects of stress. Even sleep can fail to break the cumulative stress cycle unless you've given yourself permission to deeply relax while awake.

- Increased energy level and productivity. (When under stress, you may work against yourself and become less efficient.)

- Improved concentration and memory. Regular practice of deep relaxation tends to increase your ability to focus and keeps your mind from "racing."

- Reduction of insomnia and fatigue. Learning to relax leads to sleep that is deeper and sounder.

- Prevention and/or reduction of psychosomatic disorders such as hypertension, migraines, headaches, asthma, and ulcers.

- Increased self-confidence and reduced self-blame. For many people, stress and excessive self-criticism or feelings of inadequacy go hand in hand. You can perform better, as well as feel better, when you are relaxed.

- Increased availability of feelings. Muscle tension is one of the chief impediments to an awareness of your feelings.

How can you achieve a state of deep relaxation? Some of the more common methods include:

1. Abdominal breathing

2. Progressive muscle relaxation

3. Passive muscle relaxation

4. Visualizing a peaceful scene

5. Guided visualizations

6. Meditation

7. Yoga

8. Calming music

For the purpose of this chapter, let's focus in some detail on the first four of these methods, which are quite commonly used in helping people learn to relax. The latter four methods are covered more briefly later in this chapter (see "Guided Visualizations," "Meditation," "Yoga," and "Calming Music"). Chapter 19 of this book discusses the topic of meditation, another helpful relaxation approach, in some detail.

# Abdominal Breathing

Your breathing directly reflects the level of tension you carry in your body. Under tension, your breathing usually becomes shallow and rapid, and your breathing occurs high in the chest. When relaxed, you breathe more fully, more deeply, and from your abdomen. It's difficult to be tense and to breathe from your abdomen at the same time.

Some of the benefits of abdominal breathing include:

- Increased oxygen supply to the brain and musculature.

- Stimulation of the parasympathetic nervous system. This branch of your autonomic nervous system promotes a state of calmness and quiescence. It works in a fashion exactly opposite to the sympathetic branch of your nervous system, which stimulates a state of emotional arousal and the various physiological reactions underlying a panic attack.

- Greater feelings of connectedness between mind and body. Anxiety and worry tend to keep you "up in your head." A few minutes of deep abdominal breathing will help bring yourself down into your whole body.

- More efficient excretion of bodily toxins. Many toxic substances in the body are excreted through the lungs.

- Improved concentration. If your mind is racing, it's difficult to focus your attention. Abdominal breathing will help quiet your mind.

- Abdominal breathing by itself can trigger a relaxation response.

If you suffer from phobias, panic, or other anxiety disorders, you will tend to have one or both of two types of problems with breathing:

1. You breathe too high up in your chest and your breathing is shallow.

2. You tend to hyperventilate, breathing out too much carbon dioxide relative to the amount of oxygen carried in your bloodstream. Shallow, chest-level breathing, when rapid, can lead to hyperventilation. Hyperventilation, in turn, can cause physical symptoms very similar to those associated with panic attacks.

These two types of breathing are discussed in greater detail below.

## Shallow, Chest-Level Breathing

Studies have found differences in the breathing patterns of anxious and shy people as opposed to those who are more relaxed and outgoing. People who are fearful and shy tend to breathe in a shallow fashion from their chest, while those who are more extroverted and relaxed breathe more slowly, deeply, and from their abdomens.

Before reading on, take a moment to notice how you are breathing right now. Is your breath slow or rapid? Deep or shallow? Does it center around a point high in your chest or down in your abdomen? You might also notice changes in your breathing pattern under stress versus when you are more relaxed.

If you find that your breathing is shallow and high in your chest, don't despair. It's quite possible to retrain yourself to breathe more deeply and from your abdomen. Practicing abdominal breathing (described below) on a regular basis will gradually help you shift the center of your breath downward from your chest. Regular practice of full abdominal breathing will also increase your lung capacity, helping you to breathe more deeply. A program of aerobic exercise can also be helpful.

## Hyperventilation Syndrome

If you breathe from your chest, you may tend to overbreathe, exhaling excess carbon dioxide in relation to the amount of oxygen in your bloodstream. You may also tend to breathe through your mouth. The result is a cluster of symptoms, including rapid heartbeat, dizziness, and tingly sensations that can be so similar to the symptoms of panic that they can be indistinguishable. Some of the physiological changes brought on by hyperventilation include:

- Increased alkalinity of nerve cells, which causes them to be more excitable. The result is that you feel nervous and jittery.

- Decreased carbon dioxide in the blood, which can cause your heart to pump harder and faster as well as making lights seem brighter and sounds louder.

- Increased constriction of blood vessels in your brain, which can cause feelings of dizziness, disorientation, and even a sense of unreality or separateness from your body.

All these symptoms *may* be interpreted as a developing panic attack. As soon as you start responding to these bodily changes with panic-evoking mental statements to yourself, such as "I'm losing control!" or "What's happening to me?" *you may actually start to experience panic.* Symptoms that initially only mimicked panic set off a reaction that leads to genuine panic. Hyperventilation can either 1) cause physical sensations that lead you to panic *or* 2) contribute to an ongoing panic attack by aggravating unpleasant physical symptoms.

If you suspect that you are subject to hyperventilation, you might notice whether you habitually breathe shallowly from your chest and through your mouth. Notice also, when you're frightened, whether you tend to hold your breath or breathe very shallowly and quickly. The experience of tingling or numb sensations, particularly in your hands or feet, is also a sign of hyperventilation. If any of these characteristics seem to apply to you, hyperventilation may play a role in either instigating or aggravating your panic reactions or anxiety.

The traditional cure for acute hyperventilation symptoms is to breathe into a paper bag. This technique causes you to breathe in carbon dioxide, restoring the normal balance of oxygen to carbon dioxide in your bloodstream. It is a method that works. Equally effective in reducing symptoms of hyperventilation are the abdominal breathing and calming breath exercises described below. Both of them help you slow down your breathing, which effectively reduces your intake of oxygen and brings the ratio of oxygen to carbon dioxide back into balance.

If you can recognize the symptoms of hyperventilation for what they are, then learn to curtail them by deliberately slowing your breathing, you needn't react to them with panic.

The two exercises described below can help you change your breathing pattern. By practicing them, you can achieve a state of relaxation in a short period of time. Just three minutes of practicing abdominal breathing or the calming breath exercise will usually induce a state of relaxation.

Many people have successfully used one or the other technique to abort a panic attack when they felt the first signs of anxiety coming on. The techniques are also very helpful in diminishing anticipatory anxiety you may experience in advance of facing a phobic situation. While the techniques of progressive muscle relaxation and meditation described later in this chapter take up to twenty minutes to achieve their effects, the following two methods can produce a moderate to deep level of relaxation in just three to five minutes.

## Abdominal Breathing Exercise

1.  Note the level of tension you're feeling. Then place one hand on your abdomen right beneath your rib cage.

2.  Inhale slowly and deeply through your nose into the "bottom" of your lungs—in other words, send the air as low down as you can. If you're breathing from your abdomen, your hand should actually *rise*. Your chest should move only slightly while your abdomen expands. (In abdominal breathing, the *diaphragm*—the muscle that separates the chest cavity from the abdominal cavity—moves downward. In so doing, it causes the muscles surrounding the abdominal cavity to push outward.)

3.  When you've taken in a full breath, pause for a moment and then exhale slowly through your nose or mouth, depending on your preference. Be sure to exhale fully. *As you exhale, allow your whole body to just let go* (you might visualize your arms and legs going loose and limp like a rag doll).

4.  Do ten slow, full abdominal breaths. Try to keep your breathing *smooth* and *regular*, without gulping in a big breath or letting your breath out all at once. It will help slow down your breathing if you slowly count to four on the inhale (one-two-three-four) and then slowly count to four on the exhale. Remember to pause briefly at the end of each inhalation.

5.  Count from ten down to one, counting backward one number with each *exhalation*. The process should go like this:

    Slow inhale...Pause...Slow exhale ("Ten.")

    Slow inhale...Pause...Slow exhale ("Nine.")

    Slow inhale...Pause...Slow exhale ("Eight.")

    and so on down to one. If you start to feel light-headed while practicing abdominal breathing, stop for fifteen to twenty seconds, then start again.

6.  Extend the exercise if you wish by doing two or three "sets" of abdominal breaths, remembering to count backward from ten to one for each set (each exhalation counts as one number). *Five full minutes* of abdominal breathing will have a pronounced effect in reducing anxiety or early symptoms of panic. Some people prefer to count from one to ten instead. Feel free to do this if it suits you.

## Calming Breath Exercise

The *Calming Breath Exercise* was adapted from the ancient discipline of yoga. It is a very efficient technique for achieving a deep state of relaxation quickly.

1. Breathing from your abdomen, inhale through your nose slowly to a count of five (count slowly "one...two...three...four...five" as you inhale).

2. Pause and hold your breath to a count of five.

3. Exhale slowly, through your nose or mouth, to a count of five (or more if it takes you longer). Be sure to exhale fully.

4. When you've exhaled completely, take two breaths in your normal rhythm, then repeat steps 1 through 3 in the cycle above.

5. Keep up the exercise for at least three to five minutes. This should involve going through *at least* ten cycles of in-five, hold-five, out-five. As you continue the exercise, you may notice that you can count higher when you exhale than when you inhale. Allow these variations in your counting to occur if they do, naturally, and just continue with the exercise for up to five minutes. Remember to take two normal breaths between each cycle. If you start to feel light-headed while practicing this exercise, stop for thirty seconds and then start again.

6. Throughout the exercise, keep your breathing *smooth* and *regular*, without gulping in breaths or breathing out suddenly.

7. *Optional:* Each time you exhale, you may wish to say, "Relax," "Calm," "Let go," or any other relaxing word or phrase silently to yourself. Allow your whole body to let go as you do this. If you keep this up each time you practice, eventually just saying your relaxing word by itself will bring on a mild state of relaxation.

The *Calming Breath Exercise* can be a potent technique for halting the momentum of a panic reaction when the first signs of anxiety come on. It is also useful in reducing symptoms of hyperventilation.

## Practice Exercise

Practice the *Abdominal Breathing Exercise* or *Calming Breath Exercise* for at least *five minutes every day for at least two weeks.* (Note that guided audio versions of both exercises are available on the website associated with this book. See the very end of the book for more information.) If possible, find a regular time each day to do this so that your breathing exercise becomes a habit. With practice, you can learn in a short period of time to damp down the physiological reactions underlying anxiety and panic.

Once you feel you've gained some mastery in the use of either technique, apply it when you feel stressed or anxious, or when you experience the onset of panic symptoms. By extending your practice of either exercise to a month or longer, you will begin to retrain yourself to breathe from your abdomen. The more you can shift the center of your breathing from your chest to your abdomen, the more consistently you will feel relaxed on an ongoing basis.

## Progressive Muscle Relaxation

Progressive muscle relaxation (PMR) is a systematic technique for achieving a deep state of relaxation. It was developed by Dr. Edmund Jacobson more than eighty years ago. Dr. Jacobson discovered that a muscle could be relaxed by first tensing it for a few seconds and then releasing it. Tensing and releasing various muscle groups throughout the body in sequence produces a deep state of relaxation, which Dr. Jacobson found capable of relieving a variety of conditions, from high blood pressure to ulcerative colitis.

In his original book, *Progressive Relaxation*, Dr. Jacobson developed a series of two hundred different muscle relaxation exercises and a training program that took months to complete. More recently, the system has been abbreviated to fifteen to twenty basic exercises, which have been found to be just as effective, if practiced regularly, as the original more elaborate system.

Progressive muscle relaxation is especially helpful for people whose anxiety is strongly associated with muscle tension. This is what often leads you to say that you are "uptight" or "tense." You may experience chronic tightness in your shoulders and neck, which can be effectively relieved by practicing progressive muscle relaxation. Other symptoms that respond well to progressive muscle relaxation include tension headaches, backaches, tightness in the jaw, tightness around the eyes, muscle spasms, high blood pressure, and insomnia. If you are troubled by racing thoughts, you may find that systematically relaxing your muscles tends to help slow down your mind. Dr. Jacobson himself once said, "An anxious mind cannot exist in a relaxed body."

The immediate effects of progressive muscle relaxation include all the benefits of the relaxation response described at the beginning of this chapter. Long-term effects of *regular* practice of progressive muscle relaxation include:

- A decrease in generalized anxiety

- A decrease in anticipatory anxiety related to phobias

- Reduction in the frequency and duration of panic attacks

- Improved ability to face phobic situations through exposure

- Improved concentration

- An increased sense of control over moods

- Increased self-esteem

- Increased spontaneity and creativity

These long-term benefits are sometimes called *generalization effects*: the relaxation experienced during daily sessions tends, after a month or two, to *generalize* to the rest of the day. The *regular* practice of progressive muscle relaxation can go a long way toward helping you better manage your anxiety, face your fears, overcome panic, and feel better all around.

There are no contraindications for progressive muscle relaxation unless the muscle groups to be tensed and relaxed have been injured. If you take tranquilizers, you may find that regular practice of progressive muscle relaxation will enable you to lower your dosage.

## Guidelines for Practicing Progressive Muscle Relaxation (or Any Form of Deep Relaxation)

The following guidelines will help you make the most use of progressive muscle relaxation. They are also applicable to *any* form of deep relaxation you undertake to practice regularly, including self-hypnosis, guided visualization, and meditation.

1. Practice at least *twenty minutes per day*. Two twenty-minute periods are optimal. Once a day is mandatory for obtaining generalization effects. (You may want to begin your practice with thirty-minute periods. As you gain skill in the relaxation technique, you will find that the amount of time you need to experience the relaxation response will decrease.)

2. Find a *quiet location* to practice where you won't be distracted. Don't permit your phone to ring while you're practicing. Use a fan or an air conditioner to blot out background noise, if necessary.

3. Practice at *regular times*. On awakening, before retiring, or before a meal is generally the best time. A consistent daily relaxation routine will increase the likelihood of generalization effects.

4. Practice on an *empty stomach*. Food digestion after meals will tend to disrupt deep relaxation.

5. Assume a *comfortable position*. Your entire body, including your head, should be supported. Lying down on a sofa or bed or sitting in a reclining chair are two ways of supporting your body most completely. (When lying down, you may want to place a pillow beneath your knees for further support.) Sitting up is preferable to lying down if you are feeling tired and sleepy. It's advantageous to experience the full depth of the relaxation response consciously, without going to sleep.

6. *Loosen any tight garments* and take off shoes, watch, glasses, contact lenses, jewelry, and so on.

7. *Make a decision not to worry about anything.* Give yourself permission to put aside the concerns of the day. Allow taking care of yourself and having peace of mind to take precedence over any of your worries. (Success with relaxation depends on giving peace of mind high priority in your overall scheme of values.)

8. Assume a *passive, detached attitude*. This is probably the most important element. You want to adopt a "let it happen" attitude and be free of any worry about how well you are performing the technique. Do not *try* to relax. Do not *try* to control your body. Do not judge your performance. The point is to let go.

## Progressive Muscle Relaxation Technique

Progressive muscle relaxation involves tensing and relaxing, in succession, sixteen different muscle groups of the body. The idea is to tense each muscle group hard (not so hard that you strain, however) for about ten seconds and then to let go of it suddenly. You then give yourself fifteen to twenty seconds to relax, noticing how the muscle group feels when relaxed in contrast to how it felt when tensed, before going on to the next group of muscles. You might also say to yourself, "Relax," "Letting go," "Let the tension flow away," or any other relaxing phrase during each relaxation period between successive muscle groups. Throughout the exercise, maintain your focus on your muscles. When your attention wanders, bring it back to the particular muscle group you're working on. The guidelines below describe progressive muscle relaxation in detail:

- Make sure you are in a quiet and comfortable setting. Observe the guidelines for practicing relaxation that were previously described.

- When you tense a particular muscle group, do so strongly, without straining, for seven to ten seconds. You may want to count "one-thousand-one," "one-thousand-two," and so on, as a way of marking off seconds.

- Concentrate on what is happening. Feel the buildup of tension in each particular muscle group. It is often helpful to visualize the particular muscle group being tensed.

- When you release the muscles, do so abruptly, and then relax, enjoying the sudden feeling of limpness. Allow the relaxation to develop for at least fifteen seconds before going on to the next group of muscles.

- Allow all the other muscles in your body to remain relaxed, as far as possible, while working on a particular muscle group.

- Tense and relax each muscle group once. But if a particular area feels especially tight, you can tense and relax it two or three times, waiting about ten to fifteen seconds between each cycle.

Once you are comfortably supported in a quiet place, follow the detailed instructions below:

1. To begin, take two or three deep abdominal breaths, exhaling slowly each time. As you exhale, imagine that tension throughout your body begins to flow away.

2. Clench your fists. Hold for seven to ten seconds and then release for fifteen to twenty seconds. *Use these same time intervals for all other muscle groups.*

3. Tighten your biceps by drawing your forearms up toward your shoulders and "making a muscle" with both arms. Hold…and then relax.

4. Tighten your *triceps*—the muscles on the undersides of your upper arms—by extending your arms out straight and locking your elbows. Hold…and then relax.

5.  Tense the muscles in your forehead by raising your eyebrows as far as you can. Hold… and then relax. Imagine your forehead muscles becoming smooth and limp as they relax.

6.  Tense the muscles around your eyes by clenching your eyes tightly shut. Hold…and then relax. Imagine sensations of deep relaxation spreading all around the area of your eyes.

7.  Tighten your jaw by opening your mouth so widely that you stretch the muscles around the hinges of your jaw. Hold…and then relax. Let your lips part and allow your jaw to hang loose.

8.  Tighten the muscles in the back of your neck by pulling your head way back, as if you were going to touch your head to your back. (Be gentle with this muscle group to avoid injury.) Focus only on tensing the muscles in your neck. Hold…and then relax. (Since this area is often especially tight, it's good to do the tense-relax cycle twice.)

9.  Take a few deep breaths and tune in to the weight of your head sinking into whatever surface it is resting on.

10. Tighten your shoulders by raising them up as if you were going to touch your ears. Hold… and then relax.

11. Tighten the muscles around your shoulder blades by pushing your shoulder blades back as if you were going to touch them together. Hold the tension in your shoulder blades… and then relax. (Since this area is often especially tense, you might repeat the tense-relax sequence twice.)

12. Tighten the muscles of your chest by taking in a deep breath. Hold for up to ten seconds… and then release slowly. Imagine any excess tension in your chest flowing away with the exhalation.

13. Tighten your stomach muscles by sucking your stomach in. Hold…and then release. Imagine a wave of relaxation spreading through your abdomen.

14. Tighten your lower back by arching it up. (You can omit this part of the exercise if you have lower back pain.) Hold…and then relax.

15. Tighten your buttocks by pulling them together. Hold…and then relax. Imagine the muscles in your hips going loose and limp.

16. Squeeze the muscles in your thighs all the way down to your knees. You will prob-ably have to tighten your hips along with your thighs, since the thigh muscles attach at the pelvis. Hold…and then relax. Feel your thigh muscles smoothing out and relaxing completely.

17. Tighten your calf muscles by pulling your toes toward you. (Flex carefully to avoid cramps.) Hold…and then relax.

18. Tighten your feet by curling your toes downward. Hold…and then relax.

19. Mentally scan your body for any residual tension. If a particular area remains tense, repeat one or two tense-relax cycles for that group of muscles.

20. Now imagine a wave of relaxation slowly spreading throughout your body, starting at your head and gradually penetrating every muscle group all the way down to your toes.

The entire progressive muscle relaxation sequence should take you twenty to thirty minutes the first time. With practice, you may decrease the time needed to fifteen to twenty minutes. You might want to make an audio recording of the above exercise to expedite your early practice sessions, download the version available on the website associated with this book (see the last page of this book for more details), or obtain another professionally made recording of the exercise. (See appendix 2.) Some people always prefer to use an audio recording, while others have the exercises so well learned after one or two weeks of practice that they prefer doing them from memory.

Remember—regular practice of progressive muscle relaxation once a day can produce a significant reduction in your overall level of anxiety. It can also reduce the frequency and intensity of panic attacks. Finally, regular practice will reduce anticipatory anxiety that may arise in the course of systematically exposing yourself to phobic situations (see chapter 7).

## Passive Muscle Relaxation

Progressive muscle relaxation is an excellent technique for relaxing tight muscles. Passive muscle relaxation, an alternative technique, can induce a general state of relaxation throughout your mind and body. Some people prefer it to progressive relaxation because it is effortless. There is no active tensing and relaxing of muscle groups, only focusing on each muscle group in sequence—from feet to head—and imagining each such group relaxing. Generally, it's best to lie down with your eyes closed when you practice.

The following script leads you through a passive muscle relaxation exercise. You can create your own audio recording on your smartphone using the script below. If you make a recording, it's important to read it slowly, with pauses between the sentences.

Or you can download a prerecorded version of the exercise. See the last page of this book for instructions for downloading the passive muscle relaxation exercise as well as several other exercises in this book.

*Begin by taking two or three deep, abdominal breaths and let yourself settle back into the chair, bed, or wherever you happen to be right now. Make yourself fully comfortable. Let this be a time just for yourself, putting aside all worries and concerns of the day and making this a time just for you. (Pause.)*

*Let each part of your body begin to relax, starting with your feet. Just imagine your feet letting go and relaxing right now. Let go of any excess tension in your feet. Just imagine the tension draining away. (Pause.)*

*As your feet are relaxing, imagine relaxation moving up into your calves. Let the muscles in your calves unwind and loosen up and let go. Allow any tension you're feeling in your calves to just drain away easily and quickly. (Pause.)*

*Now as your calves are relaxing, allow relaxation to move up into your thighs. Let the muscles in your thighs unwind and smooth out and relax completely. You might begin to feel your legs from your waist down to your feet becoming more and more relaxed. You might notice your legs becoming heavy as they relax more and more. (Pause.)*

*Continue now and let relaxation move into your hips. Feel any excess tension in your hips dissolve and flow away. (Pause.)*

*Soon you might allow relaxation to move into your stomach area. Just let go of any stress in your stomach area—let it all go right now, imagining deep sensations of relaxation spreading all around your abdomen. (Pause.)*

*As your stomach is relaxing, continue to allow relaxation to move up into your chest. All the muscles in your chest can unwind and loosen up and let go. Each time you exhale, imagine breathing away any remaining tension in your chest until your chest feels completely relaxed. Let the relaxation deepen and develop throughout your chest, stomach area, and your legs. (Pause.)*

*Soon you might allow relaxation to move into your shoulders—just letting deep sensations of calmness and relaxation spread all through the muscles of your shoulders. Let your shoulders drop, allowing them to feel completely relaxed. Now allow the relaxation in your shoulders to move down into your arms, spreading into your upper arms, down into your elbows and forearms, and finally all the way down to your wrists and hands. Let your arms relax, enjoying the good feeling of relaxation in your arms. (Pause.)*

*Put aside any worries, any uncomfortable, unpleasant thoughts right now. Let yourself be totally in the present moment as you let yourself relax more and more. (Pause.)*

*You can feel relaxation moving into your neck now. All the muscles in your neck just unwind, smooth out, and relax completely. Just imagine the muscles in your neck loosening up just like a knotted cord unraveling. (Pause.)*

*Then soon, the relaxation can move into your chin and jaw. Allow your jaw to relax, letting your jaw loosen up. As it is relaxing, imagine relaxation moving into the area around your eyes. Any tension around your eyes can just dissipate and flow away as you allow your eyes to relax completely. Any eyestrain just dissolves now and your eyes can fully relax. Now let your forehead relax, too—let the muscles in your forehead smooth out and relax completely, noticing the weight of your head against whatever it's resting on as you allow your entire head to relax completely. (Pause.)*

*Just enjoy the good feeling of relaxation all over now—letting yourself drift deeper and deeper into quietness and peace—getting more and more in touch with that place deep inside of perfect peace and serenity.*

## The Peaceful Scene

After completing progressive or passive muscle relaxation, it's helpful to visualize yourself in the midst of a peaceful scene. Imagining yourself in a very peaceful setting can give you a global sense of relaxation that frees you from anxious thoughts. The peaceful setting can be a quiet beach, a stream in the mountains, or a calm lake. Or it can be your bedroom or a cozy fireside on a cold winter night. Don't restrict yourself to reality; you can imagine, if you want to, floating on a cloud or flying on a magic carpet. The important thing is to visualize the scene in sufficient detail so that it completely absorbs your attention. Allowing yourself to be absorbed in a peaceful scene will deepen your state of relaxation, giving you actual physiological results. Your muscular tension lessens, your heart rate slows down, your breathing deepens, your capillaries open up and warm your hands and feet, and so on. A relaxing visualization constitutes a light form of self-hypnosis.

Here are three examples of peaceful scenes.

## The Beach

*You're walking along a beautiful, deserted beach. You are barefoot and can feel the firm white sand beneath your feet as you walk along the margin of the sea. You can hear the sound of the surf as the waves ebb and flow. The sound is hypnotic, relaxing you more and more. The water is a beautiful turquoise blue flecked with whitecaps far out where the waves are cresting. Near the horizon you can see a small sailboat gliding smoothly along. The sound of the waves breaking on the shore lulls you deeper and deeper into relaxation. You draw in the fresh, salty smell of the air with each breath. Your skin glows with the warmth of the sun. You can feel a gentle breeze against your cheek and ruffling your hair. Taking in the whole scene, you feel very calm and at ease.*

## The Forest

*You're snuggled in your sleeping bag. Daylight is breaking in the forest. You can feel the rays of the sun beginning to warm your face. The dawn sky stretches above you in pastel shades of pink and orange. You can smell the fresh, piney fragrance of the surrounding woods. Nearby you can hear the rushing waters of a mountain stream. The crisp, cool morning air is refreshing and invigorating. You're feeling very cozy, comfortable, and secure.*

## At Home

*Imagine yourself comfortably relaxing on a sofa or your bed at home. As you lie back, take some deep, abdominal breaths and set aside all of the worries and concerns of the day. The room is quiet and free of distractions. The phone is turned off and you are free of any obligations to do anything. Though people may be elsewhere in the house, they know to leave you alone. It's feeling good to be able to kick back, rest, and let your body and mind begin to slow down. You can feel your whole body starting to relax. As you continue to rest and relax, you find yourself becoming more deeply comfortable and at ease. In this quiet place, you are feeling very safe, secure, and at peace.*

Note that these scenes are described in language that appeals to the senses of sight, hearing, touch, and smell. Using multisensory words increases the power of the scene to affect you, enabling you to experience it as if you were actually there. The whole point of imagining a peaceful scene is to transport you from your normal state of restless thinking into an altered state of deep relaxation.

A version of the peaceful scene exercise using the beach setting described above is available for download at the website associated with this book. See the very back of this book for more information.

## *Exercise: Peaceful Scene*

Use a separate sheet of paper to design your own peaceful scene. Be sure to describe it in vivid detail, appealing to as many of your senses as possible. It may help to answer the following questions:

- What does the scene look like?

- What colors are prominent?

- What sounds are present?

- What time of day is it?

- What is the temperature?

- What are you in physical contact with in the scene?

- What does the air smell like?

- Are you alone or with somebody else?

Just as with progressive muscle relaxation, you may wish to record your peaceful scene so that you can conjure it up without effort. You may find it helpful to record the instructions for progressive muscle relaxation before describing your peaceful scene. You can use the script below to introduce your peaceful scene when you make your own recording:

*Just think of relaxing every muscle in your body, from the top of your head to the tips of your toes. (Pause.)*

*As you exhale, imagine releasing any remaining tension from your body, mind, or thoughts… just let that stress go. (Pause.)*

*Feel your body drifting down deeper…down deeper into total relaxation. (Pause.)*

*Now imagine going to your peaceful scene….Imagine your special place as vividly as possible, as if you were really there. (Insert your peaceful scene.)*

*You are very comfortable in your beautiful place, and there is no one to disturb you….This is the most peaceful place in the world for you….Just imagine yourself there, feeling a sense of peace flow through you and a sense of well-being. Enjoy these positive feelings….Allow them to grow stronger and stronger. (Pause.)*

*Remember, anytime you wish, you can return to this special place by just taking time to relax. (Pause.)*

*These peaceful and positive feelings of relaxation can grow stronger and stronger each time you choose to relax.*

Once you have imagined your own ideal peaceful scene, practice returning to it every time you do progressive muscle relaxation, passive muscle relaxation, an abdominal breathing exercise, or any other relaxation technique. This will help reinforce the scene in your mind. After a while, it will be so solidly established that you will be able to return to it on the spur of the moment—whenever you wish to calm yourself and turn off anxious thinking. This technique is one of the quickest and most effective tools you can use to counter ongoing anxiety or stress during the day. Fantasizing a peaceful scene is also an important part of *imagery exposure*, a visualization process for overcoming phobias described in chapter 7.

## Guided Visualizations

Many people enjoy listening to guided visualizations in order to relax. Like passive muscle relaxation, no effort is required. You simply lie down, close your eyes, and listen to a CD or download from your preferred device preferably at the same time every day. Follow the guidelines for practicing any form of deep relaxation given earlier in this chapter. See "Guidelines for Practicing Progressive Muscle Relaxation (or Any Form of Deep Relaxation)."

There are many places on the web where you can obtain relaxing visualizations. Some popular ones you can try are drmiller.com and soundstrue.com, or you can do a search for "relaxation CDs" at amazon.com. It's a good idea to purchase at least two or three different relaxation programs to see what works best for you. Also see appendix 2 for further resources.

## Meditation

From the time we awaken, until we go to bed, most of us are engaged almost continually in external activities. We tend to be only minimally in touch with our inner feelings and awareness. Even when we withdraw our senses and are falling asleep at night, we usually experience a mélange of memories, fantasies, thoughts, and feelings related to the preceding or coming day. Rarely do we get beyond all of this and experience ourselves "just being" in the present moment. For many people in Western society, in fact, the idea of doing nothing, or "just being," is difficult to comprehend.

Meditation can bring you to this place of just being. It is a process that allows you to completely stop, let go of thoughts about the immediate past or future, and simply focus on being in the here and now. It can be a helpful discipline to practice when you find that your mind is racing or excessively busy. For a detailed discussion of meditation, both as a relaxation technique and as a general strategy for coping with anxiety, please see chapter 19, Meditation.

## Yoga

The word *yoga* means to "yoke" or "unify." By definition, yoga is involved with promoting unity of mind, body, and spirit. Although in the West, yoga is usually thought of as a series of stretch exercises, it actually embraces a broad philosophy of life and an elaborate system for personal transformation. This system includes ethical precepts, a vegetarian diet, the familiar stretches or postures, specific breathing exercises, concentration practices, and deep meditation. It was originally laid out by the philosopher Patanjali in the second century BCE and is still practiced throughout the world today.

Yoga postures, by themselves, provide a very effective means to increase fitness, flexibility, and relaxation. They can be practiced alone or with a group. Many people find that yoga increases energy and vitality while simultaneously calming the mind. Yoga may be compared to progressive muscle relaxation (PMR), in that it involves holding the body in certain flexed positions for a few moments and then relaxing. Both yoga and PMR lead to relaxation. However, some people find yoga to be more effective than progressive muscle relaxation in freeing up blocked energy. It seems to get energy moving up and down the spine and throughout the body in a way that doesn't happen as readily with PMR. Like vigorous exercise, yoga directly promotes mind-body integration. However, in many ways, it is more specific. Each yoga posture reflects a mental attitude, whether that attitude is one of surrender, as in certain forward-bending poses, or of strengthening the will, as in a backward-bending pose. By emphasizing certain yoga postures and movements, you may be able to cultivate certain positive qualities or move through other negative, restrictive personality patterns.

If you are interested in learning yoga, the best place to start is with a class at a local health club or community college. If such classes are unavailable in your area, try working with a yoga video at home. The popular magazine *Yoga Journal* offers many excellent yoga videos.

## Calming Music

Music has often been called the language of the soul. It seems to touch something deep within us. It can move you into an inner space beyond your anxiety and worries. Relaxing music can help you settle down into a place of serenity deep within that is impervious to the stresses and problems of daily life. It may also uplift you from a depressed mood. If you use music to assuage anxiety, be sure to select pieces that are genuinely relaxing rather than stimulating or emotionally evocative. If the relaxing music is intended to help you get to sleep, it's best not to use it while driving. As a general rule, refrain from playing relaxation CDs while driving your car.

Your portable audio device with earphones can be particularly handy at night if you don't want to disturb others around you. You may find music to be a helpful background to relaxation techniques, such as progressive muscle relaxation or guided visualizations. See appendix 2 for a list of relaxing music selections. Doing a Google search for "relaxing music" will bring up a variety of YouTube videos intended for relaxation.

## Some Common Obstacles to a Daily Program of Deep Relaxation

There are many difficulties you may encounter in trying to practice any form of deep relaxation on a regular basis. You may start out enthusiastically, setting aside time to practice every day. Yet after a week or so, you may find yourself "forgetting" to practice. In a fast-paced society that rewards us for speed, efficiency, and productivity, it's difficult to stop everything and simply relax for twenty to thirty minutes. We are so used to "doing" that it may seem like a chore just to "be."

If you find that you've broken your personal commitment to practice deep relaxation on a daily basis, take time to examine very carefully what you are *saying to yourself*—what excuses you make—on those days when you don't relax. If you just "don't feel like it," there is usually some more specific reason for feeling that way that can be found by examining what you're telling yourself.

Some common excuses for not practicing include:

• "I don't have time to relax."

What this usually means is that you haven't given relaxation sufficient priority among all the other activities you've crowded into your schedule.

• "I don't have any place to relax."

Try creating one. You might let the kids watch their favorite TV show or play with their favorite toys while you go into another room, with instructions not to interrupt you. If you and the kids have only one room, or if they are too young to respect your privacy, then you need to practice at a time when they are out of the house or asleep. The same goes for a demanding spouse.

• "Relaxation exercises seem too slow or boring."

If you're telling yourself this, it's a good indication that you are too speeded up, too frantically pushing yourself through life. Slow down—it's good for you.

In some individuals, deep relaxation may bring up suppressed feelings, which are often accompanied by sensations of anxiety. If this happens to you, be sure to start off with relatively short periods of relaxation, working up gradually to longer periods. The moment you start feeling any anxiety, simply open your eyes and stop whatever procedure you're practicing until you feel better. With time and patience, this particular problem should diminish. If it doesn't, it would be helpful to consult a professional therapist skilled in treating anxiety disorders to assist you in exposing yourself to relaxation.

• "I just don't have the discipline."

Often this means that you haven't persisted with practicing relaxation long enough to internalize it as a habit. You may have made similar statements to yourself in the past when you were attempting to acquire a new behavior. Brushing your teeth didn't come naturally when you first started. It took some time and diligence to reach the point where it became an honored habit. If you expend the effort to practice deep relaxation five to seven days per week for at least one month, it will likely become so ingrained that you won't need to think about doing it anymore—you'll just do it automatically.

Practicing deep relaxation is more than learning a technique: it involves making a basic shift in your attitude and lifestyle. It requires a willingness to give priority to your health and internal peace of mind over the other pressing claims of productivity, accomplishment, money, or status.

# Downtime and Time Management

This chapter on relaxation would not be complete without a discussion of the concepts of downtime and time management. In fact, fully appreciating and implementing these ideas in your life is likely to be *the most important thing you can do if you would like to achieve a more relaxed lifestyle.*

You can practice deep muscle relaxation or meditation every day and feel a pleasant respite for twenty to thirty minutes. These practices can definitely enhance your overall feeling of relaxation if you practice them regularly. Yet if you're on a treadmill the rest of the time, with too much to get done and no breaks in your schedule, you're likely to remain under stress, prone to chronic anxiety or panic attacks, and ultimately headed toward burnout.

## *Downtime*

*Downtime* is exactly what it sounds like—*time out* from work or other responsibilities to give yourself an opportunity to rest and replenish your energy. Without periods of downtime, any stress you experience while dealing with work or other responsibilities tends to become *cumulative*. It keeps building without any remission. You may keep pushing yourself until finally you drop from exhaustion or experience an aggravation of your anxiety or phobias. Sleep at night doesn't really count as downtime. If you go to bed feeling stressed, you may sleep for eight hours and still wake up feeling tense, tired, and stressed. Downtime needs to be scheduled during the day, apart from sleep. Its primary purpose is simply to allow a break in the stress cycle—to prevent the stress you're experiencing from becoming cumulative. It's recommended that you give yourself the following periods of downtime:

One hour per day
One day per week
One week out of every twelve to sixteen weeks

If you don't have four weeks of paid vacation per year (fairly common in the US), then be willing to take time off without pay. During these periods of downtime, you disengage from any task you consider work, put aside all responsibilities, and don't answer the phone unless it's someone you would enjoy hearing from.

There are three kinds of downtime, each of which has an important place in developing a more relaxed lifestyle: 1) rest time, 2) recreation time, and 3) relationship time. It's important that you provide yourself enough downtime so that you have time for all three. Often recreation and relationship time can be combined. However, it's important to use rest time for just that—and nothing else.

*Rest time* is time when you set aside all activities and just allow yourself to *be*. You stop action and let yourself fully rest. Rest time might involve lying on the couch and doing nothing, quietly meditating, sitting in your recliner and listening to peaceful music, soaking in a Jacuzzi, or taking a catnap in the middle of the workday. Rest time does not mean checking your email, but it could mean reading a light magazine that doesn't focus on the news cycle. The key to rest time is that it is fundamentally passive—you allow yourself to stop doing and accomplishing and just *be*. Contemporary society encourages each of us to be productive and always accomplish more and more every moment of the waking day. Rest time is a needed counterpoint. When you're under stress, one hour of rest time per day, separate from the time you sleep, is optimal.

*Recreation time* involves engaging in activities that help "re-create" you—that is, serve to replenish your energy. Recreation time brightens and uplifts your spirits. In essence, it is doing anything that you experience as fun or play. Examples of such activities might include puttering in the garden, reading a novel, seeing a special movie, going on a hike, playing soccer, taking a short trip, baking a loaf of bread, or fishing. Recreation time can be done during the workweek and is most important to have on your days off from work. Such time can be spent either alone or with someone else, in which case it overlaps with the third type of downtime.

*Relationship time* is time when you put aside your private goals and responsibilities in order to enjoy being with another person—or, in some cases, with several people. The focus of relationship time is to honor your relationship with your spouse or partner, children, extended family members, friends, pets, and so on, and forget about your individual pursuits for a while. If you have a family, relationship time needs to be allocated equitably between time alone with your spouse, time alone with your children, and time when the entire family gets together. If you're single with a partner, time needs to be judiciously allocated between time with your partner and time with friends.

When you slow down and make time to be with others, you're less likely to neglect your basic needs for intimacy, touching, affection, validation, support, and so on (see the section called "Your Basic Needs" in chapter 15, Self-Esteem). Meeting these basic needs is vital to your well-being. Without sufficient time devoted to important relationships, you will surely suffer—and the people you most care about are bound to, as well.

How can you allow for more downtime (all three kinds) in your life? An important prerequisite is to get past workaholism. Workaholism is an addictive disorder in which work is the *only* thing that gives you a sense of inner fulfillment and self-worth. You devote all your time and energy to work, neglecting both your physical and your emotional needs. Workaholism describes an unbalanced way of life that often leads first to chronic stress, then to burnout, and ultimately to serious illness.

If you're a workaholic, it's possible to *learn* to enjoy nonwork aspects of your life, as discussed above, and achieve a more balanced approach in general. Deliberately making time for rest, recreation, and relationships may be difficult at first, but it tends to get easier and to become self-rewarding as time goes on.

Another important step is simply *to be willing to do less*. That is, you literally reduce the number of tasks and responsibilities you handle in any given day. In some cases, this may involve changing jobs; in others, it may merely involve restructuring how you allocate time for work versus rest and relaxation. For some individuals, this translates to a fundamental decision to make earning money less important and a simpler, more balanced lifestyle more important. Before you think about leaving your present job, however, consider how you can shift your values in the direction of placing more emphasis on the *process* of life ("how" you live) as opposed to accomplishments and productivity ("what" you actually do) within your current life situation.

# *Exercise: Finding More Downtime*

Take some time to reflect on how you might allocate more time for each of the three types of downtime discussed. Write your answers in the space provided below.

*Rest time:*

*Recreation time:*

*Relationship time:*

## Time Management

A very important skill to have if you want more time away from work and responsibilities is good time management. Time management describes the way in which you organize or structure your daily activities over time. Ineffective time management can lead to stress, anxiety, burnout, and, eventually, illness. Effective time management, on the other hand, will allow you more time for the three types of downtime described above: rest, recreation, and relationships.

Developing good time management skills may necessitate giving up some cherished habits. Are any of the following tendencies true for you? Check off any of the statements below that apply:

- ☐ "I tend to underestimate the amount of time it takes to complete an activity or a task. By the time I finish, I've taken up time I needed for something else."

- ☐ "I tend to squeeze too many things into too little time. As a result, I end up rushing."

- ☐ "I find it difficult to let go of something I'm involved in, so I end up not leaving myself enough time to get to (or complete) the next activity I need to do."

- ☐ "I have difficulty prioritizing activities—getting the most essential ones done before I attend to the less important ones."

- ☐ "I have difficulty delegating nonessential tasks to others, even when it is possible to do so."

If you checked off any of the above statements as true, you might benefit from learning and cultivating effective time management skills.

The skills described below—prioritization, delegation, allowing extra time, letting go of perfectionism, overcoming procrastination, and saying no—can help you work with, rather than against, time.

## Prioritization

Prioritization means learning to discriminate between tasks or activities that are essential and those that are nonessential. You attend to what's most important and put everything else on hold (or delegate tasks to other people—see below).

You may find it useful to divide your daily tasks and responsibilities into three categories: *essential, important,* and *less important* or trivial. *Essential* tasks or activities include those that require immediate attention: they are absolutely necessary—such as getting the kids off to school. Alternatively, they can be activities that are very important to you, such as physical exercise, if you're working on reducing your anxiety. *Important* tasks and activities are those that have significant value but can be delayed for a limited time, such as spending quality one-on-one time with your spouse or partner. Important tasks cannot be delayed for a long time, however. *Less important* or trivial tasks can be postponed for a long time without serious risk or can be delegated to others (tasks such as taking the stack of newspapers in the garage to the recycling center or deleting photos you don't want to keep on your computer).

You may find it helpful, perhaps when you first get up in the morning, to categorize the tasks facing you as *essential, important,* or *less important.* Actually divide a piece of paper into three columns and write everything down. Then start with tasks in the *essential* and *important* columns. Only move on to the tasks in the *less important* category when you're done with all the tasks in the first two columns. In general, consider postponing all the tasks in the *less important* column in favor of giving yourself more downtime.

If you're serious about achieving a more relaxed lifestyle, then you'll need to place downtime—time for rest, recreation, and relationships—into the *essential* category. When downtime becomes a regular and high-priority item in your schedule—something you refuse to postpone—you will begin to take life more slowly and easily. As a result, you'll feel less stressed, better able to sleep, and more capable of enjoying yourself in general. Making downtime essential requires giving up addictions to work, outer achievement, and success, as well as letting go of perfectionism.

You may also want to include under the essential column those activities that contribute to the achievement of your long-term ideals and life goals. Long-term ideals and life goals tend to remain just that for most people—postponed until the distant future—*unless* you make time to do something toward achieving them on a step-by-step basis in the present.

## Delegation

Skill in delegation means being willing to let someone else take care of a task or an activity that has lower priority for you or is an important task that *you* don't have to do personally. By delegating, you free up more time for those tasks that are essential and require your personal attention. Often delegation means paying someone else to do what you might do yourself if you had unlimited time: housecleaning, car washing, cooking, child care, basic repairs, and so on. At other times, delegation simply means distributing tasks equitably among family members: having your kids do their fair share of household chores. A key to delegation is a willingness to trust and rely on others' capabilities. Give up the idea that only you can do an adequate job, and be willing to entrust responsibility for a task to someone else.

### Allowing Extra Time

A common problem in time management is underestimating the amount of time required to complete a task. The result is that you end up rushing to try to get something done, or else run into overtime and encroach on time that was needed for the next activity in your schedule. As a general rule, it helps to allow a little more time than you would expect for each activity during the day. It's better to err in favor of overestimating the time required for a task, leaving yourself plenty of time to proceed in a leisurely manner to the next activity.

An important prerequisite for allowing extra time is to be *willing to do fewer things*—not to cram as many tasks or activities into a given time frame. This may be very difficult for people addicted to their own adrenaline, who seem to get a certain exhilaration and fulfillment from rushing around or feeling busy. However, allowing extra time has tremendous rewards in terms of letting you proceed through your day at a more relaxed and easy pace. To do so will save you a lot of stress.

### Letting Go of Perfectionism

Perfectionism essentially means setting your standards and expectations too high: there is no allowance for the inevitable mistakes, frustrations, delays, and limitations that come up in the process of working toward any goal. Perfectionism can keep you on a treadmill of overwork or overdedication, to the point that you don't allow time out for your own needs. Letting go of perfectionism requires a fundamental attitude shift. It becomes all right simply to do your best, to make some mistakes along the way, and to accept the results you get, even if your best efforts fall short. It also involves learning to laugh on occasion rather than despair at the limitations inherent to human existence. (For a more in-depth discussion about letting go of perfectionism, see chapter 11, Personality Styles That Perpetuate Anxiety.)

### Overcoming Procrastination

Procrastination is always self-defeating when you leave yourself too little time. Whether preparing for an exam or preparing to go to work, putting off the inevitable leaves you harried and stressed in the end.

One reason for procrastinating can be that you really don't want to do whatever it is that needs doing in the first place. If this is your reason for stalling, the solution lies either in delegating or in prioritizing. If you can delegate an undesirable task to someone else, then by all means do so. If you can't, then get the undesirable task done *first*—in other words, prioritize it over the other things you need to do. Promising yourself to do something fun or interesting afterward as a reward for getting the undesirable task done often works well. In overcoming procrastination, the carrot usually works much better than the stick.

Another reason for procrastinating is perfectionism. If you feel that something has to be done perfectly, you may keep postponing getting started because you fear that you can't do it "just right." The solution here is to jump in and get started, whether or not you feel you're ready to do it right. An important principle to remember is that *motivation often follows behavior.* Just getting started on a task will often generate the motivation to follow through and complete it. Then you may have enough time left over to go back and rework or refine what you did during the first round. If you keep stalling, however, you can use up all the time needed to do the kind of job you'd like to do. The worst outcome is when you don't attempt the task at all because of your impossibly high standards.

### Saying No

There are many reasons why people have difficulty saying no. You may always want to be pleasing and responsive to family and friends, no matter what they ask of you, so you have difficulty setting limits, even when their demands or needs become more than you can handle. Or you may be so bound up with your work that it's your primary source of identity and meaning. No matter how demanding and time-consuming work responsibilities become, you keep taking them on, because not to do so would leave you feeling empty.

In short, difficulty saying no is usually tied up with your self-image. If your image of yourself requires you to be nice all the time and always available to everyone, then there is probably no limit to what others will ask of you. If your work is who you are, then it will be hard for you to say no to work demands in order to make time for your personal needs.

Learning to say no requires a willingness to relinquish cherished beliefs about yourself—which can be one of the hardest things for anyone to do. This may involve expanding your identity beyond taking care of others, or taking care of business, and learning to take the time to nurture and attend to your own needs. It means accepting the reality that taking care of yourself—even at the expense of what you do for others—isn't selfish. Can you really offer your best to others or your work if you are tired, stressed, or burned out?

A sustained inability to say no can ultimately lead to burnout or even illness. In many cases, illness—whether in the form of panic attacks, depression, or some other persistent problem—may force you to reevaluate the way you live your life. Illness can be the catalyst that compels you to slow down, pay attention, and learn how to live in a simpler, more balanced fashion.

## Summary of Things to Do

1.  Reread the section on abdominal breathing and decide which breathing exercise you want to work with. Practice the exercise you prefer for five minutes per day for at least two weeks. Practice for one month or longer if you wish to change your breathing pattern from your chest downward toward your abdomen.

    Use the abdominal breathing or the calming breath exercise whenever you suddenly feel symptoms of anxiety beginning to come on.

2.  Practice progressive muscle relaxation for twenty to thirty minutes per day (two practice periods per day is even better) for at least two weeks. For the first few times, use the recordings associated with this book, have someone read you the instructions, or record

them yourself—so that you can follow them effortlessly. Eventually, you'll memorize the instructions and can dispense with the recording.

3. Visualize going to a peaceful scene following progressive muscle relaxation. It may help to record a detailed description of such a scene following your recorded instructions for progressive or passive muscle relaxation. Try going to your peaceful scene (along with doing abdominal breathing) at those times during the day when anxiety comes up.

4. After practicing progressive muscle relaxation for at least two weeks, you may enjoy its benefits so much that you decide to adopt it as your preferred deep relaxation technique. Alternatively, you may want to learn to meditate. (See chapter 19.) *The type of relaxation technique you use is less important than your willingness and commitment to practice some method of deep relaxation on a daily basis.*

5. If you encounter difficulties in maintaining your commitment to practicing deep relaxation over the long term, reread the section called "Some Common Obstacles to a Daily Program of Deep Relaxation."

6. Spend some time considering the section "Downtime and Time Management." Do you need to allocate more time in your life for rest, relaxation, and personal relationships? What changes would you need to make in your daily schedule to achieve this? Think about at least one change you could make, starting this week. Are you willing to commit to it?

## Further Reading

Benson, Herbert. *The Relaxation Response*. Updated and expanded. New York: HarperCollins, 2000.

Davis, Martha, Elizabeth Robbins Eshelman, and Matthew McKay. *The Relaxation & Stress Reduction Workbook*. 7th ed. Oakland, CA: New Harbinger Publications, 2019.

Kabat-Zinn, Jon. *Wherever You Go, There You Are*. Tenth anniversary edition. New York: Hyperion, 2005.

Lakein, Alan. *How to Get Control of Your Time and Your Life*. New York: Signet, 1989.

Mason, John. *Guide to Stress Reduction*. 2nd ed. Berkeley, CA: Celestial Arts, 2001. (This book is particularly recommended as a good resource for relaxation scripts you can record for yourself.)

# 5

# Physical Exercise

One of the most powerful and effective methods for reducing generalized anxiety and overcoming a predisposition to panic attacks is a program of regular, vigorous exercise. You have panic attacks when your body's natural fight-or-flight reaction—the sudden surge of adrenaline you experience in response to a realistic threat—becomes excessive or occurs out of context. Exercise is a natural outlet for your body when it is in the fight-or-flight mode of arousal. A majority of my clients who have undertaken a regular exercise program are less vulnerable to panic attacks and, if they do have them, find them to be less severe. Regular exercise also diminishes the tendency to experience anticipatory anxiety toward phobic situations, expediting recovery from all kinds of phobias, ranging from fear of public speaking to fear of being alone.

Regular exercise has a direct impact on several physiological factors that underlie anxiety. It brings about:

- *Reduced skeletal muscle tension*, which is largely responsible for your feelings of being tense or "uptight"

- *More rapid metabolism of excess adrenaline and thyroxine* in the bloodstream, the presence of which tends to keep you in a state of fearful arousal and vigilance

- *A discharge of pent-up frustration*, which can aggravate phobic or panic reactions

Some of the general *physiological* benefits of exercise include:

- Enhanced oxygenation of the blood and brain, which increases alertness and concentration

- Stimulation of the production of endorphins, natural substances that resemble morphine both chemically and in their effects: endorphins increase your sense of well-being

- Lowered pH (increased acidity) of the blood, which increases your energy level

- Improved circulation

- Improved digestion and utilization of food

- Improved elimination (from skin, lungs, and bowels)

- Decreased cholesterol levels

- Decreased blood pressure

- Weight loss, as well as appetite suppression, in many cases

- Improved blood sugar regulation (in the case of hypoglycemia)

Several *psychological* benefits accompany these physical improvements, including:

- Increased subjective feelings of well-being

- Reduced dependence on alcohol and drugs

- Reduced insomnia

- Improved concentration and memory

- Reduced depression

- Increased self-esteem

- Greater sense of control over anxiety

## Symptoms of Being Out of Shape

How do you know that you are out of shape and in need of exercise? Here are some common symptoms:

- Being out of breath after walking up a flight of stairs

- Long recovery time after walking up a flight of stairs

- Feeling exhausted after short periods of exertion

- Chronic muscle tension

- Poor muscle tone

- Obesity

- Muscles cramped and aching for days after participating in a sport

- General tiredness, lethargy, boredom

## Your Fitness Level

The worksheet that follows can help you assess the extent of your fitness. Think about the most strenuous physical activity you practice in an *average week*. When you have completed the questions below, determine your fitness score and evaluate your fitness level.

| INTENSITY | FREQUENCY | DURATION |
|---|---|---|
| How strenuous is your exercise per week? | How many times do you exercise each week? | How long do you exercise? |
| Heavy = 5 points (fast cycling, running, aerobic dancing) | 3 or more times = 5 points | 21 minutes to 1 hour = 5 points |
| Moderate = 3 points (jogging, cycling, very fast walking) | 1 to 2 times = 2 points | 11 to 20 minutes = 3 points |
| Light = 1 point (golf, strolling, most housework) | not at all = 0 points | 10 minutes or less = 1 point |
| Add your score: _____ | + _____ | + _____ = Total _____ |

| TOTAL SCORE | FITNESS LEVEL | RECOMMENDED ACTION |
|---|---|---|
| 13 to 15 | Very good | Congratulations! Maintain your present level of activity. |
| 8 to 12 | Average | You are moderately sedentary and could increase your level of activity. |
| 7 or less | Poor | Begin planning an exercise program now! |

An alternative way to assess your level of fitness is to measure your *resting pulse rate*, the average number of heartbeats per minute when you're at rest. As a rule of thumb, a resting pulse of eighty or above suggests that you could definitely improve your fitness. If you are in a fitness program and have an average resting pulse below seventy, you are likely to be in good shape. To measure your pulse, allow yourself to get relaxed, then take the number of pulse beats in twenty seconds and multiply by three.

# Preparing for a Fitness Program

If you've decided you would like to get more exercise, you need to ask yourself whether you are fully ready to do so. There are certain physical conditions that limit the amount and intensity of exercise you should undertake. If your answer to any of the following questions is yes, be sure to consult with your physician before beginning any exercise program. He or she may recommend a program of restricted or supervised exercise appropriate to your needs.

**YES   NO**

_____   _____   Has your physician ever said you have heart trouble?

_____   _____   Do you frequently have pains in your heart or chest?

_____   _____   Do you often feel faint or have spells of dizziness?

_____   _____   Has your physician ever told you that you have a bone or joint problem (such as arthritis) that has been or might be aggravated by exercise?

_____   _____   Has a physician ever said that your blood pressure was too high?

_____   _____   Do you have diabetes?

_____   _____   Are you over forty years old and unaccustomed to vigorous exercise?

_____   _____   Is there a physical reason, not mentioned here, why you should not undertake an exercise program?

If you answered no to all of the above questions, you can be reasonably assured that you are ready to start an exercise program. Begin slowly and increase your activity gradually over a period of weeks. If you are over forty and unaccustomed to exercise, plan to see your doctor for a physical before undertaking an exercise program.

Some individuals are reluctant to take up exercise because the state of physiological arousal accompanying vigorous exercise reminds them too much of the symptoms of panic. If this applies to you, you might want to start out doing forty-five minutes of walking on a daily basis.

Or you can *very gradually* build up to a more vigorous level of exercise. You might try just two to three minutes of jogging or cycling and then gradually increase the duration of your daily exercise a minute at a time, remembering to stop every time you feel even the slightest association with panic (see the descriptions of step-by-step exposure in chapters 3 and 7). It might also be helpful to have a support person exercise with you initially. If you feel phobic about exercise, a program of gradual exposure will help you in the same way it would with any other phobia.

## Choosing an Exercise Program

There are many types of exercise to choose from. Deciding what form of exercise to do depends upon your objectives. For reducing generalized anxiety and/or a proneness to panic, *aerobic exercise* such as running, brisk walking, cycling outdoors or on a stationary bike, swimming, aerobic dancing, or trampoline jumping can be effective for many individuals. Aerobic exercise requires sustained activity of your larger muscles. It reduces skeletal muscle tension and increases *cardiovascular conditioning*—the capacity of your circulatory system to deliver oxygen to your tissues and cells with greater efficiency. Regular aerobic exercise will reduce stress and increase your stamina. An aerobic workout should last at least twenty to thirty minutes.

Beyond aerobic fitness, you may have other objectives in taking up exercise. If increased muscle *strength* is important, you may want to include weight lifting or isometric exercise in your program. Start off easy with exercise machines or free weights and gradually increase the weight to your desired goal. An athletic trainer may be helpful when working with weight training. (If you have a heart condition or angina, you should probably *not* engage in weight lifting or body building, unless you have approval from a physician.)

If *socializing* is important, then racquetball, golf, or team sports, such as baseball, basketball, or volleyball, might be what you're looking for. Exercise that involves stretching, such as yoga, is ideal for developing muscular *flexibility*. If you want to *lose weight*, jogging or cycling is probably most effective. If *discharging aggression and frustration* is important, you might try competitive sports. Finally, if you just want to get outdoors, then hiking or gardening would be appropriate. Rigorous hiking (as done by the Sierra Club, for example) can increase both strength and endurance. For further information on the various benefits of different types of exercise, see Covert Bailey's well-known book on the subject, *The New Fit or Fat* (also published in a revised edition as *The Ultimate Fit or Fat*).

Many people find it helpful to *vary* the type of exercise they do. Popular combinations involve doing an aerobic type of exercise such as jogging or cycling three to four times a week and a socializing exercise (such as tennis) or a body-building exercise twice a week. Maintaining a program with two distinct types of exercise prevents either one from becoming too boring. What follows are brief descriptions of some of the more common types of aerobic exercise. Each type has its advantages and possible drawbacks.

## Running

For many years, running (or jogging) has been the most popular form of aerobic exercise, perhaps because of its convenience. The only equipment you need is running shoes, and in many cases, you need only step out your door to begin. Running is one of the best forms of exercise for losing weight, because it burns calories quickly. Numerous studies have shown its benefits for depression, as it raises both endorphin and serotonin levels in the brain. As mentioned above, running decreases anxiety by metabolizing excess adrenaline and releasing skeletal muscle tension. A two- to three-mile jog (up to approximately thirty minutes) four or five times per week can go a long way toward diminishing your vulnerability to anxiety.

The downside to running is that, over a period of time, it can increase your risk for injury. In particular, if you run on hard surfaces, the constant shock to your joints can lead to foot, knee, or back problems. You can minimize your risk of injury if you:

- Get proper shoes—those that minimize shock to your joints.

- Run on soft surfaces—preferably grass, dirt, a track, or a hardened beach. Avoid concrete if possible; asphalt is okay if you have good shoes and don't run every day.

- Warm up to running before you begin. Try doing a minute or two of very slow jogging.

- Avoid jogging every day—alternate it with other forms of exercise.

If running outdoors is a problem because of weather, lack of a soft surface, smog, or traffic, you may want to invest in a treadmill. To make its use less boring, put it in front of your television or media player.

## Swimming

Swimming is a popular form of exercise. It's an especially good exercise because it uses so many different muscles throughout the body. Doctors usually recommend swimming to people with musculoskeletal problems, injuries, or arthritis because it minimizes shock to their joints. It does not promote weight loss to the same degree as running, but it will help firm up your body.

For aerobic-level conditioning, it's best to swim freestyle for twenty to thirty minutes, preferably four or five times per week. For moderate, relaxing exercise, breaststroke is an enjoyable alternative. As a rule, it's best to work out in a heated pool where the water temperature is 75 to 80 degrees Fahrenheit.

The major downside with swimming is that many pools are heavily chlorinated. This may be quite irritating to your eyes, skin, or hair—as well as the membranes in your upper respiratory passages. You can counter some of this by wearing goggles and/or nose plugs. If you're fortunate, you may be able to find a pool that uses hydrogen peroxide, bubbled-in ozone, or even saline. Any of these options is preferable to chlorine. When you use a chlorinated pool, be sure to shower off with hot, soapy water afterward.

## Cycling

In recent years, cycling has become a very popular form of aerobic exercise. While having many of the same benefits as jogging, it's less shocking to your joints. To achieve aerobic conditioning, cycling needs to be done vigorously—at a rate of approximately fifteen miles per hour or more on a flat surface. When the weather is good, cycling can be quite enjoyable—especially if you have beautiful surroundings with little traffic or a designated bike trail. If weather precludes cycling, you can use a stationary bike indoors.

If you want to take up outdoor cycling, you'll need to make an initial investment in a good bike. You may want to borrow someone else's bike until you feel ready to spend several hundred dollars. In purchasing a bike, avoid racing bikes unless you decide you want to race. You'll probably find sitting upright when you cycle to be more enjoyable and less stressful than sitting hunched over. Make sure the bike you purchase is designed and sized correctly for your body—or it may cause you problems. A well-cushioned seat is a good investment.

When you undertake cycling, give yourself a few months to work up to a fifteen-miles-per-hour cruising speed—a mile every four minutes. A half hour to an hour of cycling three or four times per week is sufficient. Be sure to wear a helmet and try to avoid riding at night. Use bike lanes on roads that are preferably not too busy with traffic.

## Aerobics Classes

Most aerobics classes consist of warm-up stretches and aerobic exercises led by an instructor. These are usually done to music. Classes are generally offered by health clubs, with various levels for beginning, intermediate, and advanced participants. Since some of the exercises can be traumatic to your joints, try to find a "low-impact" aerobics class. The structured format of an aerobics class may be an excellent way to motivate you to exercise. If you are self-motivated and prefer to stay at home, there are many good aerobics videos available.

If you decide to do aerobic exercises, be sure to obtain good shoes that stabilize your feet, absorb shock, and minimize twisting. It's best to do these exercises on a wooden surface and to avoid carpets, if possible. About thirty minutes to an hour of exercise (including warm-up) three to five times per week is sufficient.

### Walking

Walking has advantages over all other forms of exercise. First, it does not require training—you already know how to do it. Second, it requires no equipment other than a pair of shoes and can be done virtually anywhere—even in a shopping mall, if necessary. The chance of injury is less than with any other type of exercise. Finally, it's the most natural exercise activity. All of us are inclined to walk. Up until society became sedentary, walking was a regular part of life.

Walking for relaxation and distraction is one thing; doing it for aerobic conditioning is another. To make walking *aerobic*, aim for doing it for about forty-five minutes to one hour at a brisk enough pace to cover three miles. A twenty-minute walk is generally not enough to obtain aerobic-level conditioning but is fine if your goal is just to do moderate exercise. If you make walking your regular form of exercise, do it four or five times per week, preferably outdoors. If you feel an hour of brisk walking is not enough of a workout, try adding hand weights or finding an area with hills.

To get the most benefit out of walking, good posture is important. If it feels natural to allow your arms to swing opposite to the stride of your legs, you'll be getting "cross-lateral conditioning," which helps integrate the left and right hemispheres of your brain. Good walking shoes are also important. Look for padded insoles, a good arch, and firm support of the heel.

Once you can comfortably walk three or four miles without stopping, consider taking group hiking trips—day or overnight—in county, state, or national parks. Hiking outdoors can revitalize your soul as much as it does your body.

## Getting Started

If you haven't been exercising, it is important not to start off too fast or hard. Doing so often results in prematurely burning out on the idea of maintaining a regular exercise program. The following guidelines for getting started are recommended:

- Approach exercise gradually. Set limited goals at the outset, such as exerting only ten minutes (or to the point of being winded) every other day for the first week. Add five minutes to your workout time each successive week until you reach thirty minutes.

- Give yourself a one-month trial period. Make a commitment to stay with your program for one month, despite aches and pains, inertia, or other resistance to exercise. By the end of the first month, you may be starting to experience sufficient benefits to make the exercise self-motivating. Be aware that achieving a high level of fitness after being out of shape can take up to three to four months.

- *Optional:* Keep a record of your daily exercise practice. Use the *Daily Record of Exercise* that follows this page to keep track of the date, time, duration, and type of exercise you engage in on a daily basis. (You may want to make copies of the *Daily Record* so you can track your exercise program beyond the first month. For a downloadable version of the *Record*, see the very back of this book.) If you're doing aerobic exercise, record your pulse immediately after completing your workout and enter it under the column labeled "Pulse Rate." Also be sure to rate your level of satisfaction, using a 1 to 10 scale, where 1 equals no satisfaction at all and 10 equals total satisfaction with your exercise experience. As you begin to get into shape, your satisfaction should increase. Finally, if you fail to exercise when you intended to, indicate your reason for not doing so. Later on it may be useful to reevaluate these reasons to see if they are truly valid or "mere excuses." (See the final section of this chapter for dealing with resistance to exercise.)

- *Expect* some initial discomfort. Aches and pains when starting out are normal if you've been out of shape. You can expect the discomfort to pass as you grow in strength and endurance.

- Try to focus on the *process* of exercise rather than the product. See if you can get into the inherently enjoyable aspects of the exercise itself. If jogging or cycling is what you like, it helps to have a scenic environment. Focusing on competition with others or yourself may tend to increase rather than reduce anxiety and stress.

- Reward yourself for maintaining a commitment to your exercise program. Give yourself a dinner out, a weekend trip, or new athletic clothes or equipment in exchange for sticking to your program during the first weeks and months.

- Warm up. Just as your car needs to warm up before you begin driving, your body needs a gradual warm-up before engaging in vigorous exercise. This is especially important if you are over forty. Five minutes of light jogging or stretching exercises will usually be sufficient.

- Give yourself a few minutes to cool down, which is important after vigorous exercise. Walking around for two or three minutes will help bring your blood back from peripheral muscles to the rest of your body.

- Avoid exercising within one hour following a meal, and don't eat until one hour after exercising.

- Avoid exercising when you feel ill or overstressed. (Try a deep relaxation technique instead.)

- Stop exercising if you experience any sudden, unexplainable bodily symptoms.

- If you find yourself feeling bored with exercising solo, find a partner to go with you or a form of exercise that requires a partner.

## Daily Record of Exercise* for _____

*(month)*

| Date | Time | Type of Exercise | Duration | Pulse Rate | Satisfaction Level | Reason for Not Exercising |
|---|---|---|---|---|---|---|
| | | | | | | |
| | | | | | | |
| | | | | | | |
| | | | | | | |
| | | | | | | |
| | | | | | | |
| | | | | | | |
| | | | | | | |
| | | | | | | |
| | | | | | | |
| | | | | | | |
| | | | | | | |
| | | | | | | |
| | | | | | | |
| | | | | | | |
| | | | | | | |
| | | | | | | |
| | | | | | | |
| | | | | | | |
| | | | | | | |
| | | | | | | |
| | | | | | | |
| | | | | | | |
| | | | | | | |
| | | | | | | |
| | | | | | | |
| | | | | | | |
| | | | | | | |

* Based on a maximum frequency of six days of exercise per week.

# Optimizing the Anxiety-Reducing Effects of Exercise

Exercise needs to be of sufficient regularity, intensity, and duration to have a significant impact on anxiety. The following standards can be viewed as goals to aim for:

- Ideally, exercise should be aerobic.

- Optimal frequency is four to five times per week.

- Optimal duration is twenty to thirty minutes or more per session.

- Optimal intensity for aerobic exercise is a heart rate of (220 – your age) x 0.75 for at least ten minutes.

The table below indicates exercise pulse rate ranges for various ages. The lower end of the range represents a desirable heart-rate goal for *moderate* exercise. The upper end of the range represents the optimal maximum heart rate for *aerobic* exercise for each age group:

| Age | Pulse (Heart) Rate |
| --- | --- |
| 20–29 | 145–164 |
| 30–39 | 138–156 |
| 40–49 | 130–148 |
| 50–59 | 122–140 |
| 60–69 | 116–132 |
| 70–79 | 108–120 |

*Avoid exercising only once per week.* Engaging in infrequent spurts of exercise is stressful to your body and generally does more harm than good (walking is an exception).

# Common Excuses for Not Exercising

If you have difficulty starting or maintaining an exercise program, ask yourself what excuses or rationalizations you are giving yourself. What are you saying to yourself that tends to make you procrastinate? If you wish, you can keep a written record of excuses you give yourself for avoiding exercise.

Below is a list of common excuses people make for avoiding exercise.

- "I don't have enough time."

What you are really saying is that you're not willing to make time. You aren't assigning enough importance to the increased fitness, well-being, and improved control over anxiety you could gain from exercise. The problem is not a matter of time but one of priorities.

- "I feel too tired to exercise."

One solution is to exercise before going to work—or on your lunch break—rather than at the end of the day. If this is simply impossible, don't give up. What many nonexercisers fail to realize is that moderate exercise can actually *overcome* fatigue. Many people exercise *in spite* of feeling tired and find that they feel rejuvenated and reenergized afterward. Exercise will grow easier once you get past the initial inertia of starting to exercise.

- "Exercise is boring—it's no fun."

Is it really true that *all* the activities listed earlier are boring to you? Have you tried out all of them? It may be that you need to find someone to exercise with in order to have more fun. Or perhaps you need to go back and forth between two different types of exercise to stimulate your interest. Exercise can begin to feel wonderful after a few months when it becomes inherently rewarding, even if it initially bored you.

- "It's too inconvenient to go out somewhere to exercise."

This is really no problem, as there are several ways to obtain vigorous exercise in the comfort of your home. Twenty minutes per day on a stationary bicycle or stair-stepper will give you a good workout. If this seems boring, try listening to a portable audio device with headphones or place your stationary bike in front of the TV set. Aerobic exercise at home is convenient and fun if you have a DVD player. There are many low-impact aerobics programs available on DVD or as podcasts or YouTube videos. Other indoor activities include jumping on a rebounder, calisthenics, using a rowing machine, and/or using a universal gym with adjustable weights. You may also find early morning exercise programs on TV. If you can't afford exercise equipment, just put on some dance music and dance for twenty minutes. In short, it is quite possible to maintain an adequate exercise program without leaving your home.

- "I'm afraid I'll have a panic attack."

Brisk walking every day for forty-five minutes is an excellent form of exercise that is very unlikely to produce symptoms you might associate with panic. If you would prefer doing something more vigorous, start off with a very short period of two or three minutes of exercise and gradually add a minute at a time. Anytime you start to feel uneasy, simply stop, wait until you fully recover, and then try completing your designated period of exercise for that day. The principles of exposure described in chapter 7 can be applied effectively to a phobia about exercise.

- "Exercise causes a buildup of lactic acid—doesn't that cause panic attacks?"

It is true that exercise increases the production of lactic acid, and that lactic acid can promote panic attacks in some people who are already prone to them. However, regular exercise also increases *oxygen turnover* in your body—that is, the capacity of your body to oxidize substances it doesn't need, including lactic acid. Any increase in lactic acid produced by exercise will be offset by your body's increased capacity to remove it. The net effect of regular exercise is an overall *reduction* in your body's tendency to accumulate lactic acid.

- "I'm over fifty—and that's too old to start exercising."

If you're over fifty and feeling that "it's too late" to take up exercise, don't give yourself that excuse. There are marathon runners who *began* running in their fifties and sixties after having not exercised at all. Unless your doctor gives you a clear medical reason for not exercising, age is not really a valid excuse. With patience and persistence, it is possible to get into excellent physical shape at almost any age.

- "I'm too overweight and out of shape" or "I'm afraid I'll have a heart attack if I stress my body by exercising vigorously."

*If you have physical reasons to worry about stressing your heart, be sure to design your exercise program with the help of your physician.* Brisk walking is a safe exercise for practically everyone and is considered by some physicians to be the ideal exercise, as it rarely causes muscle or bone injuries. Swimming is also a safe bet if you're out of shape or overweight. Be sensible and realistic in the exercise program you choose. The important thing is to be consistent and committed, whether your program involves walking for a half hour every day or training for a marathon.

- "I tried exercise once and it didn't work."

The question to ask here is this: *Why* didn't it work? Did you start off too hard and fast? Did you get bored? Did you balk at the initial aches and pains? Did you feel lonely exercising by yourself? Perhaps it is time for you to give yourself another chance to discover all the physical and psychological benefits of a regular exercise program.

Regular exercise is an essential component of a total program for overcoming anxiety, panic, and phobias presented in this workbook. If you combine regular exercise with a program of regular deep relaxation, you are undoubtedly going to experience some reduction in generalized anxiety and will likely increase your resistance to panic attacks as well. Exercise and deep relaxation are the two methods *most* effective for altering a hereditary-biochemical predisposition to anxiety. The techniques described in the remaining chapters of this workbook depend for their effectiveness on your initial commitment to and mastery of deep relaxation and a program of regular exercise.

## Summary of Things to Do

1. Evaluate your level of fitness using the worksheet in the section "Your Fitness Level."

2. Determine whether you are ready to begin a fitness program by answering the questions in the section "Preparing for a Fitness Program."

3. Choose one or more types of exercise you would prefer to do. If you're out of shape, begin with walking for periods of at least thirty minutes, or with doing a more vigorous form of exercise for ten to fifteen minutes. Increase the duration and intensity of your exercise gradually. Exercise at least four times per week.

4. Monitor your exercise program, using the *Daily Record of Exercise,* for at least one month.

5. Observe all the guidelines for maintaining a regular exercise program listed in the section "Getting Started." It's particularly important to give yourself time to warm up and cool down before and after engaging in vigorous exercise.

6. If you encounter resistance to exercise—or lose your motivation to keep exercising after the first week or so—reread the section "Common Excuses for Not Exercising." Try to identify what you're telling yourself about exercise that creates your resistance or lack of motivation. Work on countering your negative self-talk by giving yourself positive reasons to exercise the next time you have an opportunity.

## Further Reading

Bailey, Covert. *The Ultimate Fit or Fat.* New York: Houghton Mifflin Harcourt, 2000.

Cooper, Robert K. *Health and Fitness Excellence: The Scientific Action Plan.* Boston: Houghton Mifflin, 1990.

Manocchia, Pat. *Anatomy of Exercise: A Trainer's Inside Guide to Your Workout.* Richmond Hill, ON, Canada: Firefly Books, 2009.

Simon, Harvey. *The No Sweat Exercise Plan.* New York: McGraw-Hill, 2006.

# 6

# Coping with Panic Attacks

A panic attack is a sudden surge of mounting physiological arousal that can occur "out of the blue" or in response to encountering (or merely thinking about) a phobic situation. *Bodily symptoms* that occur with the onset of panic can include heart palpitations, tightening in the chest or shortness of breath, choking sensations, dizziness, faintness, sweating, trembling, shaking, and/or tingling in the hands and feet. *Psychological reactions* that often accompany these bodily changes include feelings of unreality, an intense desire to run away, and fears of going crazy, dying, or doing something uncontrollable.

Anyone who has had a full-fledged panic attack knows that it is one of the most intensely uncomfortable states human beings are capable of experiencing. Your very first panic attack can have a traumatic impact, leaving you feeling terrified and helpless, with strong anticipatory anxiety about the possible recurrence of your panic symptoms. Unfortunately, in some cases, panic does come back and occurs repeatedly. Why some people have a panic attack only once—or perhaps once every few years—while others develop a chronic condition with several attacks a week is still not understood by researchers in the field.

The *good* news is that you can learn to cope with panic attacks so well that they will no longer have the power to frighten you. Over time you can actually diminish the intensity and frequency of panic attacks *if* you are willing to make some changes in your lifestyle. Lifestyle changes that are most conducive to reducing the severity of panic reactions are described in other chapters of this workbook. They include:

- Regular practice of deep relaxation (see chapter 4)

- Regular program of exercise (see chapter 5)

- Elimination of stimulants (especially caffeine, sugar, and nicotine) from your diet (see chapter 16)

- Learning to acknowledge and express your feelings, especially anger and sadness (see chapter 13)

- Adopting self-talk and "core beliefs" that promote a calmer and more accepting attitude toward life (see chapters 8 and 9)

These five lifestyle changes vary in importance for different people. To the extent that you can cultivate all five of them, however, you will find that, over time, your problem with panic reactions will diminish.

The approach in this workbook is not strongly oriented toward medication. Yet there *are* some people who suffer from panic attacks for whom it's appropriate to take medication. If you're having panic attacks with sufficient intensity and frequency to interfere with your ability to work, your close personal relationships, or your sleep, or if such attacks persistently give you the feeling that you are losing your grip, then medication may be an appropriate intervention.

The two types of medications most frequently prescribed for panic attacks are antidepressants (such as Zoloft, Cymbalta, and Lexapro) and minor tranquilizers (for instance, Xanax or Ativan). For more information on the use of prescription medications in treating panic attacks, see chapter 18.

The remainder of this chapter will present some specific guidelines for dealing with panic attacks on an immediate basis. These are practical strategies for coping with panic attacks *at the very moment they occur.*

## Deflate the Danger

A panic attack can be a very frightening and uncomfortable experience, but it is absolutely not dangerous. You may be surprised to learn that panic is an *entirely natural bodily reaction that simply occurs out of context.* It is related to the fight-or-flight reaction—an instinctual response in all mammals (not just humans) to physiologically prepare to fight or flee when their survival is threatened. This instantaneous reaction is necessary to ensure the survival of the species in life-threatening situations. It serves to protect the lives of animals in the wild when they are faced by their predators. It also serves to protect your life by informing and mobilizing your impulse to flee from danger.

Suppose, for example, that your car stalls on the railroad tracks while a train is approaching you from about two hundred yards away. You would experience a sudden surge of adrenaline, accompanied by feelings of panic, and a very strong and sensible urge to flee your predicament. In fact, your body would undergo a whole range of reactions, including:

- An increase in your heart rate

- An increase in your respiratory rate

- A tensing of your muscles

- Constriction of your arteries and reduced blood flow to your hands and feet

- Increased blood flow to your muscles

- Release of stored sugar from your liver into your bloodstream

- Increased production of sweat

The very intensity of this reaction and the strong urge to flee are precisely what would ensure your survival. The surge of adrenaline and flow of blood to your muscles increases your alertness and physical strength. Your energy is mobilized and directed toward escape. If these reactions were less intense or less rapid, you might never get out of the way in time. Perhaps you can recall times in your life when the flight response worked properly and served you well.

In a spontaneous panic attack, your body goes through *exactly the same* physiological fight-or-flight reaction that it does in a truly life-threatening situation. The panic attack that wakes you up at night or occurs out of the blue is *physiologically indistinguishable* from your response to such experiences as your car stalling on the railroad tracks or waking to hear a robber going through your house.

What makes a panic attack unique and difficult to cope with is that these intense bodily reactions occur *in the absence of any immediate or apparent danger.* Or, in the case of agoraphobia, they occur in response to situations that have no apparent life-threatening potential (such as standing in line at the grocery store or being at home alone). In either case, you don't know why the reaction is happening. Not knowing why—not being able to make any sense out of the fact that your body is going through such an intense response—only serves to make the entire experience even more frightening. Your tendency is to react to sensations that are intense and *inexplicable* with even more fear and a heightened sense of danger.

No one fully knows all the details of why spontaneous panic attacks occur—why the body's natural fight-or-flight mechanism can come into play for no obvious reason or out of context. Some people believe that there is always *some stimulus* for a panic attack, even if this is not apparent. Others believe that sudden attacks arise from a temporary physiological imbalance. It *is* known that there is a greater tendency for panic attacks to occur when a person has been undergoing prolonged stress or has recently suffered a significant loss. However, only some people who have undergone stress or loss develop panic attacks, while others might develop headaches, ulcers, or reactive depression. It is also known that a disturbance in the part of the brain called the *locus coeruleus* is implicated in panic attacks, but it seems that this disturbance is only one event in a long chain of causes, and not the primary cause. A full understanding of what causes panic attacks awaits future research. (For a more detailed account of what is known physiologically, see chapter 2.)

Because there is no immediate or apparent external danger in a panic attack, you may tend to *invent* or *attribute danger* to the intense bodily sensations you're going through. In the absence of any real life-threatening situation, your mind may misinterpret what's going on *inside* as being life-threatening. Your mind can very quickly go through the following process: "If I feel this bad, I must be in some danger. If there is no apparent external danger, the danger must be inside of me." And so it's very common when undergoing panic to invent any (or all) of the following "dangers":

- *In response to heart palpitations:* "I'm going to have a heart attack" or "I'm going to die."

- *In response to choking sensations:* "I'm going to stop breathing and suffocate."

- *In response to dizzy sensations:* "I'm going to pass out."

- *In response to sensations of disorientation or feeling "not all there":* "I'm going crazy."

- *In response to "rubbery legs":* "I won't be able to walk" or "I'm going to fall."

- *In response to the overall intensity of your body's reactions:* "I'm going to lose complete control over myself."

As soon as you tell yourself that you're feeling any of the above dangers, you multiply the intensity of your fear. This intense fear makes your bodily reactions even worse, which in turn creates still more fear, and you get caught in an upward spiral of mounting panic.

This upward spiral can be avoided if you understand that what your body is going through is *not dangerous*. All of the above dangers are illusory, a product of your imagination when you're undergoing the intense reactions that constitute the onset of panic. *There is simply no basis for any of them in reality*. Let's examine them one by one.

**A panic attack cannot cause heart failure or cardiac arrest.** Rapid heartbeat and palpitations during a panic attack can be frightening sensations, but they are not dangerous. Your heart is made up of very strong and dense muscle fibers and can withstand a lot more than you might think. According to Claire Weekes (1991), a healthy heart can beat one hundred beats per minute for days without sustaining any damage. So, if your heart begins to race, just allow it to do so, trusting that no harm can come of it and that your heart will eventually calm down.

There's a substantial difference between what goes on with your heart during a panic attack and what happens in a heart attack. During a panic attack, your heart may race, pound, and at times miss or have extra beats. Some people even report chest pains, which pass fairly quickly, usually in the left-upper portion of their chest. None of these symptoms is aggravated by movement or increased physical activity. During a true heart attack, the most common symptom is continuous pain and a pressured, even crushing sensation in the center of your chest. Racing or pounding of the heart may occur, but this is secondary to the pain. Moreover, the pain and pressure get worse upon exertion and may tend to diminish with rest. This is quite different from a panic attack, where racing and pounding may get worse if you stand still and lessen if you move around.

In the case of heart disease, distinct abnormalities in heart rhythm show up on an electrocardiogram (EKG) reading. It has been demonstrated that during a panic attack there are no EKG abnormalities—only rapid heartbeat. (If you want to gain additional reassurance, you may want to have your doctor perform an EKG.)

In sum, there is simply no basis for the connection between heart attacks and panic. Panic attacks are not hazardous to your heart.

**A panic attack will not cause you to stop breathing or suffocate.** It is common during panic to feel your chest close down and your breathing become restricted. This might lead you to suddenly fear that you're going to suffocate. Under stress, your neck and chest muscles are tightening and reducing your respiratory capacity. Be assured that there is nothing wrong with your breathing passage or lungs, and that the tightening sensations will pass. Your brain has a built-in reflex mechanism that will eventually *force* you to breathe more if you're not getting enough oxygen. If you don't believe this, try holding your breath for up to a minute and observe what happens. At a certain point, you'll feel a strong reflex to take in more air. The same thing will happen in a panic attack if you're not getting enough oxygen. You'll automatically gasp and take a deep breath long before reaching the point where you could pass out from a lack of oxygen. (Even if you did pass out, you would immediately start breathing!) In sum, choking and sensations of constriction during panic, however unpleasant, are not dangerous.

**A panic attack cannot cause you to faint.** The sensation of light-headedness you may feel with the onset of panic can evoke a fear of fainting. What is happening is that the blood circulation to your brain is slightly reduced, most likely because you are breathing more rapidly (see the section on hyperventilation in chapter 4). This is *not* dangerous and can be relieved by breathing slowly and regularly from your abdomen, preferably through your nose. It can also be helped by taking the first opportunity you have to walk around a bit. Let the feelings of light-headedness rise and subside without fighting them. Because your heart is pumping harder and actually increasing your circulation, you are very unlikely to faint (except in rare instances if you have a blood phobia and happen to be exposed to the sight of blood).

**A panic attack cannot cause you to lose your balance.** Sometimes you may feel quite dizzy when panic comes on. It may be that tension is affecting the semicircular canal system in your inner ear, which regulates your balance. For a few moments you may feel dizzy, or it may even seem that things around you are spinning. Invariably, this sensation will pass. It is not dangerous, and very unlikely to be so strong that you will actually lose your balance. If sensations of pronounced dizziness persist for more than a few seconds, you may want to consult a doctor (preferably an otolaryngologist) to check whether infection, allergies, or other disturbances might be affecting your inner ear.

**You won't fall over or cease to walk when you feel "weak in the knees" during a panic attack.** The adrenaline released during a panic attack can dilate the blood vessels in your legs, causing blood to accumulate in your leg muscles and not fully circulate. This can produce a sensation of weakness or "jelly legs," to which you may respond with the fear that you won't be able to walk. Be assured that this sensation is just that—a sensation—and that your legs are as strong and able to carry you as ever. They won't give way! Just allow these trembling, weak sensations to pass and give your legs the chance to carry you where you need to go.

**You can't "go crazy" during a panic attack.** Reduced blood flow to your brain during a panic attack is due to arterial constriction, a *normal* consequence of rapid breathing. This can result in sensations of disorientation and a feeling of unreality that can be frightening. If this sensation comes on, remind yourself that it's simply due to a slight and temporary reduction of arterial circulation in your brain and does not have anything to do with "going crazy," no matter how eerie or strange it may feel. No one has ever gone crazy from a panic attack, even though the fear of doing so is common. As bad as they feel, sensations of unreality will eventually pass and are completely harmless.

It may be helpful to know that people do not "go crazy" in a sudden or spontaneous way. Mental disorders involving behaviors that are labeled "crazy" (such as schizophrenia or manic-depressive psychosis) develop very gradually over a period of years and do not arise from panic attacks. No one has ever started to hallucinate or hear voices during a panic attack (except in rare instances where panic was induced by an overdose of a recreational drug such as LSD or cocaine). In short, a panic attack cannot result in your "going crazy," no matter how disturbing or unpleasant your symptoms feel.

**A panic attack cannot cause you to lose control of yourself.** Because of the intense reactions your body goes through during panic, it is easy to imagine that you could "completely lose it." But what does completely losing it mean? Becoming completely paralyzed? Acting out uncontrollably or running amok? There are no reported instances of this happening. If anything, during panic, your senses and awareness are heightened with respect to a single goal: escape. Running away or trying to run away are the only ways in which you would be likely to "act out" while panicking. Complete loss of control during panic attacks is simply a myth.

The first step in learning to cope with panic reactions is to recognize that they are not dangerous. Because the bodily reactions accompanying panic feel so intense, it's easy to imagine them being dangerous. Yet in reality no danger exists. The physiological reactions underlying panic are *natural* and *protective*. In fact, *your body is designed to panic* so that you can quickly mobilize to flee situations that genuinely threaten your survival. The problem occurs when this natural, life-preserving response occurs outside the context of any immediate or apparent danger. When this happens, you can make headway in mastering panic by learning not to imagine danger where it doesn't exist.

## Breaking the Connection Between Bodily Symptoms and Catastrophic Thoughts

There is an important difference between people who have panic attacks and those who do not. *Individuals who are prone to panic have a chronic tendency to interpret slightly unusual or uncomfortable bodily sensations in a catastrophic way.* For example, heart palpitations are seen as signals of an impending heart attack, chest constriction and shortness of breath are seen as signs of imminent suffocation, or dizziness is seen as a precursor to fainting or collapse. People who do not have panic attacks may notice (and not particularly like) having such bodily symptoms, *but they do not interpret them as catastrophic or dangerous.*

If you have a tendency to interpret unpleasant bodily sensations as portending something dangerous or catastrophic, you will also tend to constantly monitor your body to see if you're having those sensations. You're probably very tuned in to your internal bodily states and over-react easily if something begins to feel slightly "off" or unusual. This increased *internalization* compounds the problem, because you're more likely to notice and magnify any sudden change in your body's internal state that is slightly unusual or unpleasant.

The variety of circumstances that might cause a sudden aberration in your body's internal physiological state is legion. Sometimes the cause lies outside of your body. For example, an argument with your spouse, seeing something unpleasant on TV, hearing your alarm clock go off, or being in a hurry to get somewhere could trigger an increase in heart rate, chest constriction, stomach queasiness, or any of a wide range of bodily symptoms associated with anxiety. At other times, the cause resides in some subtle physiological shift within your body—for example, oxygen deprivation due to underbreathing, a spontaneous shift in the neuroendocrine systems of your brain, an increase in muscle tension in your neck and shoulders, or a fall in your blood sugar level. Whether the initial cause lies primarily outside or within your body, you are usually unaware of these physiological shifts until you actually feel the resultant symptoms. The above examples illustrate only a few among many possibilities, any of which might constitute the triggering event for an increase in anxiety. Whether or not you actually develop a full-blown panic attack depends on *how you perceive and respond* to the particular increase in bodily symptoms that occurs.

To sum up, people who panic are likely to experience 1) increased internalization or preoccupation with subtle shifts in bodily symptoms or feelings and 2) an increased tendency to interpret slight aberrations or incremental changes in bodily symptoms as dangerous or catastrophic. The diagram that follows illustrates this tendency:

## Development of a Panic Attack

Phase 1    Initiating circumstances (internal or external)

↓

Phase 2    Slight increase in unusual or unpleasant bodily symptoms (i.e., heart palpitations, shortness of breath, faintness or dizziness, sweating, etc.)

↓

Phase 3    Internalization (increased focus on symptoms makes them more noticeable and easily magnified)

↓

Phase 4    Catastrophic interpretation (telling yourself the symptoms are dangerous—i.e., "I'll have a heart attack," "I'll suffocate," "I'll go completely out of control," "I must leave at once")

↓

Phase 5    Panic

The good news is that it's possible to intervene at any point in this sequence. At phase 1, it may be *generalized stress* that leads to the initial unpleasant bodily sensations—heart palpitations, chest constriction, dizziness, and so on. Incorporating regular relaxation, exercise, low-stress nutritional habits, and other stress management techniques into your lifestyle (see chapters 4, 5, and 16, respectively) on a daily basis can go a long way toward reducing the propensity for sudden increases in your body's state of sympathetic nervous system arousal. Beyond generalized stress, you may be able to identify the particular initiating circumstances that cause your panic attacks by noting carefully what was going on just before—or in the several hours before—a panic attack occurred. You can use the *Panic Attack Record* later in this chapter to help you determine what initial circumstances may have led to a particular panic attack. (The *Panic Attack Record*, and most of the other worksheets in this chapter, is available for download at the website associated with this book. See the very last page of the book for details and instructions.) You can then try to avoid or eliminate these circumstances so that they don't cause you trouble in the future. Interventions that reduce the propensity for having unpleasant bodily sensations in the first place (phases 1 and 2 in the above diagram) all require making changes in your lifestyle and attitudes.

Phase 3 of the panic cycle consists of internalization—being too focused on your internal bodily state. When you actually feel panic coming on, you can reduce internalization by using any of the active coping techniques described later in this chapter in the section "Coping Strategies to Counteract Panic at an Early Stage." These techniques serve to divert your attention away from internal bodily symptoms, and they also can have a directly relaxing effect.

Perhaps the most important change you can make to defuse panic attacks, however, is to intervene at phase 4. That is, you can learn to stop interpreting unpleasant bodily sensations as being dangerous or potentially catastrophic. In fact, research in both the United States and

England has determined that eliminating catastrophic interpretations of bodily symptoms can, *in and of itself alone*, be sufficient to relieve panic attacks. If you can learn to tolerate sensations of dizziness, tightness in your chest, rapid heartbeat, and so on as innocuous bodily symptoms— rather than read them as signs of imminent danger—you will very likely have fewer, if any, panic attacks. That is not to say that stress management techniques and coping strategies for panic are unimportant; it does imply, though, that eliminating catastrophic interpretations by itself can go a long way toward relieving panic.

To assist you in breaking the connection between bodily symptoms and catastrophic interpretations, please refer to the three worksheets that follow in a couple of pages. The first worksheet is a list of bodily symptoms that can trigger panic attacks. Rate each bodily symptom on a 0 to 5 scale, according to how much it affects you when you panic. The second worksheet is a list of common catastrophic self-statements that people who panic make in response to unpleasant bodily symptoms. Rate each of these catastrophic statements on a 1 to 4 scale, according to how much you feel it contributes to your panic attacks.

Finally, using the worksheet *Connecting Bodily Symptoms and Catastrophic Thoughts*, try to connect the two lists from *Panic Attack Worksheet 1* and *Panic Attack Worksheet 2*—that is, see if you can connect specific body symptoms with specific catastrophic thoughts that occur for you during a panic attack. For each troublesome bodily symptom you rated a 4 or 5, list the specific catastrophic thoughts likely to be triggered by that symptom. For example, you might connect heart palpitations with "I'm having a heart attack" and "I'm going to die," or dizziness with "I'm going to pass out" or "I'm going to lose control."

When you're finished, you should have a better idea of what particular bodily symptoms and associated catastrophic interpretations trigger your panic attacks. This knowledge will likely help you break the false connection you've made between your unpleasant bodily symptoms and mistaken interpretations. Keep in mind throughout this exercise that *none of the bodily symptoms you've listed is actually dangerous. However unpleasant such symptoms might feel, they are completely harmless.* Equally important, keep in mind that *none of the catastrophic thoughts you have checked off is true or valid, even though you might have convinced yourself that it is. Every one of these catastrophic thoughts is simply false—a mistaken belief that you can learn to let go of.*

What else can you do to break the automatic connection between unpleasant body sensations and false, catastrophic thoughts? The following three processes can help:

- Recognition

- Writing down alternative explanations of symptoms

- Interoceptive exposure

## Recognition

Just recognizing your tendency to believe that harmless body symptoms are signs of imminent danger is the first step. Awareness of specific connections between particular symptoms and particular catastrophic thoughts, which you can gain from the worksheet *Connecting Bodily Symptoms and Catastrophic Thoughts*, will help you begin defusing the danger when those symptoms come up in day-to-day life.

## *Writing Down Alternative Explanations for Bodily Symptoms*

The catastrophic thoughts (self-statements) you make in an attempt to make sense of unpleasant bodily sensations during a panic attack are simply false. It's just not true, for example, that rapid heartbeat or palpitations occur because you are having a heart attack. Nor is constriction in your chest or shortness of breath happening because you're about to suffocate. Nor are dizziness and light-headedness occurring because you're about to faint or "go crazy." In each of these cases, there is an alternative explanation that is not catastrophic and based in fact. Alternative logical explanations might go something like this:

- An increase in heartbeat and/or heart palpitations is very likely caused by increased output of adrenaline and sympathetic nervous system activity that accompany the early stage of an anxiety reaction. Such reactions are part of the body's normal means of handling any *perceived* threat—they are part of the "fight-or-flight response." They are in no way dangerous, even if they continue for some time. For example, a healthy heart can beat rapidly for many hours without putting you at any risk.

- An increase in chest constriction and shortness of breath can be explained in terms of contraction of the muscles surrounding your chest cavity, also due to increased sympathetic nervous system activity. Such symptoms have nothing to do with the process of suffocating. Your chest muscles cannot contract to the point where you would be at risk of suffocating, no matter how unpleasant the tightness in your chest happens to feel.

- Becoming dizzy and becoming light-headed, common symptoms that can occur when you become anxious, are not caused by the fact that you are about to faint. They are caused by minor constrictions in the arteries of your brain, which lead to a slight reduction in blood circulation. It's extremely unlikely that you would faint, even if you feel quite light-headed. Fainting typically occurs during a drop in blood pressure. When you start to feel anxious, you usually experience an *increase* in blood pressure due to increased adrenaline and sympathetic nervous system activity. Even less plausible is the idea that dizziness and light-headedness are caused by the fact that you're about to go crazy. The development of serious mental disorders has nothing to do with panic attacks and takes place over a much longer period of time than the duration of any panic attack.

These examples can serve as guidelines for developing your own alternative, *noncatastrophic* explanations for troublesome body symptoms. You'll likely find it helpful to refer to the first section of this chapter, "Deflate the Danger," in coming up with your own alternative explanations. The process of writing down such explanations will help strengthen your conviction that uncomfortable body symptoms are truly harmless rather than signs of imminent danger.

You might want to put your alternative explanations of body symptoms on 3 by 5 index cards—one explanation of a particular symptom per card. Keep the cards with you in your purse or backpack and take them out and read them if you feel symptoms coming on.

## *Panic Attack Worksheet 1*
### *Bodily Symptoms*

Any of the following bodily symptoms can occur during a panic attack. Please evaluate each one according to its effect when you are having an attack and indicate your answers on the 0 to 5 scale in the right-hand column.

| | |
|---|---|
| 0 = No effect | 3 = Strong effect |
| 1 = Mild effect | 4 = Severe effect |
| 2 = Medium effect | 5 = Very severe effect |

| | 0 | 1 | 2 | 3 | 4 | 5 |
|---|---|---|---|---|---|---|
| 1. Sinking feeling in stomach | 0 | 1 | 2 | 3 | 4 | 5 |
| 2. Sweaty palms | 0 | 1 | 2 | 3 | 4 | 5 |
| 3. Warm all over | 0 | 1 | 2 | 3 | 4 | 5 |
| 4. Rapid or heavy heartbeat | 0 | 1 | 2 | 3 | 4 | 5 |
| 5. Tremor of the hands | 0 | 1 | 2 | 3 | 4 | 5 |
| 6. Weak or rubbery knees or legs | 0 | 1 | 2 | 3 | 4 | 5 |
| 7. Shaky inside and/or outside | 0 | 1 | 2 | 3 | 4 | 5 |
| 8. Dry mouth | 0 | 1 | 2 | 3 | 4 | 5 |
| 9. Lump in throat | 0 | 1 | 2 | 3 | 4 | 5 |
| 10. Tightness in chest | 0 | 1 | 2 | 3 | 4 | 5 |
| 11. Hyperventilation | 0 | 1 | 2 | 3 | 4 | 5 |
| 12. Nausea or diarrhea | 0 | 1 | 2 | 3 | 4 | 5 |
| 13. Dizzy or light-headed | 0 | 1 | 2 | 3 | 4 | 5 |
| 14. A feeling of unreality—as if "in a dream" | 0 | 1 | 2 | 3 | 4 | 5 |
| 15. Unable to think clearly | 0 | 1 | 2 | 3 | 4 | 5 |
| 16. Blurred vision | 0 | 1 | 2 | 3 | 4 | 5 |
| 17. A feeling of being partially paralyzed | 0 | 1 | 2 | 3 | 4 | 5 |
| 18. A feeling of detachment or floating away | 0 | 1 | 2 | 3 | 4 | 5 |
| 19. Palpitations or irregular heartbeat | 0 | 1 | 2 | 3 | 4 | 5 |
| 20. Chest pain | 0 | 1 | 2 | 3 | 4 | 5 |
| 21. Tingling in hands, feet, or face | 0 | 1 | 2 | 3 | 4 | 5 |
| 22. Feeling faint | 0 | 1 | 2 | 3 | 4 | 5 |
| 23. Fluttery stomach | 0 | 1 | 2 | 3 | 4 | 5 |
| 24. Cold, clammy hands | 0 | 1 | 2 | 3 | 4 | 5 |

*Panic Attack Worksheet 2*
*Catastrophic Thoughts\**

Catastrophic thoughts play a major role in aggravating panic attacks. Using the scale below, rate each of the following thoughts according to the degree to which you believe that each thought contributes to your panic attacks.

| | |
|---|---|
| 1 = Not at all | 3 = Quite a lot |
| 2 = Somewhat | 4 = Very much |

|  |  | 0 | 1 | 2 | 3 | 4 | 5 |
|---|---|---|---|---|---|---|---|
| 1. | I'm going to die. | 0 | 1 | 2 | 3 | 4 | 5 |
| 2. | I'm going insane. | 0 | 1 | 2 | 3 | 4 | 5 |
| 3. | I'm losing control. | 0 | 1 | 2 | 3 | 4 | 5 |
| 4. | This will never end. | 0 | 1 | 2 | 3 | 4 | 5 |
| 5. | I'm really scared. | 0 | 1 | 2 | 3 | 4 | 5 |
| 6. | I'm having a heart attack. | 0 | 1 | 2 | 3 | 4 | 5 |
| 7. | I'm going to pass out. | 0 | 1 | 2 | 3 | 4 | 5 |
| 8. | I don't know what people will think. | 0 | 1 | 2 | 3 | 4 | 5 |
| 9. | I won't be able to get out of here. | 0 | 1 | 2 | 3 | 4 | 5 |
| 10. | I don't understand what's happening to me. | 0 | 1 | 2 | 3 | 4 | 5 |
| 11. | People will think I'm crazy. | 0 | 1 | 2 | 3 | 4 | 5 |
| 12. | I'll always be this way. | 0 | 1 | 2 | 3 | 4 | 5 |
| 13. | I'm going to throw up. | 0 | 1 | 2 | 3 | 4 | 5 |
| 14. | I must have a brain tumor. | 0 | 1 | 2 | 3 | 4 | 5 |
| 15. | I'll choke to death. | 0 | 1 | 2 | 3 | 4 | 5 |
| 16. | I'm going to act foolish. | 0 | 1 | 2 | 3 | 4 | 5 |
| 17. | I'm going blind. | 0 | 1 | 2 | 3 | 4 | 5 |
| 18. | I'll hurt someone. | 0 | 1 | 2 | 3 | 4 | 5 |
| 19. | I'm going to have a stroke. | 0 | 1 | 2 | 3 | 4 | 5 |
| 20. | I'm going to scream. | 0 | 1 | 2 | 3 | 4 | 5 |
| 21. | I'm going to babble or talk funny. | 0 | 1 | 2 | 3 | 4 | 5 |
| 22. | I'll be paralyzed by fear. | 0 | 1 | 2 | 3 | 4 | 5 |
| 23. | Something is really physically wrong with me. | 0 | 1 | 2 | 3 | 4 | 5 |
| 24. | I won't be able to breathe. | 0 | 1 | 2 | 3 | 4 | 5 |
| 25. | Something terrible will happen. | 0 | 1 | 2 | 3 | 4 | 5 |
| 26. | I'm going to make a scene. | 0 | 1 | 2 | 3 | 4 | 5 |

\* Adapted from "Panic Attack Cognitions Questionnaire" in *Coping with Panic: A Drug-Free Approach to Dealing with Anxiety Attacks* by G. A. Clum. Copyright 1990 by Brooks/Cole Publishing Company, a division of International Thomson Publishing Inc., Pacific Grove, CA 93950. Reprinted by permission of the publisher.

## *Connecting Bodily Symptoms and Catastrophic Thoughts*

In the left-hand column below, list bodily symptoms you rated 5 or 4 on the first *Panic Attack Worksheet*. Describe your most troublesome bodily symptoms, one at a time. Then list catastrophic self-statements from the second worksheet that you rated 4 or 3. List those catastrophic statements you would be most likely to make in response to each particular bodily symptom. For example, "rapid heartbeat" is a bodily symptom that might elicit such catastrophic self-statements as "I'm having a heart attack" and "I'm going to die."

Bodily symptom:                                   Catastrophic thoughts:

Bodily symptom:                                   Catastrophic thoughts:

Bodily symptom:                                   Catastrophic thoughts:

Bodily symptom:                                   Catastrophic thoughts:

## Interoceptive Exposure

A very effective treatment for panic attacks involves voluntarily inducing the very bodily symptoms that can trigger panic. Many therapists refer to this technique as *interoceptive exposure,* a process of *exposing yourself to internal bodily symptoms associated with panic* (such as those listed in the *Panic Attack Worksheet 1*), to help you learn that the symptoms are not harmful. Interoceptive exposure is typically done in a therapy session. For example, if dizziness and shortness of breath are troublesome symptoms, the therapist might have you hyperventilate for two minutes and then stand up suddenly, to actually bring on these symptoms. This might sound like an unusual and extreme therapeutic procedure, but, in fact, it is harmless and often quite helpful. Unless you have a respiratory disorder, hyperventilating for two minutes is harmless. Deliberately hyperventilating gives you an opportunity to *actually experience uncomfortable bodily symptoms without anything negative or dangerous happening.* The key here is that you learn on a "gut" or experiential level that nothing terrible follows body sensations that you used to interpret as dangerous. Repeated inductions of dizziness in this way help a panic-prone person develop a strong conviction that dizziness is not dangerous.

Please note that interoceptive exposure can be a useful technique for taming internal anxiety sensations that come up during exposure therapy (see chapter 7, Exposure for Phobias) or when you are worrying excessively (see chapter 10, Overcoming Worry). Cognitive behavioral therapy, which may include changing your catastrophic self-talk to constructive self-talk, can be quite helpful in dealing with all types of anxiety disorders. Likewise, interoceptive exposure can help you normalize any intense internal body sensations (rapid heartbeat, sweating, even the sensation of "being not all there") that may arise not only during panic attacks but also during exposure to phobias or excessive worrying.

You may want to try symptom induction techniques with a professional therapist who has had experience using them. On the other hand, some people have tried these techniques on their own and found them to be quite helpful. If you decide that you want to include these techniques in your self-help program, please observe the following guidelines:

- *Check with your doctor if you are over forty or suspect that you might have any physical condition that would preclude using symptom induction procedures.* For example, you wouldn't try three minutes of hyperventilation if you have a chronic respiratory problem like asthma or emphysema. You also wouldn't run up and down stairs if you have any kind of heart condition that restricts physical exercise. Nor would you do induction procedures if you were pregnant or had epilepsy.

- Although the techniques are harmless, it's a good idea to have a friend or family member present when you first do them to provide support and encouragement. If you can get your support person to do the procedure with you, so much the better.

- You need to persist in doing each induction procedure long enough so that the sensations produced are unpleasant and/or cause an increase in anxiety. Usually, this is anywhere from thirty seconds to two minutes. You *want* to simulate, if possible, the actual sensations you experience during a panic attack. The point is to expose yourself to unpleasant bodily sensations and learn that they are not harmful. As a general rule, keep doing the procedure for about thirty seconds *after* you first notice it producing unpleasant sensations and/or anxiety. If you stop the moment you start to feel unpleasant symptoms, you'll tend to reinforce your fear of them.

- Review the *Panic Attack Worksheet 1* and identify those bodily symptoms that are most troublesome for you. Then practice any of the induction techniques below that can produce those symptoms. Practice each induction technique three or four times in a row, then repeat the practice each day for several days until it loses its ability to make you anxious. With practice, the symptoms you experience from induction procedures will lose their capacity to cause anxiety. This is precisely what you want.

## Induction Techniques

After obtaining clearance from your physician, try practicing the following six symptom induction techniques:

1. Hyperventilate continuously for two minutes. This involves breathing deeply and rapidly with your mouth open. At the end of two minutes, stand up. (Symptoms: dizziness, disorientation, light-headedness)

2. Breathe through a straw while holding your nose for one minute—don't allow any air through your nose. (Symptoms: shortness of breath, suffocation)

3. Walk up and down some stairs rapidly for about ninety seconds or until your heart rate increases noticeably. Stop if you experience dizziness or your heart rate exceeds 140 beats per minute. Alternatively, you can use a stationary bike or stair-stepper to increase your heart rate. (Symptoms: rapid heartbeat, heart pounding)

4. Spin—preferably in a desk chair or while standing up—for thirty seconds to one minute. It's not necessary to go a full minute if you find yourself getting significantly dizzy. Be near a chair or couch where you can sit back down easily. (Symptoms: dizziness, disorientation)

5. Tense every part of your body and hold yourself tight for one minute before releasing. (Symptom: muscle tension)

6. Put on warm clothes and turn up the heat or sit in a sauna. (Symptom: sweating)

Remember to persist with each of these procedures long enough to produce unpleasant sensations. It's ideal if you allow yourself to feel these unpleasant sensations for at least thirty seconds, although you may want to start out with a shorter period when you first try the induction. You'll get the most from this exercise if the procedure actually makes you somewhat uncomfortable or anxious. Again, the idea is to teach yourself that you can have unpleasant bodily symptoms without anything terrible or dangerous happening. To the extent that this learning carries over to real-life panic symptoms, you can likely overcome having full-blown panic attacks—that is, you'll be able to withstand the unpleasant body sensations during the early stage of panic without reacting to them as dangerous. Keep in mind that you may need to practice the symptom induction procedures many times before you get to the point at which the symptoms don't cause you anxiety.

After you've produced unpleasant symptoms and anxiety for thirty seconds, you can practice some coping skills that you'll learn later in this chapter. These skills include abdominal breathing, repeating coping statements, moving around, or talking to someone. You want to fully experience the unpleasant symptoms and anxiety so that you can get used to them, but you also can practice these coping skills to bring your anxiety down. Symptom inductions provide an excellent opportunity to gain confidence in your mastery of coping skills.

What if the inductions don't produce any anxiety, even from the beginning? This might happen for at least two reasons. It could happen because you feel safe doing the procedure in the comfort of your own home or with your support person. Possibly, the process of inducing body symptoms *voluntarily* may give you a sense of control over what is happening that isn't present when a real-life panic situation occurs. In order to give the symptom induction procedures a little more "charge," you can modify the conditions in which you do them as follows:

- Do the procedures alone.

- Do the procedures away from your home or safe place.

- Do them while *visualizing* yourself having a full-blown panic attack.

As mentioned, induction techniques also work for neutralizing anxious internal body sensations that can come up while facing a phobia. If you want to completely master your phobia, you might deliberately attempt to induce uncomfortable symptoms in a phobic situation (unless it could be potentially dangerous to do so, such as when driving on a busy highway).

For a more in-depth discussion of how to use and benefit from symptom inductions, please see the books by David Barlow and Michelle Craske and by Denise Beckfield listed at the end of this chapter.

## Don't Fight Panic

Resisting or fighting initial panic symptoms is likely to make them worse. It's important to avoid tensing up in reaction to panic symptoms or trying to make them go away by suppressing them or gritting your teeth. Although it's important to act rather than be passive (as discussed below), you still shouldn't fight your panic. Claire Weekes, in her iconic, popular books *Hope and Help for Your Nerves* and *Peace from Nervous Suffering*, describes a four-step approach for coping with panic:

1. *Face the symptoms—don't run from them.* Attempting to suppress or run away from the early symptoms of panic is a way of telling yourself that you can't handle a particular situation. In most cases, this will only create more panic. A more constructive attitude to cultivate is one that says, "Okay, here it is again. I can allow my body to go through its reactions and handle this. I've done it before."

2. *Accept what your body is doing—don't fight against it.* When you try to fight panic, you simply tense up against it, which only makes you more anxious. Adopting just the opposite attitude,

one of *letting go* and *allowing* your body to have its reactions (such as heart palpitations, chest constriction, sweaty palms, dizziness, and so on) will enable you to move through panic much more quickly and easily. The key is to be able to *watch* or *observe* your body's state of physiological arousal—no matter how unusual or uncomfortable it feels—without reacting to it with further fear or anxiety.

3. *Float with the wave of a panic attack rather than try to force your way through it.* Claire Weekes makes a distinction between *first fear* and *second fear.* First fear consists of the physiological reactions underlying panic; second fear is when you make yourself afraid of these reactions by saying scary things to yourself like "I can't handle this!" "I've got to get out of here right now!" or "What if other people see this happening to me?" While you can't do much about first fear, you can eliminate second fear by learning to flow with the rise and fall of your body's state of arousal rather than fighting or reacting fearfully to it. Instead of scaring yourself about your body's reactions, you can move with them and make reassuring statements to yourself, such as "This, too, will pass," "I'll let my body do its thing and move through this," or "I've handled this before and I can handle it now." A list of such positive coping statements follows in the next section.

4. *Allow time to pass.* Panic is caused by a sudden surge of adrenaline. If you can allow and float with the bodily reactions caused by this surge, much of this adrenaline will metabolize and be reabsorbed in three to five minutes. As soon as this happens, you'll start to feel better. *Panic attacks are time limited.* In most cases, panic will peak and begin to subside after a few minutes. It is more likely to pass quickly if you don't aggravate it by fighting against it or reacting to it with even more fear (causing "second fear") by saying scary things to yourself.

## Coping Statements

Use any or several of the following positive statements to help yourself cultivate attitudes of accepting, "floating," and allowing time to pass during a panic attack. You may find it helpful to repeat a single statement, or two or three statements, over and over during the first minute or two when you feel panic symptoms coming on. You may also want to do deep abdominal breathing in conjunction with repeating a coping statement. If one statement gets tiresome or seems to stop working, try another.

- This feeling isn't comfortable or pleasant, but I can accept it.

- I can be anxious and still deal with this situation.

- I can handle these symptoms or sensations.

- This isn't an emergency. It's okay to think slowly about what I need to do.

- This isn't the worst thing that could happen.

- I'm going to go with this and wait for my anxiety to decrease.

- This is an opportunity for me to learn to cope with my fears.

- I'll just let my body do its thing. This will pass.

- I'll ride this through—I don't need to let this get to me.

- I deserve to feel okay right now.

- I can take all the time I need in order to let go and relax.

- There's no need to push myself. I can take as small a step forward as I choose.

- I've survived this before and I'll survive this time, too.

- I can do my coping strategies and allow this to pass.

- This anxiety won't hurt me—even if it doesn't feel good.

- This is just anxiety—I'm not going to let it get to me.

- Nothing serious is going to happen to me.

- Fighting and resisting this isn't going to help—so I'll just let it pass.

- These are just thoughts—not reality.

- I don't need these thoughts—I can choose to think differently.

- This isn't dangerous.

- So what.

- Don't worry—be happy. *(Use this to inject an element of lightness or humor.)*

## Ways to Work with Coping Statements

Select your favorite coping statements from the preceding list and try working with them in any of the following ways. This will help you reinforce them in your mind.

1. *Write* up to five of your favorite coping statements in large, bold print on a large index card or an 8½ by 11-inch sheet of paper. If available, use a felt-tipped pen to make the print for each statement stand out. Make copies of this list and post them in a few prominent places around your house. If you have anxiety associated with driving, post the list on your dashboard. Take your list with you in a pocket or purse when you experience the onset of panic symptoms or confront a phobic situation. Then review it as needed.

2. *Recite* your coping statements out loud from your written list. Say each statement slowly, with emphasis, allowing time between each consecutive statement.

3. *Listen* to your favorite coping statements on an audio recording in your own voice (or in a friend's voice). Explicit instructions for making a recording of your voice on a laptop or smartphone can be found by doing a Google search for "How to record your voice."

The instructions are easy and simple for most types of computers and handheld devices. Record your coping statements slowly, leaving time between each consecutive statement. Then play back the recording of your coping statements twice a day, first while relaxing and eventually when entering an anxiety-provoking situation.

# Explore the Antecedents of Your Panic Attacks

You can increase your mastery over panic attacks by investigating the types of circumstances that tend to precede them. If you are agoraphobic, you are very familiar with these circumstances. You know that you are more likely to panic, for example, if you are far from home, driving over a bridge, or sitting in a restaurant, and so you systematically avoid these particular situations. If you have spontaneous panic attacks that come "out of the blue," you might find it helpful to monitor their occurrence for two weeks and take careful note of what was going on immediately—as well as for several hours—before each one occurred. You might observe whether any of the following conditions makes a difference in the likelihood of your having a panic reaction:

- Were you under stress?

- Were you by yourself or with someone?

- If with someone, was it a family member, a friend, or a stranger?

- What kind of mood were you in for several hours before panic came on? Anxious? Depressed? Excited? Sad? Angry? Other?

- Were you engaging in negative or fearful thoughts just before you panicked?

- Did you feel tired or rested?

- Were you experiencing some kind of loss?

- Were you feeling hot or cold?

- Were you feeling restless or calm?

- Had you consumed caffeine or sugar before panic came on?

- Are there any other circumstances that appear to correlate with your panic reactions?

You can use the *Panic Attack Record* that follows to monitor every panic attack you experience over a two-week period. Make copies of the form and fill one out for each separate panic attack. Answer all the questions for the entire day from the time you awoke until the time you panicked. If the attack happens at night, answer for the day preceding that night.

By making the effort to record your panic attacks and carefully observing any circumstances that consistently precede them, you are taking an important step. You are learning that you need not be a passive victim of an event that seems totally outside your control. Instead, you can begin to alter the circumstances of your daily life in a direction that significantly reduces the odds of having panic attacks.

# *Panic Attack Record*

Fill out one form for each separate panic attack during a two-week period.

Date: _____

Time: _____

Duration (minutes): _____

Intensity of panic (rate 5 to 10 using the *Anxiety Scale* that follows): _____

## *Antecedents*

1.  Stress level during preceding day (rate on a 1 to 10 scale where 1 is the lowest stress level and 10 is the highest): _____

2.  Alone or with someone? _____

3.  If with someone, was it a family member, friend, stranger? _____

4.  Your mood for three hours preceding panic attack.

    Anxious _____    Depressed _____    Excited _____    Angry _____

    Sad _____    Other (specify) _____

5.  Were you facing a challenge _____ or taking it easy _____?

6.  Were you engaging in negative or fearful thoughts before you panicked?

    Yes \_\_\_\_ No \_\_\_\_ If so, what thoughts? _____

7.  Were you tired _____ or rested _____?

8.  Were you experiencing some kind of emotional upset or loss?   Yes \_\_\_\_ No \_\_\_\_

9.  Were you feeling hot _____, cold _____, neither _____?

10. Were you feeling restless and impatient?   Yes        No

11. Were you asleep before you panicked?   Yes        No

12. Did you consume caffeine or sugar within eight hours before you panicked?

    Yes \_\_\_\_ No \_\_\_\_ If yes, how much? _____

13. Have you noticed any other circumstances that correlate with your panic reactions? (specify)

_____

_____

# Learn to Discriminate Early Symptoms of Panic

With practice, you can learn to identify the preliminary signs that a panic attack may be imminent. For some individuals, this might be a sudden quickening of the heartbeat. For others it might be a tightening in the chest, sweaty hands, or queasiness. Still others might experience a slight dizziness or disorientation. Most people experience some preliminary warning symptoms before reaching the "point of no return," when a full-blown panic attack is inevitable.

It's possible to distinguish among different levels or degrees of anxiety leading up to panic by using the 10-point *Anxiety Scale* (see below).

## *Anxiety Scale*

| | | |
|---|---|---|
| 7–10 | *Major Panic Attack* | All of the symptoms in level 6 exaggerated; terror; fear of going crazy or dying; compulsion to escape |
| 6 | *Moderate Panic Attack* | Palpitations; difficulty breathing; feeling disoriented or detached (feeling of unreality); panic in response to perceived loss of control |
| 5 | *Early Panic* | Heart pounding or beating irregularly; constricted breathing; spaciness or dizziness; definite fear of losing control; compulsion to escape |
| 4 | *Marked Anxiety* | Feeling uncomfortable or "spacey"; heart beating fast; muscles tight; beginning to wonder about maintaining control |
| 3 | *Moderate Anxiety* | Feeling uncomfortable but still in control; heart starting to beat faster; more rapid breathing; sweaty palms |
| 2 | *Mild Anxiety* | Butterflies in stomach; muscle tension; definitely nervous |
| 1 | *Slight Anxiety* | Passing twinge of anxiety; feeling slightly nervous |
| 0 | *Relaxation* | Calm; a feeling of being undistracted and at peace |

The symptoms at various levels of this scale are typical, although they may not correspond exactly to your specific symptoms. The important thing is to identify what constitutes a level 4 for *you*. This is the point at which—whatever symptoms you're experiencing—*you feel your control over your reaction beginning to diminish.* Up to and through level 3, you may be feeling very anxious and uncomfortable, but you still feel that you're coping. Starting at level 4, you begin to wonder whether you can manage what's happening, which can lead to further panic. With practice, you can learn to "catch yourself"—abort a panic reaction *before* it rises above this point of no return. The more adept you become at recognizing the early warning signs of panic, up through level 4 on the scale, the more control you will gain over your panic reactions. Mark this page in some fashion, as the *Anxiety Scale* will be referred to frequently here and in subsequent chapters.

# Coping Strategies to Counteract Panic at an Early Stage

First you must learn to identify your own preliminary warning signs of a potential panic attack. What are your own level 4 symptoms? Once you learn the signs, it is time to *do something* about them. *Fighting* panic is not a good idea, but doing nothing and just remaining passive can be even less helpful. The best solution is to utilize a number of tried-and-true coping strategies.

If you've been able to detect the early symptoms of emerging panic before they get out of control (before they exceed level 4 on the *Anxiety Scale*), any of the following coping strategies can be used to prevent a full-fledged panic reaction.

## Practice Abdominal Breathing

Breathing slowly from your abdomen can help reduce the bodily symptoms of panic in either of two ways:

- By slowing down your respiration and breathing from your abdomen, you can reverse two of the reactions associated with the fight-or-flight response—increased respiratory rate and increased constriction of your chest wall muscles. After three or four minutes of slow, regular, abdominal breathing, you are likely to feel that you have slowed down a "runaway reaction" that was threatening to get out of control.

- Slow, abdominal breathing, especially when done through your nose, can reduce symptoms of hyperventilation that may cause or aggravate a panic attack. The dizziness, disorientation, and tingly sensations associated with hyperventilation are produced by rapid, shallow, chest-level breathing. Three or four minutes of slow, abdominal breathing reverses this process and will eliminate hyperventilation symptoms.

Review the section on abdominal breathing in chapter 4 along with the *Abdominal Breathing* and *Calming Breath* exercises. Pick the exercise you prefer and practice it for five minutes every day until you feel that you've mastered it. (Practicing abdominal breathing every day will also help you retrain yourself to naturally breathe from a lower area of your lungs.) Once you feel comfortable and confident with a particular technique, try using it anytime you feel the initial symptoms of panic coming on. Remember to keep up slow abdominal breathing for three to five minutes or longer until you can feel your panic symptoms beginning to subside. If the breathing exercise itself causes you to feel light-headed, stop for thirty seconds and then start again.

An alternative practice that helps some people offset panic is simply to take a deep breath and hold it as long as you can at the moment you feel panic symptoms coming on. If you still feel anxious after this, repeat the procedure two or three times.

## Repeat Positive Coping Statements

One of the central points of this chapter has been to emphasize the role of negative self-talk and catastrophic thoughts in aggravating a panic attack. While the physical, bodily reactions associated with panic (first fear) may come out of the blue, your interpretation of these bodily symptoms (second fear) does not. It is based on *what you tell yourself* about these symptoms. If you tell yourself that your physiological symptoms are horrible and very threatening, you can't stand them, you're going to lose control, or you might die, you can likely scare yourself into a high state of anxiety. On the other hand, to the extent you can accept what's happening and make calming, reassuring statements to yourself, such as "It's only anxiety—I'm not going to let it get to me," "I've been through this before and it's not dangerous," or "I can handle this until it passes," you can minimize or eliminate the escalation of your symptoms.

Use any of the positive coping statements listed earlier in this chapter when you feel the first symptoms of panic coming on. This will help divert your mind away *both* from the bodily symptoms of panic *and* from fear-inducing self-talk that can only make things worse. Choose any of the strategies listed in the section "Ways to Work with Coping Statements" (above) to practice your coping statements two or more times per day, when you're not feeling panic or anxiety. Keep practicing them until they become almost automatic. Then use them when a panic episode occurs (or while entering or enduring a phobic situation). Keep up the practice for a minute or two until you feel the physiological intensity of your anxiety begin to subside.

Learning to use coping statements effectively to overcome panic will take practice and perseverance. You need to rehearse your preferred coping statements many times to fully internalize them. If you make the effort, you will be surprised how well coping statements can work to reduce the likelihood of your anxiety symptoms from going above level 4 on the *Anxiety Scale*. Constructive self-talk also can help to limit a panic attack that has already gone *above* level 4 (see the section later in this chapter, "What to Do When Panic Goes Above Level 4").

In sum, the way you respond to early physical symptoms of panic will be determined largely by *what you say to yourself,* as illustrated below.

| **First Fear** | *Negative Self-Talk* | **Second Fear** | |
| --- | --- | --- | --- |
| | "Oh no—here it comes." | Immediate Emotional | |
| | "I'm losing control." | Reaction to $\longrightarrow$ | Panic |
| | "I can't stand this." | Bodily Symptoms | |
| | "What will others think if I lose it?" | | |

*Bodily Symptoms*
Rapid Heartbeat
Sweaty Palms
Constricted Breathing
Dizziness

*Constructive Self-Talk*
*or Coping Statements*

| | | | |
| --- | --- | --- | --- |
| "I can handle these symptoms." | | Disengagement or: | |
| "This is just anxiety— $\longrightarrow$ I'll let it pass." | | witnessing: $\longrightarrow$ Flowing with | Coping |
| "I can ride this through." | | bodily symptoms | |

The choice is up to you.

## Use Abdominal Breathing in Combination with Coping Statements

You might find that a *combination* of abdominal breathing and repeating positive coping statements will work best in limiting your panic. Generally, it's best to address the physical sensations of panic first with an abdominal breathing exercise and to follow up shortly thereafter with methodical repetition of coping statements. You may prefer to completely overlap the two types of techniques or, alternatively, you may want to work exclusively on reducing your physiological arousal for a minute or two and then start working with constructive statements. Experiment to see what works better for you. It's best if you gain some skill and familiarity with each type of strategy by itself, initially, before attempting to put them together.

## Talk to a Supportive Person Nearby or on the Phone

Talking to someone can help get your mind off your anxious bodily symptoms and thoughts. Whether you are driving in a car, standing in line at the grocery store, standing in an elevator, or flying on a plane, this can work very well. If you are driving, talk with a passenger or pull over and stop to use your cell phone. In a public speaking situation, confiding in your audience that you feel a bit nervous can often help dispel initial anxiety. Talking to someone is a way you *disrupt* the early onset of a panic attack. It should not be used as a way to *escape and avoid* panic symptoms by seeking reassurance. This is a subtle but important distinction if you utilize talking to someone as a coping strategy.

## Move Around or Engage in Some Physical Activity

Moving and doing something physical helps dissipate the extra energy or adrenaline created by the fight-or-flight reaction that occurs during acute anxiety. Instead of resisting the normal physiological arousal that accompanies anxiety, you move with it. At work, you can walk to the bathroom and back or walk outdoors for ten minutes. At home, you can do household chores requiring physical activity or work out on your stationary bike or rebounder. Gardening is an excellent way to channel the physical energy of an anxiety reaction.

## Stay in the Present

Focus on concrete objects around you in your immediate environment. In a grocery store, for example, you might look at the people standing around or the various magazines next to the cash register. While driving, you might focus on the cars in front of you or on the other details of the surrounding environment (as long as you don't look away from the road, of course). Staying in the present and focusing on external objects will help minimize the attention you give to troublesome physical symptoms or catastrophic "what-if" thoughts. If possible, you might try actually touching objects nearby to reinforce staying in the immediate present. Another good way to ground yourself is to focus on your legs and feet. As you're standing or walking, pay attention to your legs and feet and imagine that you are connected to the ground.

## Use Simple Disruption Techniques

There are many simple disruption techniques that can help divert some of your attention away from your anxiety. The attitude you take in enacting these techniques is important. You are disrupting the onset of a panic attack, *not trying to escape it*. Here are a few examples:

- Unwrap and chew a piece of gum.

- Count backward from one hundred in threes: 100, 97, 94, and so on.

- Count the number of people in line (or all of the lines) at the grocery store.

- Count the money in your wallet.

- While driving, count the bumps on the steering wheel.

- Take a cold shower.

- Sing.

**Note:** Disruption techniques are fine for helping you cope with the sudden onset of anxiety or worry. However, don't let disruption become a way of avoiding or running away from your anxiety. Ultimately, you need to directly experience anxiety and let it pass in order to learn that it is not harmful or potentially dangerous. Every time you experience a surge of anxiety and allow it to pass without trying to get away from it, you learn that you can survive whatever your nervous system dishes out. In doing so, you build confidence in your ability to manage your anxiety in any and all situations.

## Relinquish Safety Behaviors

Safety behaviors are self-protective maneuvers you undertake to avoid fear. Usually they tend to backfire and aggravate your fear. Fleeing fear begets fear. Relinquishing safety behaviors means taking a stance where you accept and endure panic sensations. The payoff is that you ultimately learn you can handle your unpleasant sensations.

Some common types of safety behaviors follow.

**Reassurance seeking.** For example, your heart is beating hard or fast because you've been under excessive stress for the past few hours or all day. This is a normal occurrence for many people. You fear you might have some serious heart affliction or even be susceptible to a heart attack. For reassurance, you call a friend on your smartphone, or maybe even try to get in touch with your primary care physician.

**Overchecking.** Suppose you are having an episode of rapid heartbeat or even tachycardia (your heart beat exceeds one hundred beats per minute). Even though your heart muscle is designed to beat at up to hundred beats a minute for even a day or two with no real danger, you resort to checking your pulse to check your heart rate. Each time you check, you add to your anxiety when you notice your heartbeat has not slowed down. The more checking you do, the more anxiety you'll have. During a panic attack, your heart may beat over a hundred beats a minute for as long as perhaps fifteen to twenty minutes, but over time it will gradually start to slow down. By repeatedly checking your pulse, you can increase your anxiety and postpone the natural tendency of your heart to eventually slow down. You may even resort to calling a friend or trying to reach a doctor on your phone, which only further aggravates your anxiety by creating more uncertainty.

**Overreliance on a support person.** When anxiety arises while, for example, facing a long-standing phobia, it often helps at the outset to have a support person go with you. If you're making your first flight after many years of avoiding flying, having someone accompany you on your first flight can provide both diversion and reassurance to help mitigate anxiety. Or perhaps you have a phobia of going to the doctor for a routine exam, and you've let yourself stay away from medical practitioners for a few years. It may be quite helpful to have someone accompany you when you make your first visit to the doctor in a long time. Just having the support person sit in the waiting room while you're having the checkup may be sufficient.

Support people are a kind of "crutch" that can help you manage anxiety or even panic when you *first* face a phobic situation you've avoided for a long time. However, if you keep taking your support person with you in every case of facing the fear, you will never learn that you can become capable of handling the fear on your own. In order to *complete* exposure to most phobias, it becomes necessary to relinquish the safety behavior of bringing a support person along. Then can you learn to be fully confident about your ability to overcome the fear.

**Rituals.** When strong anxiety or panic comes up, you may try to assuage it with a ritual such as saying a prayer four times or continually snapping a rubber band against your wrist. The ritual serves to foster the false belief that you can *only* handle the situation by performing the ritual. Ultimately, you can only gain confidence in your ability to *fully* handle the fearful sensations and thoughts by relinquishing the ritual and learning that nothing terrible happens if you omit it.

To reduce reliance on safety behaviors, utilize the following three guidelines.

1. *Notice* you are engaging in safety behavior(s) in order to protect yourself from anxiety.

2. *Face (or accept) rather than resist.* Desist from fighting or fleeing uncomfortable body sensations or fearful thoughts. The key to overcoming safety behaviors is *full acceptance* of the situation and an ability to *tolerate discomfort* (as long as discomfort doesn't soar to an overwhelming degree, which is usually unlikely).

3. *Cope.* Rely on your most helpful *coping strategies*, described in this section, to move through the experience of panic and tolerate the discomfort.

## Get Angry with Anxiety

Anger and anxiety are incompatible responses. It's impossible to experience both at the same time. In some cases, it turns out that symptoms of anxiety are a stand-in for deeper feelings of anger, frustration, or rage. If you can get angry at your anxiety the moment it arises, you may stop it from building any further. You can do this either verbally or physically. You might say things to your symptoms such as "Get out of my way. I have things to do!" "To hell with this—I don't care what other people think!" or "This reaction is ridiculous—I'm going into this situation anyway!" This approach can be effective for some people.

Time-honored techniques for physically expressing anger include these:

- Pounding on a pillow on your bed with both fists

- Screaming into a pillow—or in your car alone with the windows rolled up

- Hitting a bed or a couch with a plastic baseball bat

- Throwing eggs into the bathtub (if the remains will wash away)

- Chopping wood

Please keep in mind that it's very important in expressing anger to direct it either into empty space or toward an object, *not at another person.* If you find yourself quite angry with someone, vent the physical charge of your anger first in one of the above ways before you attempt to communicate with that person. Rise above physical and verbal expressions of anger toward other human beings.

### Experience Something Immediately Pleasurable

The feeling of pleasure is also incompatible with an anxiety state. Any of the following may help offset anxiety, worry, or even panic:

- Have your significant other or spouse hold you (or give you a back rub).

- Take a hot shower or relax in a hot bath.

- Have a pleasurable snack or meal.

- Engage in sexual activity.

- Read humorous books or watch a comical DVD.

## Learn to Observe Rather Than React to Bodily Sensations of Anxiety

You can take a major step forward by learning to detach emotionally from the first physical symptoms of panic: simply *observe* them. To the extent that you are able to *witness* the intense reactions your body goes through when anxious, and not interpret them as a threat, you will be able to save yourself considerable distress. Several of the strategies described in the previous section can help you adopt this detached stance. By doing deep abdominal breathing, you can slow down the physiological mechanisms responsible for panic, giving yourself *time* to gain some detachment. By using constructive self-talk, you replace the scare-talk, which can aggravate your anxiety, with coping statements specifically designed to foster an attitude of observing and "flowing with" the experience.

You'll find that it takes some practice to learn how to use breathing techniques or constructive coping statements. Consistently working with them will in time enable you to reach a point where, rather than just react, you can observe and go with the bodily reactions associated with panic. This kind of detachment is the key to being able to master your panic.

## What to Do When Panic Goes Above Level 4

If you are unable to arrest a panic reaction before it goes beyond your personal point of no return (level 5 or higher on the *Anxiety Scale*), observe the following guidelines:

- Get out of the panic-provoking situation if possible.

- Don't try to control or fight your symptoms—accept them and ride them out as best you can; remind yourself that panic is not dangerous and will pass.

- Call someone—express your feelings to them.

- Move around or engage in physical activity.

- Focus on simple objects around you.

- Touch the floor, touch the physical objects around you, or "ground" yourself in some other way. Feel free to sit on the floor if that helps.

- Discharge tension by pounding your fists, crying, or screaming into a pillow, if you are in a place where you can do so.

- Breathe slowly and regularly through your nose to reduce possible symptoms of hyperventilation.

- Use positive self-talk (coping statements) in conjunction with slow breathing.

- As a last resort, take an extra dose of a minor tranquilizer (with the general approval of your doctor).

During an intense panic attack, you may feel very confused and disoriented. Try asking yourself the following questions to increase your objectivity (you may want to write these out on an index card to carry with you at all times):

- *Are these symptoms I'm feeling truly dangerous?* (Answer: "No.")

- *What is the absolute worst thing that could happen?* (Usual answer: "I might have to leave this situation quickly, or I might have to ask for assistance.")

- *Am I telling myself anything that is making this worse?*

- *What is the most supportive thing I can do for myself right now?*

## Putting It All Together

In general, when anxiety symptoms start to come on, use the following three-step technique to manage them:

1. *Accept your symptoms.* Don't fight or resist them. Resisting or fleeing symptoms of anxiety tends to make them worse. The more you can adopt an attitude of acceptance, no matter how unpleasant the symptoms may be, the better your ability to cope will be. Acceptance prepares you to do something proactive about your anxiety rather than get caught up in reactions to it.

2. *Practice abdominal breathing.* When anxiety first comes up, always go to abdominal breathing first. If you've been practicing abdominal breathing regularly, merely initiating it provides a cue to your body to relax and disengage from a potential fight-or-flight response.

3. *Use a coping strategy.* After you begin to feel more centered in abdominal breathing, use a coping strategy or a disruption technique (for example, talking to another person or repeating coping statements) to continue to manage your feelings. Any coping strategy will reinforce the basic stance of not giving attention or energy to negative thoughts and/ or uncomfortable bodily sensations. By regularly practicing coping techniques, you reinforce an attitude of mastery—instead of passive submission and victimization—in the face of your anxiety. Be aware that abdominal breathing is itself a coping strategy, and sometimes it alone will be enough.

## Sharing About Your Condition

A good way to minimize the likelihood of panic in social or public situations is simply to inform someone in charge that you have a problem with panic attacks and/or agoraphobia.

This is especially critical if you are afraid of panic attacks interfering with your capacity to perform your job. If you try to work without letting anyone know about your problem, you may come to feel increasingly trapped in the situation—trapped by your fear of what other people might think of you if you "lose it." This is likely to increase, rather than decrease, the probability of actually panicking.

If you say a little bit about your problem to your boss or a coworker, you will make your workplace into more of a "safe place." You'll worry less about what others might think if you panic, because someone important already knows. More importantly, you will have given yourself permission to temporarily leave work in the event that you do experience panic. With this permission, you are much less likely to feel trapped, and any fears you might have developed about going to work are likely to dissipate.

The same applies to any other situations in which you're afraid of panicking and yet where there is someone in charge you might talk to. This includes classrooms, doctors' and dentists' offices, parties (talk to the host or hostess), or group meetings (talk to the facilitator).

# Summary of Things to Do

1.  Reread the section "Deflate the Danger" in this chapter one or more times to reinforce the idea that the various symptoms of a panic attack are not dangerous.

2.  Complete the first two panic attack worksheets in this chapter. Then use the third worksheet to make connections between physical sensations or symptoms that accompany your panic reactions and any catastrophic interpretations you tend to make of those sensations. Remember that it's your catastrophic thoughts that are mainly responsible for triggering panic attacks.

3.  Reread the section "Don't Fight Panic" on Claire Weekes's four-step approach to coping with panic attacks to help you cultivate attitudes of acceptance and nonresistance toward panic symptoms. Learn to flow with panic rather than fight it.

4.  Monitor your panic attacks for two weeks, using the *Panic Attack Record* to look for conditions and stimuli that precede your panic reactions.

5.  Work on learning to recognize your own early symptoms of panic. Identify what symptoms constitute a level 4 for you on the *Anxiety Scale* (the point at which you feel like you're beginning to lose control).

6.  Experiment with different coping strategies when you feel panic symptoms coming on. Which strategies work best for you?

7.  Give special attention to the following coping strategies:

    *   *Practice abdominal breathing* (using either the *Abdominal Breathing* or the *Calming Breath* exercise from chapter 4) for five minutes per day until you've mastered the technique. Then use it to reduce body sensations of anxiety when you feel the initial physical symptoms of panic emerging.

    *   *Choose one or more coping statements and practice using them* at the moment when you notice that you're starting to scare yourself with negative self-talk. Rehearse your coping statements until you are able to overcome any fearful self-talk going on in your mind.

    *   *After you've gained mastery in the use of abdominal breathing and coping statements, try combining them.* Start with abdominal breathing and follow this up with the repetition of one or more coping statements. The right combination of these techniques can be even more effective than either one of them alone.

8.  Experiment with coping strategies for panic reactions *above* level 4 on the *Anxiety Scale* to find out which ones work best for you.

9.  If you feel so inclined, try the symptom induction procedures. These procedures will expose you to physical sensations that you associate with panic. If you're working with a therapist, you may wish to ask him or her to assist you in carrying out symptom inductions.

10. Talk about your condition with a relative, a friend, or your supervisor at work.

## Further Reading

Barlow, David, and Michelle Craske. *Mastery of Your Anxiety and Panic: Workbook.* 4th ed. New York: Oxford University Press, 2007. (Detailed presentation of the cognitive behavioral approach to treating panic.)

Beckfield, Denise F. *Master Your Panic and Take Back Your Life.* 3rd ed. Atascadero, CA: Impact Publishers, 2004. (Thorough and useful self-help guide.)

Weekes, Claire. *Hope and Help for Your Nerves.* New York: Signet, 1990.

———. *Peace from Nervous Suffering.* New York: Signet, 1990. (An excellent resource for learning to deal with panic and other forms of anxiety.)

Wilson, Reid. *Don't Panic: Taking Control of Anxiety Attacks.* 3rd ed. New York: Harper Perennial, 2009.

Zuercher-White, Elke. *An End to Panic.* 2nd ed. Oakland, CA: New Harbinger Publications, 1998.

# 7

# Exposure for Phobias

The most effective way to overcome a phobia is simply to face it. Continuing to avoid a situation that frightens you is, more than anything else, what keeps the phobia alive.

Having to face a particular situation you have been avoiding for years may at the outset seem an impossible task. Yet this task can be made manageable by breaking it down into sufficiently small steps. Instead of entering a situation all at once, you can do it very gradually in small increments.

One theory of how phobias develop is as a result of *sensitization*. This is a process of becoming sensitized to a particular stimulus. In essence, you learn to associate anxiety with a particular situation. Perhaps you once panicked while sitting in a restaurant or by yourself at home. If your anxiety level was high, it's quite possible that you acquired a strong association between being in that particular situation and being anxious. Thereafter, being in, being near, or perhaps just thinking about that situation automatically triggered your anxiety: a connection between the situation and a strong anxiety response was established. Because this connection was automatic and seemingly beyond your control, you probably did all you could to avoid putting yourself in the situation again. Your avoidance was rewarded because it saved you from reexperiencing your anxiety. At the point where you began to *always* avoid the situation, you developed a full-fledged phobia.

*Exposure* is the process of *unlearning* the connection between anxiety and a particular situation. Over the years, there has been an evolution in thinking about how exposure works. For exposure to occur, you typically need to enter a phobic situation gradually through a series of steps. With *real-life* exposure, you confront a phobic situation directly, letting your anxiety rise and enduring the anxiety for a period of time in order to learn that you can actually *handle* your anxiety in a situation you've been accustomed to avoiding. The point is to 1) *unlearn a connection* between a phobic situation (such as driving on a freeway) and an anxiety response and 2) *gain confidence* in your ability to handle the situation regardless of whether anxiety comes up. Repeatedly entering the situation will eventually allow you to overcome your previous avoidance.

Exposure is the single most effective available treatment for phobias. In many controlled studies, direct exposure to phobic situations has consistently been found to be more effective than other, nonbehavioral treatments, such as insight therapy, cognitive therapy by itself, or medication. Nothing works better toward overcoming a fear than facing it—especially when this is done systematically through a series of steps. Furthermore, improvement resulting from real-life exposure does not typically disappear weeks or months later. Once you've fully completed exposure to a phobic situation in real life, you tend to remain free of the fear. In some cases, however, you might need to complete a periodic "booster" exposure session to retain the results of your original exposure, particularly if the situation is one that you don't deal with often (such as seeing snakes at the zoo, for example).

Exposure is the treatment of choice for agoraphobia, social phobias, and many specific phobias. It's useful in overcoming the *territorial phobias* that are common in agoraphobia—for example, fear of entering grocery stores or shopping malls, driving on bridges or freeways, riding on buses, trains, or planes, scaling heights, and being alone.

*Social phobias* that respond to direct exposure include fears of public speaking, making presentations, being in groups, attending social functions, dating, using public restrooms, and taking examinations.

*Specific phobias* can range from a fear of spiders to a fear of water or dentists. All of these can be overcome by direct exposure. See chapter 12 of this book, Ten Common Specific Phobias, for more information on specific phobias and their treatment.

*Worry exposure* involves repeatedly facing situations you are prone to worry about, first through detailed imagery and, if possible, later in real life. By enduring anxiety during worry exposure sessions, and eliminating subtle avoidance techniques known as "safety behaviors," you gradually learn that you can reduce or eliminate your worry about almost any topic you previously worried or even obsessed about. For more information on worry exposure, see chapter 10 in this book, Overcoming Worry.

If exposure is such an effective treatment, why are there still so many phobic people around? Why hasn't everybody availed themselves of a treatment that is so powerful? The answer is simple. For all its effectiveness, exposure isn't a particularly easy or comfortable process to go through. Not everyone is willing to tolerate the unpleasantness of facing phobic situations or to persist with doing so on a regular basis. *Exposure therapy demands a strong commitment on your part.* If you're genuinely committed to your recovery, then you'll be willing to:

- *Take the risk* to start facing situations you may have been avoiding for many years.

- *Tolerate the initial discomfort* that entering phobic situations—even in increments—often involves.

- *Persist in practicing exposure* on a consistent basis, despite possible setbacks, over a long enough period of time to allow your complete recovery (generally this can take from weeks to up to a year or more, depending on the pace you prefer and the number of phobias you have to deal with).

If you're ready to make a consistent commitment to exposure for as long as it takes, you *will* recover from your phobias.

## Coping Exposure vs. Full Exposure

The exposure process can generally be divided into two stages, coping and full exposure. The coping stage involves relying on various anxiety management strategies to help you get started with exposure and negotiate the early steps in the process. Such strategies might include a person to accompany you (referred to as a "support person"), a low dose of a tranquilizer, practicing deep abdominal breathing, or rehearsing positive *coping statements*. (See, for example, the list of coping statements in the "Coping Statements" section of chapter 6.) As you progress beyond the early steps of your *hierarchy* (an incremental series of approaches to your phobic situation), you need to gradually wean yourself away from such anxiety management—for short, "coping"—strategies.

The second, "full exposure" stage follows. Full exposure means you enter into your phobic situation without relying on supports or coping strategies. Full exposure is necessary *because it teaches you that you can handle a situation you previously avoided under any circumstances.* Instead of learning "I can only handle driving on freeways if I take medication," you learn that "I can handle driving on freeways regardless of my anxiety or anything I might use to mitigate it." Full exposure leads to complete *mastery* of a previously phobic situation.

Full exposure, without reliance on any coping strategies, such as a support person or a smartphone on which you can call a friend during exposure, is the fastest and most efficient way to overcome a phobia. Quite a few people courageously undertake full exposure to a phobia—for example, staying home alone, traveling to high places, or driving to the local supermarket—*without using supportive coping strategies*. Other people prefer the gentler approach of utilizing coping strategies to help them get started with exposure and negotiate its early stages. Gradually, as they proceed, they wean themselves away from these coping strategies in order to fully master the situation.

Throughout the last few decades of the twentieth century, it was thought that the mechanism behind exposure was a process of desensitization or habituation. The idea was that if you repeatedly faced a phobic situation, you would gradually habituate to it and unlearn any connection between the situation and anxiety. Basically, repeated exposure would enable you to get used to the situation to the point of boredom rather than anxiety.

In the last fifteen years, research has shown that the most important mechanism behind effective exposure is *new learning*. What overcomes the phobia is the new learning that entering a difficult situation is less threatening or catastrophic than you previously thought it might be. In short, with phobias, you tend to *overestimate the risk of threat or danger* and *underestimate your ability to cope when actually encountering the phobic situation* (whether flying, public speaking, encountering spiders, going to the dentist, and any of a long list of possible phobias). This new understanding of how exposure works through new learning (technically called "inhibitory learning") is based primarily on research by Michelle Craske at UCLA (Craske 2008).

## Coping vs. Mastery Approach to Exposure

The distinction just made between "coping exposure" and "full exposure" implies that there are really two approaches to dealing with phobias: simply coping versus full mastery. Complete mastery of a phobia—for example, flying, riding elevators, or driving freeways—is definitely desirable. In actual practice, however, some people opt for simply *coping*—being able to negotiate their phobic situation with the use of whatever aids they feel they need. Their aim is just to cope with the situation, not to fully master it.

In short, for many phobic people, the ability to fully negotiate a challenging situation without a support person, deep abdominal breathing, or medication, is a significant accomplishment. However, in practice, people vary quite a bit in their willingness to give up these kinds of assistance. Often, as would be expected, the critical variable is the *frequency* with which a situation needs to be confronted. If you have to deal with a situation frequently, such as driving on a freeway daily to save considerable time in getting to your work (versus using surface streets), you're likely to aim for full mastery of the situation. If you want to maintain your job, mastery of the most direct drive to get there becomes a necessity. Doing the exposure over and over every single day for weeks on end will make full mastery (without need of supportive coping strategies) more achievable.

Phobic situations you encounter rarely, perhaps only once or twice per year, are different. If flying or giving a presentation is a relatively rare event, then reliance on whatever resource is needed just to cope with the situation may be sufficient for some people. For these people, coping exposure is as far as they wish to proceed.

# How to Practice Exposure

You can use the guidelines below to design your exposure therapy.

## Set Goals

Start out by clearly defining your goals. What situations would you most like to stop avoiding? Do you want to be able to drive on the freeway alone? Buy the week's groceries by yourself? Give a presentation at work? Fly on a jet?

Be sure to make your goals specific. Instead of aiming for something as broad as being comfortable with all types of shopping, define a specific goal such as "buying the week's groceries at the local grocery store by myself" or "making a one-hour flight." Eventually, you will want to remove all restrictions—in other words, be comfortable in any store or on any flight. Once you've defined goals, set up timelines. By what date would you like to be able to give a speech, drive on the freeway, or make a flight? Two months from now? One year from now? Give yourself a time frame within which to work and then make a commitment to stick with it. It's often useful to differentiate between short- and long-term goals. Use the space below to define where you would like to be with your recovery process at various points in the future. Make a copy of this statement of your goals and post it in a conspicuous place to remind yourself of your plan for overcoming your fears.

## Goals

In three months:

In six months:

In one year:

## Create a Hierarchy for Each Goal

For each goal you've defined, you need to create a hierarchy of exposures. A *hierarchy* is an incremental series of approaches to your phobic situation. You start off with a very limited exposure to the situation and then gradually, in small increments, increase your degree of exposure. For example, if you're afraid of riding in elevators, you might start out simply approaching an elevator without getting on. The next step might be to get on and off the elevator without riding it up. Then the next step would be to ride up one floor and return. After that, you would proceed to go up two floors, and so on. You can use the following guidelines, as well as sample hierarchies that appear later in the chapter, to develop your own exposure hierarchy.

1.  Choose a particular phobic situation you want to work on, whether this involves going to the grocery store, driving on the freeway, having a blood draw, or giving a talk before a group.

2.  Imagine having to deal with this situation in a very limited way—one that hardly bothers you at all. In the case of going to the grocery store, this might be driving to the parking lot in front of the store and then returning home. In the case of giving a talk, this might be giving a one-minute talk to a friend in the comfort of your home. On a scale of 1 to 10, such exposures would be a 1 or 2 in intensity.

3.  Now imagine what would be the strongest or most challenging exposure relating to your phobia, and place it at the opposite extreme as the highest step in your hierarchy. For example, if you're phobic about grocery stores, your highest step might be waiting in a long line at the checkout counter by yourself. For flying, such a step might involve taking off on a transcontinental flight and encountering severe air turbulence in transit. For public speaking, you might imagine presenting to a large crowd, giving a long presentation, or speaking on a very demanding topic. On a scale of 1 to 10, such exposures would be a 9 or 10.

4.  Now take some time to imagine six or more exposures of graduated intensity related to your phobia and rank them, on a scale of 1 to 10, according to their anxiety-provoking potential. Place these situations in ascending order between the two extremes you've already defined. Use the sample hierarchies that follow in a few pages to assist you. Then write down your list of scenes on the *Hierarchy Worksheet* later in this chapter.

## Determine Scenes of Varying Intensity

Try to identify what specific parameters of your phobia make you more or less anxious and use them to develop situations of varying intensity. In the case of driving, such variables might include distance from home, whether you're driving alone or have someone with you, traffic congestion, number of stoplights, or ease of getting on and off the highway. In the case of public speaking, the variables might include length of the talk, the number of people you're presenting to, or how well you know the people you're presenting to.

For every phobia, there are usually one or more parameters you can use to vary the intensity of your exposure. Common variables include:

- Distance from the feared situation

- Duration of the exposure

- Proximity of an exit or way out of the situation

- General complexity of the situation (such as number of cars or people)

- Time of day

Becoming aware of the specific elements of any phobic situation that make you anxious will increase your sense of control over that situation, and accelerate learning a new and adaptive response to the situation.

**Note:** If you are having difficulty moving from one step to the next in your hierarchy, you can always add an additional step. For example, suppose you're exposing yourself to grocery shopping. You've reached the point where you can stay in the store for several minutes, but you can't bring yourself to buy an item and go through the express checkout line. One intermediate step you could add would be taking an item in your basket up to the checkout line, waiting in line as long as your anxiety level remains mild, and then returning the item to where you found it. You could repeat this step without buying anything until the action becomes monotonous. The next intermediate step would be to buy only one item in the store and go through the express checkout line. After one or two repetitions of this, you would then buy two or three items and go through the express checkout line, or, if you feel ready, a regular checkout line. After you become accustomed to this, you would then be ready to buy a larger number of items and go through a regular checkout line.

If you have difficulty getting started with exposure therapy, that is, your first attempt at exposure leads to very high anxiety or even a panic attack, you might try beginning with an even less challenging step than your original first step. For example, you might have a phobia about flying and you don't feel ready even to drive to the airport. As a preliminary step, watch a video that shows jets taking off and in flight, or get used to looking at photos of planes in a magazine. If you still can't make it to the airport, drive *by* it repeatedly until you feel able to drive to the airport parking lot, turn around, and return home.

The flip side of this is if you find your early exposures are too easy. If you aren't feeling any anxiety to early exposures in your hierarchy, you can dispense with those exposures. You want to begin with an exposure that leads you to feel some anxiety (specifically sensations like increased heartbeat, light-headedness, or muscle tension). New learning that a phobic situation is not as threatening as you thought it might be only occurs when you are experiencing some anxiety during exposure.

## Incremental vs. Random Exposure

An alternative way to do exposure is *not* to work through a series of *incremental* steps from the bottom to the top of your hierarchy. Instead you choose exposures *randomly* at various levels of your hierarchy and do them in random order. So you might start with an exposure of intermediate difficulty first, then do an easier exposure, then follow it up with a difficult exposure. It's quite possible that you may surprise yourself by disconfirming much sooner your expectation that bad things will happen when you face your phobia. This can expedite the entire process of mastering your phobia (as opposed to working up incremental steps of your hierarchy from bottom to top). You can do random exposures with the assistance of anxiety management coping strategies, or you can completely "go for it" by doing random exposures without the assistance of any coping strategies. Research has shown that some people can do this latter, "fast track" form of exposure, starting off with more difficult exposures without any coping techniques. If you are one of those people, exposure can take a whole lot less time.

In sum, there are actually four ways to do exposure: 1) incremental steps through your hierarchy with the assistance of coping strategies, gradually weaning yourself off the coping strategies until you fully master the phobia, 2) incremental steps through your hierarchy without using anxiety management coping strategies, 3) random steps at various levels of your hierarchy with the assistance of coping strategies first, then weaning off of them, and 4) the "go for it " approach of doing exposures in random order of difficulty without using any coping strategies.

Everybody is different. If you are working with a therapist, you and your therapist need to decide which approach to exposure is best for you. If you are working through exposure hierarchies on your own, you will learn with experience whether you prefer a more gradual approach or whether you are sufficiently motivated to use a rapid approach (i.e., random order of exposure without any anxiety management strategies).

## Optional: Try Imagery Exposure First

Some people practice a technique called imagery exposure before navigating a phobic situation in real life. This involves visualizing the experiences outlined in your hierarchy rather than confronting them in real life. If you wish to use this as a precursor to real-life exposure, see the section "Imagery Exposure" at the end of this chapter. For some people, first doing exposure in imagery enhances their ability to undertake real-life exposure.

## Examples of Hierarchies

Three examples of hierarchies developed for real-life exposure follow. Please note that these are only sample hierarchies; your own hierarchy of phobic scenes involving elevators, grocery stores, or flying may differ depending on what aspects of the situations elicit your greatest anxiety. Note that the first two examples, elevators and grocery stores, illustrate *both the coping and the full exposure stages of the process.* The hierarchy includes relying on a support person during the coping stage of exposure, while coping strategies are relinquished during full exposure.

The third example, a hierarchy for flying, illustrates undertaking exposure alone without a support person but utilizing some coping strategies in the early stages.

In accordance with my own preferred way of conducting exposure, all three of the hierarchies illustrate the possibility of undertaking a coping exposure phase *before* proceeding to full exposure. Many of my clients seem to prefer such an approach, as they've had full-blown panic attacks during exposure attempts in the past. However, *the coping phase is optional and not necessary or essential to completing exposure.* Some therapists utilize only full exposure with their clients, with the expectation that even prolonged anxiety in the phobic situation is not harmful but actually conducive to learning that facing a fear is not so overwhelming or threatening as anticipated. Clients learn they can negotiate the situation without any supportive strategies and in spite of uncomfortable levels of anxiety. If you and/or your therapist feel inclined to do this, then work with only the full exposure portions of the hierarchies listed below.

**Note:** All of the examples below use an *incremental* approach to exposure. As mentioned, for some people, the sequence of moving through a hierarchy can be *randomized*, starting with mid-range steps first. It is a matter of your—or your and your therapist's—preference. Using a random sequence of exposures usually shortens the time necessary to complete exposure.

## Elevators

### Coping Exposure

1. Look at elevators, watching them come and go.

2. Stand in a stationary elevator with your support person.

3. Travel up and down one and then two floors with your support person. You might also add in abdominal breathing as a coping strategy in addition to having your support person accompany you.

4. Stand in a stationary elevator alone.

5. Travel up or down one floor alone, with your support person waiting outside the elevator on the floor where you will arrive. Feel free to use abdominal breathing to manage your anxiety if you wish.

6. Travel up and down two or three floors first with your support person, then without your support person. At this stage, you need not exit the elevator when it reaches the intended floor. You can use abdominal breathing (or another coping strategy, such as coping statements) in the absence of having your support person go along. You can ask your support person to wait for you outside the elevator at the ground floor if you wish.

7. Now, travel up and down five to ten floors, either with your support person accompanying you or with them waiting outside the elevator on the ground floor. Use abdominal breathing or coping statements to assist your exposure at first, then try doing the exposures without these coping techniques.

**Full Exposure**

1. Travel up or down one floor alone, with your support person waiting in a car outside the building.

2. Travel up and down one floor alone without your support person at all (that is, you've visited the building on your own).

3. Travel up and down two or three floors alone without your support person.

4. Continue to incrementally increase the number of floors you ascend on the elevator without the presence of your support person or any other aid, such as abdominal breathing or coping statements, until you are able to reach the top of a five- to ten-story building.

5. Continue to incrementally increase the number of floors you ascend without a support person or any other anxiety management strategies until you are able to reach the top of a twenty-story building, or the tallest building in your city with an elevator. Practicing every day will increase the rate of your progress.

6. Travel on two different elevators in two different buildings of varying height on your own.

7. Travel on a variety of different elevators in a variety of different buildings in your city (or nearest city) on your own.

## Grocery Stores

**Coping Exposure**

1. Drive to the grocery store with your support person and spend one minute in the parking lot.

2. Drive to the grocery store with your support person and spend five to ten minutes in the parking lot.

3. Walk up to the entrance of the grocery store and walk around outside for two minutes with your support person.

4. Enter the grocery store for fifteen to thirty seconds with your support person and then walk out.

5. Enter the grocery store for one to two minutes with your support person and then walk out.

6. Walk to the back of the store with your support person and spend up to five minutes in the store.

7.    Enter the store with your support person and go along while he or she buys one or two items.

8.    Enter the store with your support person and buy one or two items yourself.

9.    Enter the store with your support person parked in the parking lot outside; use other anxiety management strategies such as abdominal breathing and/or coping statements if you wish.

10.   Enter the store *without* your support person waiting outside, but still have access to your preferred anxiety management strategies.

### Full Exposure

1.    Go the grocery store and park for five minutes near the main entrance, without your support person or using any anxiety management strategies. Repeat this approach for all subsequent steps.

2.    Go to the grocery store and enter the store for ten to thirty seconds without your support person.

3.    Go to the grocery store and stay there for up to a minute, walking up and down one of the aisles.

4.    Go to the grocery store, walk to the back of the store, and stay in the store for two to five minutes on your own (divide this into substeps if you need to).

5.    Go to the grocery store and stay there for five minutes, walking throughout the store up and down the aisles (divide into substeps if necessary).

6.    Go to the grocery store, stay there for five to ten minutes, and purchase one item using the express checkout line.

7.    Visit the grocery store, stay there for five to ten minutes, and buy two or three items using the express checkout line.

8.    Visit the grocery store, stay for fifteen minutes, buy several items, and use one of the regular checkout lines.

9.    Visit the grocery store, stay in the store for a minimum of fifteen to twenty minutes, and buy a dozen or more items, using a grocery cart, and check out at one of the regular checkout lines.

10.   Shop at two or three different grocery stores in your town, buying a dozen or more items and using one of the regular checkout lines.

## Flying

### Coping Exposure

1. Approach the airport and drive around it.

2. Park at the airport for five to ten minutes.

3. Enter the terminal and walk around for five minutes, utilizing coping strategies such as a support person, abdominal breathing, and/or coping statements. Continue to rely on any coping strategies that you find helpful to negotiate steps 4 through 7.

4. Go to the security checkpoint and stand in line for five minutes.

5. Purchase a *refundable ticket* (usually more expensive than a nonrefundable ticket) for a flight, preferably a night or two before you go to the airport. Obtain your boarding pass for your specific flight. You can download the pass to a smartphone or obtain a pass at one of the kiosks in the check-in area of the airport. Go through the security checkpoint with your boarding pass and walk to the gate in the airport for your chosen flight. Then, assuming you plan to defer actually flying until a later exposure, return to the ticketing counter to obtain a refund for the ticket you previously purchased. If anyone asks why you are requesting a refund, you can say you had a sudden change of plans. Note that you will likely need to go through security without your support person, unless they are also willing to purchase a refundable ticket for the same flight as yours.

6. When you feel ready, after having made it to an airport gate once or twice, take a short flight (no more than a half hour to an hour, if possible). Utilize coping strategies such as abdominal breathing, coping statements, and/or a low dose of a tranquilizer on your first flight.

7. Take a longer flight (an hour or longer) utilizing coping strategies like those in the previous step. Try using fewer coping strategies, even though the flight is longer.

### Full Exposure

1. If you feel you need some additional exposure to airport environments, approach and enter your local, largest airport until you feel comfortable standing in line, purchasing a refundable ticket a day or two ahead of the flight, and finally going through the security checkpoint (as in steps 1 to 5 of the coping exposure above, but without utilizing anxiety management coping techniques).

2. Take a short flight, if possible no more than a half hour to an hour, without relying on any coping strategies such as a support person or medication.

3. Take a longer flight, if possible one to two hours, without relying on any coping strategies. You might read a magazine or look out the window to avert boredom, but it's important

that you don't use such activities as a way to escape or avoid your experience of exposure to the situation. That way, you expedite the process of overcoming your phobia. If you feel anxiety rising to a near-panic level, get up and walk around the cabin, maybe going to the bathroom and then back to your seat.

4. Schedule a long flight (five or more hours, or transcontinental). Refrain from using coping strategies.

5. Schedule long flights with layovers and two or more separate "legs" to the total trip. Refrain from using coping strategies.

6. Fly to a new destination you've never been to before without utilizing coping strategies.

## Designing Your Own Hierarchies

You can design your own hierarchy of steps for a particular phobia using the *Hierarchy Worksheet* that follows. Make several copies of this page and write down hierarchies for the specific phobias you wish to work on. (You can also download a PDF version online; see the very back of this book for more details.) For each phobia, you can use one hierarchy for the coping phase of exposure and a second hierarchy for the full exposure phase. With each hierarchy, you may not need to create twenty steps, but try to create a minimum of seven or eight different steps, proceeding from the least to the most challenging step. For each particular phobia, your coping exposure hierarchy and full exposure hierarchy should have close to the same number of steps. For a few further examples of hierarchies, see my website: Helpforanxiety.com.

Keep in mind, once again, that some people do fine with full-on mastery exposure without going through a preliminary coping exposure phase. You just do various exposures without the aid of anxiety management techniques, such as abdominal breathing, calling a support person on your smartphone, or relying on a low dose of a tranquilizer. Since the fundamental basis of exposure is learning that a feared situation is less difficult or challenging than you anticipated, you can expedite exposure by jumping head-on into the full mastery phase.

Also keep in mind that if you feel motivated and ready to endure and stay with any anxiety that might arise, you can do the steps of your hierarchy in a random rather than incremental order. You are likely to complete exposure more rapidly this way. If you feel more comfortable proceeding from low-anxiety steps in the hierarchy toward higher-anxiety steps, by all means do the steps in an incremental order of difficulty.

# *Hierarchy Worksheet*

Hierarchy for _____

(specify phobia)

*Instructions:* Start with a relatively easy or mild instance of facing your phobia. Develop at least seven or eight steps that involve progressively more challenging exposures. The final step should be your goal or even a step beyond what you've designated as your goal. For each phobia, make a separate hierarchy for the coping exposure phase and for the full exposure phase. If you feel ready to proceed to full exposure without going through a coping exposure phase, then just write a single hierarchy involving incremental steps of facing your fear without the assistance of anxiety management techniques. Make a number of copies of the *Hierarchy Worksheet* from this page. Or you can download it from the website and make copies. (See the last page of the book for more information about the website for downloading worksheets in this book.) Use separate worksheets for the coping and full exposure phases for each of your phobias.

*Step*                                                                                  *Date Completed*

1. _____

2. _____

3. _____

4. _____

5. _____

6. _____

7. _____

8. _____

9. _____

10. _____

11. _____

12. _____

13. _____

14. _____

15. _____

16. _____

17. _____

18. _____

19. _____

20. _____

**Note:** Remember to make at least two copies of the *Hierarchy Worksheet* for *each* of your phobias (one for coping exposure and one for full exposure) before filling in the one in the book.

# Basic Procedure for Exposure

## Incremental Exposure

1. *Approach and eventually enter your phobic situation.* Proceed into your phobic situation, beginning with the first step on your hierarchy or with the one at which you last left off. Continue to proceed into the situation, staying there even if your anxiety begins to feel somewhat uncomfortable. If your anxiety feels uncomfortable but manageable, great. It's necessary to feel some anxiety during exposure in order for new learning to occur. *Just stay in your fearful situation and endure your anxiety, giving it time to pass.* Even if you are uncomfortable in the situation, stay with it as long as your anxiety level doesn't reach a point of panic or where it feels out of control. *Allow time to pass.* During the early, coping phase of exposure, it can be helpful to utilize a support person or practice one of the abdominal breathing techniques described in chapter 4. Breathing from your abdomen can help diffuse some of the anxiety that might come up. Or you might practice coping statements from the list in chapter 6 to help maintain your confidence to proceed.

   Later, during full exposure, you should refrain from utilizing coping strategies so that you don't become overly dependent upon them. During the second "full exposure" phase of mastering your phobia, make your best effort to stay in the exposure situation without retreating. Research by Michelle Craske and associates (2008, 2014) has found that a willingness to endure anxiety during exposure, even at high and uncomfortable levels, actually improves and expedites a good outcome. You learn that you can remain in a situation you previously feared while at the same time tolerating anxiety. This rapidly builds your confidence to continue progressing up your hierarchy.

2. *Continue working up your hierarchy.* Work through your hierarchy step by step. If you have to retreat and return to a step, that's fine; just continue to proceed up the steps of your hierarchy during your exposure session for the day. Accept anxiety symptoms if they come up, and do your best to endure them as they arise and pass. Do not chastise yourself if your performance one day turns out to be less spectacular than it was initially. This is a common experience. In a day or two, you'll find that you'll be able to continue in your progression up your hierarchy. Continue to progress through as many steps in your hierarchy as you feel able to. This constitutes one practice session, and it will typically take you from thirty minutes up to an hour.

In general, longer exposure sessions achieve more rapid results than short sessions do, but go at your own pace. For most people, one practice session per day, three to five days per week, is enough. Be aware that your progress through the steps in your hierarchy is likely to be uneven. On some days, you'll enjoy excellent progress, perhaps going through several steps. On other days, you will have to repeat the same step several times. Other days you may hardly progress at all, and on still others you will not go as far as you did on preceding days. On a given Monday, you might spend five minutes alone in the grocery store for the first time in years. On Tuesday, you may endure five minutes again but no more. Then on Wednesday, you may be unable to go into the store at all. On Thursday or Friday, however, you may then discover that you can last ten minutes in the store. This up-and-down, two-steps-forward, one-step-back phenomenon is typical of exposure therapy. Don't let it discourage you!

### Randomized Exposure

To expedite the exposure process, you can do your hierarchy in random order. Start with an exposure that is midrange in your hierarchy, then proceed to do different steps in a random order, sometimes doing steps at a lower anxiety level and sometimes steps at higher anxiety levels. You disconfirm your expectation that facing your phobia will be threatening or overwhelming much more rapidly. With randomized exposure, you can choose to do a coping exposure hierarchy first, relying on anxiety management techniques, followed by a full exposure hierarchy. Or, if you feel motivated, you may choose the "go for it" strategy of doing full-on, mastery level exposure without the aid of coping techniques as you complete different exposures in random order.

## What to Do If You Start to Panic During Coping Exposure

Some anxiety experts advocate continuing to expose to a phobic situation no matter how high anxiety rises, even to the point of panic. The problem with this is that, in the author's experience, if you actually progress to a full-blown panic attack during exposure, you could risk reinforcing your fear of the phobia. A severe panic attack, in some instances, may reduce your confidence in undertaking exposure to your phobia(s). This is particularly true during the early stages of practicing exposure. While it's always best to try to endure the discomfort you feel with exposure, it's also helpful to be able to have an "exit strategy" if a full-blown panic attack comes on. If you suddenly feel you're heading toward a full-blown panic attack, consider temporarily retreating from the situation *and then returning to it as soon as possible* after your anxiety settles down to manageable proportions.

Retreat is a "fallback strategy" to be used only if you feel your anxiety seems to be truly getting out of control. It's always best to try to stay in the situation, accept and endure the discomfort you feel, and wait for the anxiety to pass. (Recall Claire Weekes's four-step process for dealing with high anxiety from chapter 6: face the symptoms, accept what your body is doing, float with the wave of anxiety, and allow time to pass.) However, if you feel you simply can't endure your anxiety and are starting to move into a full-blown panic attack, you can retreat and then subsequently return to the situation as soon as possible. In many situations, this is easy to do. If you're driving on the freeway, you can pull over onto the shoulder or get off at the nearest exit. If you're sitting in a restaurant, you can retreat to the restroom and then return. If you're flying, you can't leave the plane, but you can retreat to a safe place in your mind (using a recorded visualization—see chapter 4) or get up and walk to the plane's restroom. Remember that retreat is not the same thing as escape—*with retreat, the idea is to temporarily leave the situation and then return.*

During the full exposure stage, most often you are sufficiently accustomed to the situation that a full-blown panic attack is unlikely to occur. In the unlikely instance that you start to panic during full exposure, you can choose to stop the exposure temporarily. Give yourself a few minutes to recover, but don't go home. Once you are calmer, finish the exposure session. Also, it's optimal if you can repeat an exposure to the same situation within the next day or two.

# Making the Most of Exposure

These instructions are intended to help you get the most out of real-life exposure:

1. *Be willing to take risks.*

   Entering a phobic situation that you've been avoiding for a long time is going to feel risky. There's simply no way to face your fears and recover without feeling that you're taking on a risk. Risk taking is easier, however, when you start with small, limited goals and proceed incrementally. Establishing a hierarchy of phobic situations allows you to take this incremental approach toward mastering your phobias.

2. *Deal with resistance.*

   Undertaking exposure to a situation that you've been avoiding may bring up resistance. Notice if you delay getting started with your exposure sessions or find reasons to procrastinate. The mere thought of actually entering a phobic situation may elicit strong anxiety, a fear of being trapped, or self-defeating statements to yourself, such as "I'll never be able to do it" or "This is hopeless." Instead of getting stuck in resistance, try to regard the process of exposure as a major therapeutic opportunity. By plunging in, you will learn about yourself and work through long-standing avoidance patterns that have held up your life. Give yourself pep talks about how much your life and relationships can improve when you are no longer plagued by your phobias. You might also want to review the section on motivation under "Necessary Ingredients for Undertaking Your Own Recovery Program" in chapter 3. Consider whether there are any secondary gains (that is, subtle rewards) that might be contributing to your resistance. Once you get through any initial resistance to real-life exposure, the going gets easier. If you feel you're having problems with resistance at any point, you may want to consult a therapist who is familiar with exposure therapy.

3. *Be willing to tolerate some discomfort.*

   Facing situations that you've been avoiding for a long time is not particularly comfortable or pleasant. It's inevitable that you will experience some anxiety in the course of practicing exposure. In fact, it is common to feel *worse initially*, at the outset of exposure therapy, before you feel better. Recognize that feeling worse is *not* an indication of regression but rather that exposure is really *working*. Feeling worse means that you're laying the foundation to feel better. As you gain more skill in handling symptoms of anxiety when they come up during exposure, your practice sessions will become easier and you'll gain more confidence.

4. *Avoid flooding—be willing if necessary to retreat.*

   During the early, coping stage of exposure, you can resort to the option to retreat from and return to your phobic situation if your anxiety suddenly becomes unmanageable and headed for panic. While enduring uncomfortable anxiety during exposure can expedite your progress, having a full-blown panic attack *might* set you back. So, if necessary, consider retreat *followed by a return to the situation as soon as possible* if you feel like you're headed for full-blown panic. This is most important during the initial coping exposure phase of negotiating your hierarchy. During the later full exposure phase, you want to make your best effort to remain in the exposure situation without retreat. Of course, retreat and return is always an option in an "emergency situation" (for example, if you're driving in heavy traffic and start to feel dizziness and depersonalization feelings that affect your capacity to drive). Still, it's preferable to utilize retreat primarily early in your exposure process and minimize it during the full exposure phase. A willingness to endure anxiety during full exposure ensures you will fully master the phobia.

5. ***Utilize coping strategies during the early, coping exposure phase to get started.***
   If you can start exposure without using any coping strategies (including a support person to accompany you), it can expedite your progress. If not, there are a number of coping strategies that can help you begin exposure and carry you through the early stages of your hierarchy. These strategies will help give you confidence to undertake exposure and negotiate the early stages of your hierarchy:

   - *Do deep abdominal breathing* (see chapter 4).

   - *Use coping statements* to prepare for and first confront your phobia (see chapter 6 for examples of coping statements).

   - *Have a support person accompany you.* Having a support person, usually a good friend or relative, accompany you as you begin to face a phobia can provide reassurance and safety, comfort (by talking with you), encouragement to persist, and praise for your incremental successes. You need to educate your support person on how best to work with you. (See the section "Coping Exposure: What Your Support Person Needs to Know" below.)

6. ***Get angry with your anxiety.***
   As described in chapter 6, anger and fear are incompatible responses. If you can get angry with your anxiety, it will tend to diminish. You can get angry verbally by strongly expressing statements such as "Get out!" or "This is ridiculous—I'm going to enter into this situation anyway!" or "Okay, the anxiety is there; just do it (enter the phobic situation) anyway!"

7. ***Use a low dose of a tranquilizer (such as no more than 0.25 mg of Xanax, Ativan, or Klonopin).***
   It's preferable *not* to use a tranquilizer at all during exposure; however, a low dose may be useful in getting started with exposure to a situation you have avoided for a long time. Keep in mind that exposure won't be successful if the medication *masks* your anxiety. It's necessary to feel anxiety during exposure, even to an uncomfortable degree, for the exposure to be fully effective.

8. ***Plan for contingencies when first undertaking exposure.***
   Suppose you're practicing on an elevator and the worst happens—it stops between floors. Or suppose you are just beginning to drive on the freeway and you start to panic when

you're far away from an exit. Especially at the outset, during the coping stage of exposure, it's good to have an action plan for those worst-case scenarios. In the first example, give yourself some insurance by practicing on an elevator that has a functioning emergency phone. Or in the case of the freeway, tell yourself in advance that it will be all right to retreat to the shoulder or at least to drive slowly with your emergency flashers on until you reach an exit. During the coping exposure stage for flying phobia, you might keep a set of "emergency strategies" on hand (such as talking to a flight attendant, getting up and walking to the restroom, listening to a portable media player with headphones, or using medication). Once again, during the full exposure phase, you want to curtail such strategies.

9. *Plan your exposures in advance.*

   When you first begin to practice exposure, you may be inclined to do it spontaneously, only when you most feel like it. Practicing only when you want to—on your so-called "good" days—may certainly help you get started in facing situations you've been avoiding for a long time. However, once you've made a start, it's best to plan your exposure practices ahead of time. Make the effort to do them on both your "good" and "bad" days alike. If you wait only for good days to practice, you'll tend to put it off until you feel better, which will slow your progress. While you may have more anticipatory anxiety when facing planned exposures, this anxiety will recede as you begin to have successes with your practice.

10. *Trust your own pace.*

    It's important not to regard real-life exposure as some kind of race. The goal is not to see how fast you can overcome the problem: pressuring yourself to make great strides quickly is generally not a good idea. Decide on the pace you wish to adopt in exposing yourself to a difficult situation, realizing that very small gains count for a lot in this type of work.

11. *Let go of the need for complete control.*

    Work on accepting the fact that some things are under your control while others are not. You can control a car when you're the driver, but you need to relinquish control when you're a passenger on a bus or an airplane. You can control how far you choose to drive from home, but you can't control traffic, lines in the store, or how an elevator works. During the coping exposure phase, you can use strategies like abdominal breathing or coping statements, such as "Let go and trust," "I'll do the best I can," or even "God is with me," to help you accept both the external situations and/or the physical symptoms that you can't completely control. As mentioned throughout this chapter, though, full exposure ultimately involves relinquishing such strategies.

12. *Reward yourself for small successes.*

    It's common for people going through real-life exposure to castigate themselves for not making sufficiently rapid progress. Bear in mind that it's important to consistently reward yourself for small successes. For example, being able to go into a phobic situation slightly further than the day before is worthy of giving yourself a reward, such as a trip to the ice cream parlor, a new plant for your garden, or a dinner out. So is being able to stay in the situation a few moments longer—or being able to tolerate anxious feelings a few moments longer. Rewarding yourself for small successes will help sustain your motivation to keep practicing.

13. ***Practice regularly.***
Practicing methodically and regularly—rather than hurrying or pressuring yourself—will do the most to expedite your recovery. Ideally, it is good to practice real-life exposure *three to five days per week*, if possible. Longer practice sessions (an hour or longer), with several trials of exposure to your phobic situation, tend to produce more rapid results than shorter sessions. As long as you endure your anxiety in the situation, it's impossible to undergo too much exposure in a given practice session. The worst that can happen is that you might end up feeling tired or drained at the end of your exposure for the day. The *regularity* of your practice will determine the rate of your recovery. If you're not practicing regularly, notice what excuses you're making to yourself and sit down with someone else to evaluate them. Then find arguments for refuting those excuses the next time they come up. Regular practice of exposure is *the key* to a full and lasting recovery.

14. ***Expect and know how to handle setbacks.***
For some people, progressing up the steps of their hierarchy is not always a smooth, linear process. It's possible you may have "good" days and "bad" days. A setback simply means that one day you might not be able to progress as far up the steps of your hierarchy as you did the day before, despite your best efforts and spending more time at it. Don't be discouraged by a setback, if it happens. View it as just temporary. Resume working up the steps of your hierarchy the following day.

For example, one day you may be able to drive to a store three miles away from your home, and the next day, no matter how much effort and time you put in, you can only drive to a store two miles away.

Similarly, one day you may be able to stay home alone without your support person for six hours. The next day you start to feel panicky after three hours, so you call your support person or ask him or her to return home. Perhaps even then you still remain anxious for a while. You can't seem to get past feeling anxious no matter what you do.

During the early phases of exposure, learn to accept brief setbacks when they occur. Don't allow yourself to get discouraged and disheartened. Just resume working with your hierarchy—incrementally or randomly—the next day. If setbacks start to happen frequently, it's a good idea to speak with a therapist who is experienced in working with anxiety and phobias.

During the mastery phase of exposure, the aim is to strive to do the very best you can with each exposure practice—within the limits of fatigue and exhaustion. If an unavoidable setback still occurs during the mastery phase, again, speak to a therapist who is skilled in treating phobias and who understands exposure.

15. ***Pay attention fully to the emotions and sensations that come up during exposure.***
During exposure, observe all of the sensations and feelings that come up. You might even try naming each emotion or sensation you experience to enhance your awareness

of it. As you continue with exposure, refrain from any "safety behaviors" where you attempt to avoid or numb yourself from your feelings and sensations. Examples of safety behaviors include seeking reassurance by calling someone, performing a ritual such as saying a prayer, taking along a stuffed animal, or distracting yourself by taking your pulse or listening to music on a smartphone. By paying full attention to the sensations and feelings that come up during exposure, you expedite the process. There is a subtle distinction between coping strategies and safety behaviors. Coping strategies are proactive techniques you use to help you negotiate the coping phase of exposure. They help you move forward. Safety behaviors, on the other hand, are escape tactics you use to avoid or distract yourself from the physical sensations or fearful thoughts that come up during exposure.

16. *Be prepared to experience stronger emotions.*
    Facing phobic situations you've been avoiding for a long time often stirs up suppressed feelings—not only of anxiety but of anger and sorrow as well. Recognize that this is a normal and expected part of the recovery process. *Allow* these feelings to surface and let yourself express them. Let yourself know that it's okay to have these feelings even though you may be uncomfortable with them. An important part of recovery from a phobic condition is learning to accept, express, and communicate your feelings (see chapter 13).

17. *Follow through to completion.*
    Finishing exposure therapy means that you reach a point where you are no longer afraid of panic attacks in *any* situation that was formerly a problem (obviously this does not include extreme situations that anyone would be afraid of). The recovery process can generally take as little as a month or up to a year or more to complete, depending on how many phobias you wish to confront. Getting comfortable with most situations but still having one or two that you are afraid of is generally insufficient. To attain lasting freedom from your phobias, it's important to keep working until you get to the point where 1) you can go into any situation that nonphobic people would regard as safe and 2) you regard panic reactions themselves as manageable and not at all dangerous.

18. *Make a worst-case scenario plan.*
    In *The CBT Anxiety Solution Workbook,* authors Matthew McKay, Michelle Skeen, and Patrick Fanning suggest that you imagine what you would do if your worst-case scenario associated with facing a phobia came to pass. The point of doing so is to get past catastrophic thoughts that interfere with exposure, such as "I couldn't handle it if I completely fell apart" or "What if I totally collapsed from fear during exposure?" These ideas are patently false because the notions of totally falling apart or collapsing are just scary ideas rather than reality. You might collapse if you were suddenly subjected to a severe physical trauma, but not from facing a fear!

    So, you may want to write up a "worst-case scenario plan" with an emphasis on how you would *cope* in the event that you encountered difficulties with exposure. The plan should emphasize behavioral, emotional, and cognitive coping. As an example of behavioral coping, let's say you're facing driving on a freeway, and you start to panic while driving. What could you do? Practical behavioral coping strategies might include pulling off the highway onto the shoulder of the road, if there is a shoulder available. If not, you could move over to the far right lane, slow down your speed so you feel you can manage the car better even with high anxiety, and put your flashers on to let other people know you are driving more slowly than the usual speed. For emotional coping, imagine how you would persist through uncomfortable feelings, striving to endure them rather than flee them. In the unlikely instance you had a full-blown panic attack, you could temporarily retreat from the situation, give yourself fifteen or twenty minutes to calm down, then make your best effort to return to it. Review the guideline above: "Be prepared to experience stronger emotions," which basically means letting yourself know it's okay to have challenging emotions and bodily sensations, even if they are uncomfortable. Cognitive coping has already been covered in the guideline on utilizing coping strategies. In response to fearful, catastrophic thoughts that might have a tendency to creep up during exposure, you counter them with coping statements, such as those listed in chapter 6 of this book or from your own list of customized constructive coping statements. Also from chapter 6, the list of guidelines of what do to when panic rises above "level 4" on the *Anxiety Scale*, that is, rises above a feeling of manageability, can round out your "worst-case scenario plan."

19. **Combine exposures.**

When you become more confident with doing exposure, try combining exposures to more than one situation in a single session or day. For example, you could combine both driving on freeways and driving far from home in the same session. Or you could combine going to crowded shopping mall as well as making a trip to the dentist in the same day. Proceeding with several different exposures in close succession increases the tendency *to replace your anticipation of harm of threat with an understanding that facing what you fear is manageable and doable.*

## Coping Exposure: What Your Support Person Needs to Know

As mentioned, having a support person to accompany you can be helpful when you first undertake exposure as well as during the entire early, coping phase of exposure. Support people come in many guises, including spouses, partners, relatives, friends, other people with phobias, recovered phobics, and therapists. The most important characteristics of an effective support person include an attitude of caring and support, the ability to be nonjudgmental and patient, and a willingness to encourage you to face your fears with persistence. You need to educate your support person about how to work with you if they are willing to assist you in facing a phobia:

- Encourage your support person to read chapter 6 and especially chapter 7 of The Anxiety & Phobia Workbook so they are familiar with the nature of exposure for phobias as well as the nature and remedies for panic attacks. They might also want to read the book *How to Help Your Loved One Recover from Agoraphobia* by Karen Williams (1993).

- Let them know how you want them to assist you with your exposure. For example, do you want them to stay with you the entire time, follow you from behind, wait outside a store while you go inside, or wait at the top floor or bottom floor of a tall building when you are working on exposure to elevators, and so on.

- Encourage them not to push you to complete an exposure. Whatever you accomplish during a particular exposure session is entirely up to you. If you fall short of what you expected, that's just part of the process, not an occasion for either of you to be disappointed. *Setbacks during exposure are normal and expected.*

- Let them know you would like them to stay calm in the possible instance that you become highly anxious or even panic. They are there to be a supportive presence, not to mirror your particular reactions. If your support person is inclined to get rattled by seeing you become anxious or panicky, that will not serve your success with exposure. Check with them ahead of time about how they would feel if you suddenly had a full-blown panic attack. If they don't have experience with panic attacks, refer them to chapter 6 of *The Anxiety & Phobia Workbook.*

- Request reliability. Your support person needs to show up on time, and it's particularly important that your support person be where you expect them to be. If you temporarily separate from your support person as part of the exposure, make sure both of you have a prearranged time and place for getting back together. Both of you should have a watch or smartphone so you can know exactly what time it is.

- Be sure your support person is up to the commitment involved in helping you. Coping exposure may involve many sessions over a long period of time. Is your support person willing to stick with you throughout the entire process, which could potentially take up to a few days per week for a few months?

- Perfection is not expected. If your support person has limits on how much time or energy they have available to assist you, it's important that both of you communicate fully and clearly about this in advance.

## Maintaining the Right Attitude

Approaching fearful situations with the *right attitude* is as important as (if not more important than) learning specific strategies for exposure. If you begin with the right attitude, then utilizing appropriate techniques becomes much easier. The following five attitudes are particularly important in increasing your ability to effectively face and overcome your fears.

### Accept Bodily Symptoms of Anxiety

Recall Claire Weekes's four points, stated in chapter 6: 1) *face* your symptoms, 2) *accept* your body's reaction, 3) *float* with the wave of anxiety, and 4) *allow time to pass.* Struggling with bodily symptoms of anxiety that arise while facing something difficult will make them worse. Trying to deny or run away from them will also make them worse. *Acceptance* of the bodily symptoms of anxiety is the first thing you need to do when anxiety comes up, whether spontaneously or in a phobic situation. It's an attitude you can learn and cultivate.

## Stay Grounded in the Present Moment

Anxiety begins as a physical reaction and is aggravated further by "what-if" or catastrophic thoughts. The more you can stay grounded in your body in the present moment, the less you'll be carried away by such thoughts.

During the coping phase of exposure, abdominal breathing is an excellent way to stay grounded in your body. Breathing is a process that is centered in your body rather than your mind. Another helpful strategy is to focus on your arms and legs while you breathe. The more attention you can bring down to your arms and legs, the less involved you're likely to be in your thoughts.

Again, rely on abdominal breathing if you need it during the early coping phase of exposure. Relinquish it along with other coping strategies by the time you reach the full mastery phase.

## Know That Fear Always Passes

No state of anxiety is permanent—it always passes. The body usually metabolizes excess adrenaline in five to ten minutes, so the worst degree of panic you might ever experience is not likely to last beyond this. Lesser degrees of heightened anxiety may persist longer than a few minutes, but they, too, will eventually pass. *Sooner or later, whatever you have constructed in your mind as threatening disappears because your mind stops focusing on it and moves on to something else.*

## If You're Anxious About Something, You're Already Beginning Exposure to It

When you face something you fear, you almost inevitably experience some anxiety. Rather than magnifying the anxiety with further anxious thoughts, reframe it with the attitude "This anxiety is a good sign: it means I'm already experiencing exposure." Or you can say, "I need this anxiety—I can't complete exposure to the situation without feeling it." It's true—you cannot overcome anxiety to a phobic situation without first feeling it in the situation to some extent. The path out of anxiety starts with directly experiencing it. If you know this, facing what you fear becomes easier. Every time your anxiety recurs, you can confidently remind yourself you are a step closer to being done with it.

## Exposure Always Works—with Practice

There is no fear that cannot be overcome by repeated exposure. Exposure always defeats fear, if you're willing to persevere with facing what you fear again and again. Anxiety is based on the projection of frightening outcomes in the face of something not fully known. Once that "something" becomes fully known and familiar, it invariably loses its ability to evoke fear. Exposure always works—with practice. Truly knowing that fact will help give you courage to persist in facing your fear, no matter how challenging it may appear at the outset.

## Factors That Can Promote or Impede Your Success

Numerous studies have examined the conditions affecting the success of exposure therapy. This section summarizes the findings of this research. For a more detailed discussion, see David Barlow's book *Anxiety and Its Disorders: The Nature and Treatment of Anxiety and Panic* (especially chapter 11).

### What Promotes Success

- *Cooperation of your partner or spouse.* When your partner or spouse supports your recovery and is willing to assist you in the exposure process itself, results are often excellent. Conversely, if your partner is indifferent, is uncooperative, or consciously or unconsciously opposes your recovery, success with exposure may be difficult to attain. If you feel that your partner is interfering with your progress in overcoming your phobias, you both may want to consult a competent couples therapist who is knowledgeable about the treatment of phobias.

- *Willingness to tolerate discomfort.* As discussed in the previous section, it is inevitable that you will feel more anxiety when you begin to confront phobic situations in real life. Practicing exposure therapy is hard work and requires a willingness to tolerate discomfort. It may be tempting not to begin or not to follow through with exposure because you dread the unpleasantness involved. That is why it is so important to reward yourself for your efforts. As previously mentioned, in some cases, *low* doses of a minor tranquilizer may be a useful adjunct in the early coping stages of exposure therapy. Medication doses should always be low enough to ease but not blunt or mask the experience of anxiety during exposure.

- *Ability to handle the initial symptoms of panic.* Fear of having a panic attack is perhaps the greatest deterrent to undertaking a course of exposure. If you've learned to handle your panic symptoms through interoceptive exposure (as detailed in chapter 6, "Interoceptive Exposure"), you can approach exposure with more confidence. These days, many phobia treatment programs train clients to cope with physical symptoms associated with panic *before* beginning a program of gradual exposure.

- *Ability to handle setbacks.* Some people stop their program of exposure after experiencing one or two setbacks, failing to recognize that setbacks are a normal and predictable part of the process. Your ability to tolerate setbacks and still persist in your daily practice sessions will be a crucial determinant of your success.

- *Willingness to practice regularly.* Regular, consistent practice—in other words, three to five days per week—is unquestionably the *strongest* predictor of success with exposure. There is simply no substitute for regular practice. It has been my experience over the years that the clients who practice regularly are the ones who recover. There is no phobia that cannot be overcome by a steady and persistent commitment to practicing exposure. This is definitely an area of human experience where "persistence wins the race."

- *Doing follow-up exposures and varying the context of exposure.* According to Michelle Craske and colleagues (2008), the success of exposure can be further strengthened by two conditions: 1) conducting *"follow-up"* exposures at periodic intervals after the initial exposure therapy treatment (which reinforces what you learned during the initial exposure) and 2) *varying the context* of exposure (that is, the attributes of the exposure situation itself). For example, if you have a freeway phobia, you would drive on a variety of freeways rather than just increasing the distance you drive on a single freeway. Or, if you were afraid of snakes, you would confront a variety of different snakes rather than just approaching a single snake more closely. Or, finally, in the case of fear of heights, you would look out of high windows and take rides to high elevations, as well as walk up more and more flights of a single inner (as well as outer) stairway, and so on.

## What Interferes with Success

The opposite of any of the above-mentioned conditions will tend to impede your success with exposure: lack of cooperation from your partner, your own inability to tolerate some discomfort, a lack of skills for coping with panic, an inability to handle setbacks, and/or an unwillingness to practice consistently. In addition, clinical research has shown that these two factors can impede success with exposure therapy:

1.  *Depression.* People who suffer from clinical depression associated with agoraphobia or social phobia are generally less motivated to practice exposure. They also have a tendency to discount successes and progress when they do practice. These are common symptoms of clinical depression:

    - *Fatigue and lack of energy*

    - *Self-reproach and feelings of worthlessness*

    - *Loss of interest or pleasure in usual activities*

    - *Difficulty concentrating*

    - *Reduced appetite*

    - *Difficulty sleeping*

    - *Suicidal thoughts*

If you feel you're experiencing three or more of the above symptoms, it would be advisable to have a clinical consultation before undertaking a self-paced program of exposure. Cognitive behavioral therapy is an extremely effective treatment for depression. In more serious cases, antidepressant medication, taken under a doctor's supervision, can help lift your mood enough to allow you to practice real-life exposure.

2. *Alcohol and tranquilizers.* Alcohol or standard doses of minor tranquilizers tend to interfere with exposure. It's necessary to experience *some* anxiety during exposure to a phobic situation if you are to learn new and more adaptive responses to it. People who undergo exposure therapy while on high doses of minor tranquilizers often relapse when they go off the medication. If you can undertake exposure without the use of medication, this is optimal. However, if you and your doctor decide to rely on a tranquilizer just to enable you to be willing to undertake exposure in the first place, then be sure to utilize a low dose (for example, 0.25 mg of Ativan or Klonopin), as mentioned above. Tranquilizers are a temporary "crutch" during the early stages of exposure but eventually need to be relinquished.

## Utilizing Medications

The emphasis of this chapter up to this point has been to offer practical strategies you can use to help you face and overcome your phobias in real life. If practiced regularly and conscientiously, these strategies can be very effective. Direct exposure has repeatedly proven itself to be the most helpful method for overcoming phobias.

Sometimes, however, it is difficult for some people to get started with exposure. When your anxiety level is very high, facing your phobia in the past has brought on panic attacks, or if you've been avoiding particular situations for a long time, your initial resistance to beginning the first few sessions of exposure may be strong. You may, quite literally, have difficulty "getting out the door." It's in this situation that medication can sometimes be useful. While not providing a long-term solution, medication can sometimes help you get over initial blocks and barriers to getting started. It can also help you negotiate the early, coping phase of exposure—initially moving up the steps of your hierarchy. Once you've gained more confidence about being able to handle a previously avoided situation, your medication can and should gradually be phased out.

Two types of medication may be useful in facilitating early exposure. Both types can reduce the frequency and intensity of panic attacks sufficiently to help you get past your initial resistance. In so doing, they will also tend to reduce anticipatory anxiety.

- The SSRI antidepressant medications, such as Lexapro, Celexa, or Zoloft (see the section "SSRI Antidepressant Medications" in chapter 18), often help by reducing both anxiety and depression. This can certainly help increase motivation to undertake exposure. It's usually necessary to take these medications for three to four weeks before therapeutic benefits occur. Start with a low dose of the SSRI medication and gradually increase the dose.

- A *low* dose of a benzodiazepine tranquilizer, such as 0.25 to 0.5 mg Klonopin (clonazepam) or 0.25 mg Xanax (alprazolam), can be taken about one half hour prior to your practice session. With benzodiazepines, two conditions need to be observed. First, it's important that the dose be low, since if you take a dose high enough to mask your anxiety, you will not experience exposure. It's always necessary to experience some anxiety for exposure to be effective. Second, if possible, use the medication *only* before you go out to practice. Taking the medication several times per day and/or daily for several weeks, although this is often the way benzodiazepines are prescribed, is more likely to lead to dependence and eventual addiction.

See chapter 18 for further guidelines on how to use either antidepressant medications or tranquilizers.

# Imagery Exposure

The original procedure for treating phobias, developed by Joseph Wolpe in the 1950s, involved visualizing incremental exposures to a phobia using imagery. Wolpe, a psychiatrist from South Africa, referred to this process as "imagery desensitization" and had some success with it. The anxiety field shifted from imagery to "real-life" desensitization (facing the phobia in real life), usually referred to simply as "exposure," in the 1970s. There are certain types of phobias that are difficult to face in real life because of infrequent opportunities for direct exposure, such as thunderstorms or transcontinental flights. In such cases, rather than using traditional imagery desensitization, video exposures (for example, watching videos of lightning and thunderstorms) or high-tech reenactments of the situation called "virtual exposures" (see the section on treatment of specific phobias in chapter 1) are used.

In some cases, you may find it useful to visualize entering your phobic situation in imagery before you face it in real-life exposure. This provides a gentler way to deal with the situation initially before you confront it directly.

## How Imagery Exposure Works

To work with imagery exposure, choose a particular phobic situation you want to work on—for example, flying. Then create a hierarchy of exposures. Imagine having to deal with this situation in a very limited way—one that hardly bothers you at all. You can create this scenario by imagining yourself somewhat removed in space or time from full exposure to the situation, such as parking in front of the airport without going in or imagining your feelings one month before you have to make a flight. Or you can diminish the difficulty of the situation by visualizing yourself with a supportive person at your side. Try using these ways to create a very mild instance of your phobia and designate it as the first step in your hierarchy. It's helpful to write out a detailed scene for this first step.

Then imagine what would be the strongest or most challenging scene relating to your phobia and place it at the opposite extreme, as the highest step in your hierarchy. For flying, such a step might involve taking off on a transcontinental flight and/or encountering severe air turbulence midflight. Again, develop your most challenging scene by writing it out in full detail.

Now take some time to imagine eight or more scenes of graduated intensity related to your phobia and rank them according to their anxiety-provoking potential. The scenes for flying might include any of the following, with the first scenes being "lower" in the hierarchy (that is, less anxiety provoking) and the later scenes typically being "higher" in the hierarchy:

1. Arriving at the airport the day of your flight

2. Checking in your bags

3. Passing through security

4. Waiting at the gate for your flight

5. Boarding the plane

6. Finding your seat on the plane

7. Strapping yourself into your seat

8. Hearing the flight attendant lock the door to the plane before takeoff (this may be the most challenging exposure for many people)

9. Taxiing to the runway

10. Accelerating on the runway for takeoff

11. Feeling the plane lift off the ground

12. Ascending to cruising altitude while strapped in your seat

(The following steps are needed only if you perceive landing to be more difficult than takeoff.)

13. Hearing the flight attendant announce preparation for landing

14. Hearing the landing gear deploy as the plane approaches the runway for landing

15. Experiencing the jolt of ground impact as the plane hits the runway upon landing

If you are planning to eventually face the fear in real life, it is desirable to describe the scenes as closely as possible to their real-life counterparts. Place your scenes in ascending order between the two extremes you've already defined. Again, develop each scene by writing it out in as much detail as possible.

Just writing the scenes out in detail is actually a mild form of exposure. In order to do imagery exposure, start by relaxing for about ten minutes at first. You can use progressive muscle relaxation or a guided visualization for this purpose (see chapter 4 for details). Then visualize each successive scene in your hierarchy in detail, spending about a minute with each scene. If you feel anxiety coming up, that's fine. Stay with it and allow it to pass. In the unlikely circumstance that you think you're headed toward a panic attack, stop visualizing the scene, take a break, and then return to it when you feel better. Then continue progressing up your hierarchy step by step, visualizing each scene one or more times until you feel comfortable or minimally anxious about it. Spend fifteen to twenty minutes per day with this process of imagining your phobic scenes in succession until you have completed the highest step of your hierarchy.

For more detailed information on imagery exposure, see the author's website Helpforanxiety. com.

## Summary of Things to Do

1.  Decide on those phobias for which you're ready to undertake exposure.

2.  Establish a hierarchy with at least eight steps for each phobia you wish to work on. If you haven't yet constructed any hierarchies for your phobias, use the examples in this chapter as models. If you are doing coping exposure followed by full exposure, create a separate hierarchy of incremental steps for each.

3.  Review the section "Basic Procedure for Exposure" so that you're thoroughly familiar with the correct procedure for exposure.

4.  Practice exposure three to five days per week. Regular practice is the best way to ensure your success.

5.  Consider whether you feel confident and ready to simply do *full exposure* (without the aid of anxiety management techniques) to your phobia, whether it is driving on freeways, staying home alone, or confronting snakes. With full exposure, you still face your phobia in a series of progressive or randomized steps from your exposure hierarchy. However, you dispense with relying on coping strategies, such as using a support person, repeating affirmations, or taking a low dose of a tranquilizer.

6.  If you decide you want to begin your exposure with the assistance of coping strategies before proceeding to full exposure, choose whether you want to utilize a support person (your spouse, your partner, a close friend, a recovered phobic, or a therapist) to accompany you. Having a support person with you can help make early stages of exposure easier unless you have a strong preference for doing exposure on your own. Be willing to relinquish reliance on your support person when you advance to the mastery phase of exposure.

7.  Review the section "Making the Most of Exposure" so that you fully understand all of the ingredients that contribute to success with exposure. Your willingness to deal with initial resistance, tolerate discomfort, learn to retreat and return to the situation in the unlikely instance of panic, practice regularly, and handle any setbacks are particularly important.

8.  You may wish to visualize entering your phobic situation first before you actually confront it in real life. If so, utilize the guidelines presented in the section "Imagery Exposure" above.

9.  If you've utilized everything in this book up to and including this chapter and you're still having a difficult time getting started with exposure, consult with your doctor or a psychiatrist well versed in treating anxiety disorders about the possibility of using *low doses of medication* to help you move forward.

# Further Reading

Barlow, David. *Anxiety and Its Disorders: The Nature and Treatment of Anxiety and Panic.* 2nd ed. New York: Guilford Press, 2004.

Beckfield, Denise F. *Master Your Panic and Take Back Your Life.* 3rd ed. Atascadero, CA: Impact Publishers, 2004.

Bourne, Edmund J. *Overcoming Specific Phobia: Therapist Protocol and Client Manual* (two-book set). Oakland, CA: New Harbinger Publications, 1998.

Craske, Michelle G., Katharina Kircanski, Moriel Zelikowsky, Jayson Mystkowski, N. Chowdhury, and Aaron Baker. 2008. "Optimizing Inhibitory Learning During Exposure Therapy." *Behaviour Research and Therapy* 46: 5–27.

———, Michael Treanor, Chris Conway, Tomislav Zbozinek, and Brian Vervliof. 2014. "Maximizing Exposure: An Inhibitory Learning Approach." *Behaviour Research and Therapy* 55: 10–23.

Feninger, Mani. *Journey from Anxiety to Freedom.* New York: Three Rivers Press, 1997.

McKay, Matthew, Michelle Skeen, and Patrick Fanning. *The CBT Anxiety Solution Workbook.* Oakland, CA: New Harbinger Publications, 2017.

McNally, Richard J. 2007. "Mechanisms of Exposure Therapy: How Neuroscience Can Improve Psychological Treatments for Anxiety Disorders." *Clinical Psychology Review* 27: 750–59.

Ross, Jerilyn. *Triumph over Fear.* New York: Bantam Books, 1994.

Williams, Karen. *How to Help Your Loved One Recover from Agoraphobia.* Far Hills, NJ: New Horizon Press, 1993.

Zuercher-White, Elke. *An End to Panic.* 2nd ed. Oakland, CA: New Harbinger Publications, 1998.

# 8

# Self-Talk

Imagine two individuals sitting in stop-and-go traffic at rush hour. One perceives himself as trapped, and says such things to himself as "I can't stand this," "I've got to get out of here," and "Why did I ever get myself into this commute?" What he feels is anxiety, anger, and frustration. The other perceives the situation as an opportunity to sit back, relax, and listen to music. She says, "I might as well just relax and adjust to the pace of the traffic" or "I can unwind by doing some deep breathing." What she feels is a sense of calm and acceptance. In both cases, the situation is exactly the same, but the feelings in response to that situation are vastly different because of each individual's internal monologue, or *self-talk*.

The truth is that it's *what we say to ourselves* in response to any particular situation that mainly determines our mood and feelings. Often we say it so quickly and automatically that we don't even notice, and so we get the impression that the external situation "makes" us feel the way we do. But it's really our interpretations and thoughts about what is happening that form the basis of our feelings. This sequence can be represented as a timeline:

| External Events | → | Interpretation of Events and Self-Talk | → | Feelings and Reactions |

In short, you are largely responsible for how you feel (barring physiological determinants, such as illness). This is a profound and very important truth—one that sometimes takes a long time to fully grasp. It's often much easier to blame the way you feel on something or someone outside yourself than to take responsibility for your reactions. Yet it is through your willingness to accept that responsibility that you begin to take charge and have mastery over your life. The realization that you are mostly responsible for how you feel is empowering once you fully accept it. It's one of the most important keys to living a happier, more effective, and anxiety-free life.

## Anxiety and Self-Talk

People who suffer from phobias, panic attacks, and general anxiety are especially prone to engage in negative self-talk. Anxiety can be generated on the spur of the moment by repeatedly making statements to yourself that begin with the two words "what if." Any anxiety you experience in anticipation of confronting a difficult situation is manufactured out of your own "what-if statements" to yourself. When you decide to avoid a situation altogether, it is probably because of the scary questions you've asked yourself: "What if I panic?" "What if I can't handle it?" "What will other people think if they see me anxious?" Just noticing when you fall into "what-if think-ing" is the first step toward gaining control over negative self-talk. The real change occurs when you begin to *counter* and *replace* negative what-if statements with positive, self-supportive state-ments that reinforce your ability to cope. For example, you might say, "So what," "These are just thoughts," "This is just scare-talk," "I can handle this," or "I can breathe, let go, and relax."

Consider some basic facts about self-talk. Following these facts is a discussion of the different types of self-defeating inner monologues.

## Some Basic Points About Self-Talk

Self-talk is usually so automatic and subtle that you don't notice it or the effect it has on your moods and feelings. You react without noticing what you told yourself right before you reacted. Often it's only when you relax, take a step back, and really examine what you've been telling yourself that you can see the connection between self-talk and your feelings. What is important is that *you can learn to slow down and take note of your negative internal monologue.*

*Self-talk often appears in telegraphic form.* One short word or image contains a whole series of thoughts, memories, or associations. For example, you feel your heart starting to beat faster and say to yourself, "Oh no!" Implicit within that momentary "Oh no!" is a whole series of asso-ciations concerning fears about panic, memories of previous panic attacks, and thoughts about how to escape the current situation. Identifying self-talk may require unraveling several distinct thoughts from a single word or image.

*Anxious self-talk is typically irrational but almost always sounds like the truth.* What-if thinking may lead you to expect the worst possible outcome in a given situation, one that is highly unlikely to occur. Yet because the association takes place so quickly, it goes unchallenged and unquestioned. It's hard to evaluate the validity of a belief you're scarcely aware of—you just accept it as is.

*Negative self-talk perpetuates avoidance.* You tell yourself that a situation such as the freeway is dangerous and so you avoid it. By continuing to avoid it, you reinforce the thought that it's dangerous. You may even project images of catastrophe around the prospect of confronting the situation. In short, anxious self-talk leads to avoidance, avoidance begets further anxious self-talk, and around and around the cycle goes.

Avoidance ⟷ Self-Talk

*Self-talk can initiate or aggravate a panic attack.* A panic attack often starts out with symptoms of increasing physiological arousal, such as a more rapid heartbeat, tightness in the chest, or sweaty palms. Biologically, this is the body's *natural* response to stress—the fight-or-flight response that all mammals, including humans, normally experience when subjected to a perceived threat. There is nothing inherently abnormal or dangerous about it. Yet these symptoms can remind you of previous panic attacks. Instead of simply allowing your body's physiological reaction to rise, peak, and subside in its own good time, you scare yourself into a considerably more intense panic attack with scary self-talk: "Oh no, it's happening again," "What if I lose control?" "I *have* to get out of here now," or "I'm going to fight this and make it go away." This scare-talk aggravates the initial physical symptoms, which in turn elicits further scare-talk. A severe panic attack might have been aborted or rendered much less intense had you made reassuring statements to yourself at the onset of your first symptoms: "I can accept what's happening even though it's uncomfortable," "I'll let my body do its thing," "This will pass," "I've gotten through this before and I will this time, too," or "This is just a burst of adrenaline that can metabolize and pass in a few minutes." See the section "Coping Statements" in chapter 6 for further examples of this kind of reassuring, constructive statements.

*Negative self-talk is a series of bad habits.* You aren't born with a predisposition to fearful self-talk: you *learn* to think that way. Just as you can replace unhealthy *behavioral* habits, such as smoking or drinking excess coffee, with more positive, health-promoting behavior, so can you replace unhealthy thinking with more positive, supportive *mental* habits. Bear in mind that acquiring positive mental habits takes the same persistence and practice required for learning other new behaviors.

## Types of Negative Self-Talk

Not all negative self-talk is the same. Human beings are not only diverse but also complex, with multifaceted personalities. These facets are sometimes referred to as "subpersonalities." Our different subpersonalities each play their own distinct role and possess their own voice in the complex workings of consciousness, memory, and dreams. Below you will find four of the more common subpersonality types that tend to be prominent in people who are prone to anxiety: the Worrier, the Critic, the Victim, and the Perfectionist.[1] Since the strength of these inner voices varies for different people, you might find it useful to rank them from strongest to weakest in yourself.

### The Worrier (promotes anxiety)

*Characteristics.* This usually is the strongest subpersonality in people who are prone to anxiety. The Worrier creates anxiety by imagining the worst-case scenario. It scares you with fantasies of disaster or catastrophe when you imagine confronting something you fear. It also aggravates panic by reacting to the first physical symptoms of a panic attack. The Worrier promotes your fears that what is happening is dangerous or embarrassing ("What if I have a heart attack?!" "What will they think if they see me?!").

In short, the Worrier's dominant tendencies include 1) anticipating the worst, 2) overestimating the odds that something bad or embarrassing will happen, and 3) creating grandiose images of potential failure or catastrophe. The Worrier is always vigilant, watching with uneasy apprehension for any small symptoms or signs of trouble.

---

1   These subpersonalities are based on Reid Wilson's descriptions of the Worried, Critical, and Hopeless Observers in his book *Don't Panic: Taking Control of Anxiety Attacks.*

*Favorite expression.* By far, the favorite expression of the Worrier is "What if...?"

*Examples.* Some typical dialogue from the Worrier might be: "Oh no, my heart's starting to beat faster! What if I panic and lose complete control of myself?" "What if I start stammering in the middle of my speech?" "What if they see me shaking?" "What if I'm alone and there's nobody to call?" "What if I just can't get over this phobia?" or "What if I'm restricted from going to work for the rest of my life?"

## The Critic (promotes low self-esteem)

*Characteristics.* The Critic is that part of you that is constantly judging and evaluating your behavior (and in this sense may seem more "apart" from you than the other subpersonalities). It tends to point out your flaws and limitations whenever possible. It jumps on any mistake you make to remind you that you're a failure. The Critic generates anxiety by putting you down for not being able to handle your panic symptoms, for not being able to go places you used to go, for being unable to perform at your best, or for having to be dependent on someone else. It also likes to compare you with others and usually sees them coming out favorably. It tends to ignore your positive qualities and emphasizes your weaknesses and inadequacies. The Critic may be personified in your own dialogue as the voice of your mother or father, a dreaded teacher, or anyone who wounded you in the past with their criticism.

*Favorite expressions.* "What a disappointment you are!" "That was stupid!"

*Examples.* The following would be typical of the Critic's self-talk: "You stupid _____." (The Critic relishes negative labels.) "Can't you ever get it right?" "Why are you always this way?" "Look at how capable _____ is," or "You could have done better." The Critic holds negative self-beliefs, such as "I'm inferior to others," "I'm not worth much," "There's something inherently wrong with me," or "I'm weak—I should be stronger."

## The Victim (promotes depression)

*Characteristics.* The Victim is that part of you that feels helpless or hopeless. It generates anxiety by telling you that you're not making any progress, that your condition is incurable, or that the road is too long and steep for you to have a real chance at recovering. The Victim also plays a major role in creating depression. The Victim believes that there is something inherently wrong with you: you are in some way deprived, defective, or unworthy. The Victim always perceives insurmountable obstacles between you and your goals. Characteristically, it bemoans, complains, and regrets things as they are at present. It believes that nothing will ever change.

*Favorite expressions.* "I can't." "I'll never be able to."

*Examples.* The Victim will say such things as "I'll never be able to do that, so what's the point in even trying?" "I feel physically drained today—why bother doing anything?" "Maybe I could have done it if I'd had more initiative ten years ago—but it's too late now." The Victim holds such negative self-beliefs as "I'm hopeless," "I've had this problem too long—it will never get better," or "I've tried everything—nothing is ever going to work."

## The Perfectionist (promotes chronic stress and burnout)

*Characteristics.* The Perfectionist is a close cousin of the Critic, but its concern is less to put you down than to push and goad you to do better. It generates anxiety by constantly telling you that your efforts aren't good enough, that you *should* be working harder, that you *should* always have everything under control; that you *should* always be competent, *should* always be pleasing, *should* always be _____ (fill in whatever you keep telling yourself that you "should" do or be). The Perfectionist is the hard-driving part of you that wants to be best and is intolerant of mistakes or setbacks. It has a tendency to try to convince you that your self-worth is dependent on *externals*, such as vocational achievement, money and status, acceptance by others, being loved, or your ability to be pleasing and nice to others, regardless of what they do. The Perfectionist isn't convinced by any notions of your inherent self-worth, but instead pushes you into stress, exhaustion, and ultimately burnout in pursuit of its goals. It likes to ignore warning signals from your body.

*Favorite expressions.* "I should." "I have to." "I must."

*Examples.* The Perfectionist may provide such instructions as "I should always be on top of things," "I should always be considerate and unselfish," "I should always be pleasant and nice," or "I *have to* (get this job, make this amount of money, receive _____'s approval, and so on)," or "I'm not worth much." (See the discussion of "should statements" at the end of the next section.)

## Exercise: What Are Your Subpersonalities Telling You?

Take some time to think about how each of the above subpersonalities plays a role in your thinking, feelings, and behavior. First, estimate how much each one affects you by rating its degree of influence from "not at all" to "very much" on a six-point scale (see the worksheets over the next few pages). Which subpersonality is strongest and which is weakest for you? Then think about what each subpersonality is saying to you to create or aggravate anxiety in each of the following four situations.

1. *Work* (on your job, at school, or in other performance situations)

2. *Personal relationships* (with your spouse or partner, parents, children, and/or friends)

3. *Anxiety symptoms* (on occasions when you experience panic, anxiety, or obsessive-compulsive symptoms)

4. *Phobic situations* (either *in advance* of facing a phobia or while actually *confronting* the phobic situation)

Here are some examples for the Worrier:

## The Worrier

*Work:*  "What if my boss finds out that I have agoraphobia? Will I get fired?"

*Relationships:*  "My husband is getting tired of having to take me places. What if he refuses? What if he leaves me?"

*Anxiety symptoms:*  "What if they see me panic? What if they think I'm weird?"

*Phobic situation:*  "What if I get into an accident the first time I try to drive on the freeway?"

You may find that the Worrier's self-talk in the latter two situations is by far the most common source of your anxiety. If you have panic attacks, the Worrier is prone to create anxiety about when and where your next one might occur. Should the bodily symptoms of panic actually start to come on, the Worrier may magnify them into something dangerous, which only creates more panic. Many of the coping strategies described in chapter 6 (in particular, the use of positive coping statements) are designed to help you deal with the Worrier during a panic attack.

If you have phobias, the Worrier is typically busy telling you about all kinds of things that might happen if you were to actually face your fear. As a result, you often experience "anticipatory anxiety" (anxiety in advance of facing a phobia) and try to avoid dealing with whatever your phobia may be. You'll find it helpful to do a separate analysis of what your Worrier is telling you (in other words, your "what-ifs") for *each* of your specific phobias. Ask yourself what you're afraid could happen if you face each phobia.

Here are some examples of how other subpersonalities operate:

## The Critic

*Work:*  "I'm incompetent because of my condition."

*Relationships:*  "I'm a burden to my spouse."

*Anxiety symptoms:*  "I'm such a weakling—I go to pieces when I panic."

*Phobic situation:*  "Everybody else can drive—I feel like a loser."

## The Victim

*Work:*  "My situation at work is hopeless—sooner or later I'll be fired."

*Relationships:*  "My parents really messed me up" or "I can't make it without my partner."

| | |
|---|---|
| *Anxiety symptoms:* | "I'll *never* get over these panic attacks—there must be something very wrong with me." |
| *Phobic situation:* | "It's useless going on any more job interviews. No one's going to hire me when they see that I'm so anxious." |

## The Perfectionist

| | |
|---|---|
| *Work:* | "I should be able to make sales like I used to, no matter how anxious I feel." |
| *Relationships:* | "I shouldn't need to depend on my spouse or anyone else to take me places." |
| *Anxiety symptoms:* | "I *have to* be able to stop these thoughts from going through my mind." |
| *Phobic situation:* | "I *have to* learn to drive like anyone else." |

Use the worksheets that follow to write down the anxiety-provoking statements that each of your subpersonalities are using in each type of situation. (You can also find downloadable digital versions at the website associated with this book. See the back page of the book for details.) You don't need to do this for all four subpersonalities or for all four types of situations in each case. Only include those subpersonalities and situations that you suspect are the greatest problem for you.

Monitor what your subpersonalities are telling you for at least one week. Just complete the left-hand columns for now. (You'll be filling in the right-hand columns of the worksheets later. Use additional sheets of paper if you need more room.) Pay attention especially to occasions when you are feeling anxious (panicky), depressed, self-critical and ashamed, or otherwise upset. Look for the thoughts that were going through your mind that led you to feel the way you did. "I felt scared" is not a clear example of self-talk because it doesn't indicate what you were thinking (telling yourself) that caused you to feel scared. On the other hand, the self-statement "What if I panic on the job today?" is an example of a thought that could have led you to feel scared.

See step 4 in the section later in this chapter called "Summary: Guidelines for Identifying and Countering Self-Talk" for further suggestions about separating thoughts from feelings.

# *Subpersonality Worksheet: The Worrier*

Affects me: not at all _____ very much

1  2  3  4  5  6

| Negative Self-Talk | Positive Counterstatements |
| --- | --- |
| **Situation** | |
| *Work/School* | |
| *Relationships* | |
| *Anxiety Symptoms* | |
| *Phobias* | |
| (Determine the Worrier's self-talk for each of your phobias—use a separate sheet if necessary.) | |

# Subpersonality Worksheet: The Critic

Affects me: not at all _____ very much

 1   2   3   4   5   6

| Negative Self-Talk | Positive Counterstatements |
|---|---|
| **Situation** | |
| *Work/School* | |
| *Relationships* | |
| *Anxiety Symptoms* | |
| *Phobias* | |
| (Identify critical self-talk for each of your phobias—use a separate worksheet if needed.) | |

# Subpersonality Worksheet: The Victim

Affects me: not at all _____ very much

1  2  3  4  5  6

| Negative Self-Talk | Positive Counterstatements |
| --- | --- |
| **Situation** | |
| *Work/School* | |
| *Relationships* | |
| *Anxiety Symptoms* | |
| *Phobias* | |
| (Identify the Victim's self-talk for each of your phobias on a separate worksheet.) | |

# *Subpersonality Worksheet: The Perfectionist*

Affects me: not at all _____ very much
           1  2  3  4  5  6

| Negative Self-Talk | Positive Counterstatements |
| --- | --- |
| **Situation** | |
| *Work/School* | |
| *Relationships* | |
| *Anxiety Symptoms* | |
| *Phobias* | |
| (Identify the Perfectionist's self-talk for each of your phobias on a separate worksheet.) | |

# Countering Negative Self-Talk

The most effective way to deal with the negative self-talk of your Worrier and other subpersonalities is to *counter* it with positive, supportive statements. Countering involves *writing down* and *rehearsing* positive statements that directly refute or invalidate your negative self-talk. If you're creating anxiety and other upsetting emotional states through negative mental programming, you can begin to change the way you feel by substituting positive programming. Doing this will take some *practice*. You've had years to practice your negative self-talk and naturally have developed some very strong habits. Your Worrier and other subpersonalities are likely to be very well entrenched. By starting to notice when you're engaging in negativity and then countering it with positive, supportive statements to yourself, you'll begin to turn your thinking around. With practice and consistent effort, you'll change both the way you think *and the way you feel* on an ongoing basis.

Sometimes countering comes naturally and easily. You are ready and willing to substitute positive, reasonable self-statements for ones that have been causing you anxiety and distress. You're more than ready to relinquish negative mental habits that aren't serving you. On the other hand, you may object to the idea of countering and say, "But what if what my Worrier (Critic, Victim, or Perfectionist) says is true? It's hard for me to believe otherwise." Or you may say, "How can I substitute positive self-statements for negative ones if I don't really believe them?"

Perhaps you're strongly attached to some of your negative self-talk. You've been telling yourself these things for years and it's difficult to give up both the habit and the beliefs. You're not someone who's easily persuaded. If that's the case, and you want to do something about your negative self-talk, it's important that you subject it to rational scrutiny. You can weaken the hold of your negative self-statements by exposing them to any of the following Socratic questions, or rational investigation.

- What is the evidence for this?

- Is this *always* true?

- Has this been true in the past?

- What are the odds of this really happening (or being true)?

- What is the very worst that could happen? What is so bad about that? What would you do if the worst happened?

- Are you looking at the whole picture?

- Are you being fully objective?

The validity of your negative self-statements has nothing to do with how attached you are to them or how ingrained they might be. Rather, it has to do with whether they stand up under careful, objective scrutiny. Consider the following examples:

**Worrier:**  "What if I have a heart attack the next time I panic?"

*Questioning:*  "What is the evidence that panic attacks cause heart attacks?" (Answer: None—see the section "Deflate the Danger" at the beginning of chapter 6.)

*Counterstatement:*  "A panic attack, however uncomfortable, is not dangerous to my heart. I can let panic rise, fall, and pass, and my heart will be fine."

**Critic:**  "You're weak and neurotic because of your stupid phobias."

*Questioning:*  "What is the evidence for this?" (Answer: Phobias are caused by a conditioning process that occurs in a high-anxiety state— see chapter 2. "Weak" and "neurotic" are pejorative labels that explain nothing.)

*Counterstatement:*  "My phobias developed because of a conditioning process that caused me to be sensitized to certain situations. I'm learning to overcome my phobias through a process of gradual exposure."

**Victim:**  "I'll never get over this problem. I'll be limited in my mobility for the rest of my life."

*Questioning:*  "What is the evidence that agoraphobia is a lifelong condition? What other outcomes are possible?" (Answer: A great majority of agoraphobics recover with effective treatment.)

*Counterstatement:*  "My condition isn't hopeless. I can overcome it by establishing and committing myself to a program for recovery."

**Perfectionist:**  "I have to receive my parents' acceptance and approval or I'll be devastated."

*Questioning:*  "Am I being fully objective? Is it actually true that my parents' approval is absolutely necessary for my well-being? What is the worst that could happen?" (Answer: I could still survive and have people who care for and support me even without my parents' approval.)

*Counterstatement:*  "I'm willing to go forward with my life and try to better myself regardless of what my parents think."

If you feel attached to your negative self-talk, use any of the above Socratic questions to evaluate the validity of what you're telling yourself. In most cases, you'll find that the negative statements of your Worrier, Critic, Victim, and Perfectionist have little basis in reality. At worst, they will be only partially or occasionally true. Once you've discredited a particular subpersonality's views, you will be ready to counter with positive, supportive statements.

## Rules for Writing Positive Counterstatements

- *Avoid negatives* in writing your counterstatements. Instead of saying, "I'm not going to panic when I board the plane," try "I am confident and calm about boarding the plane." Telling yourself something will *not* happen is more likely to create anxiety than giving yourself a direct affirmation.

- Keep counterstatements in the *present tense* ("I can practice a relaxation technique and let these feelings pass" is preferable to "I will feel better in a few minutes"). Since much of your negative self-talk is in the here and now, it needs to be countered by statements that are also in the present tense. If you're not ready to *directly* affirm something, try beginning your positive statement with "I am willing to…" or "I am learning to…" or "I can…"

- Whenever possible, keep your statements in the *first person*. Begin them with an "I-statement" or refer to yourself somewhere in the statement. It's okay to write a sentence or two explaining the basis for your counterstatement (see the previous examples of counterstatements for the Worrier and Critic), but try to end with an "I-statement."

- It's important that you have some *belief* in your positive self-talk. Don't write something down just because it's positive if you don't actually believe it. If appropriate, use Socratic questions to challenge your negative self-talk first, and then follow this up with a positive counterstatement that holds some personal credibility for you.

To get you started, here are some more examples of positive counterstatements you can use with each of the above subpersonalities:

### The Worrier

Instead of "What if…," you can say, "So what," "I can handle this," "I can be anxious and still do this," "This may be scary, but I can tolerate a little anxiety, knowing that it will pass," or "I'll get used to this with practice."

### The Critic

Instead of putting yourself down, you can say, "I'm okay the way I am," "I'm lovable and capable," "I'm a unique and creative person," "I deserve the good things in life as much as anyone else," "I accept and believe in myself," or "I am worthy of the respect of others."

### The Victim

Instead of feeling hopeless, you can say, "I don't have to be all better tomorrow," "I can continue to make progress one step at a time," "I acknowledge the progress I've made and will continue to improve," "It's never too late to change," or "I'm willing to see the glass as half full rather than half empty."

### The Perfectionist

Instead of demanding perfection, you can say, "It's okay to make mistakes," "Life is too short to be taken too seriously," "Setbacks are part of the process and an important learning experience," "I don't have to always be…" or "My needs and feelings are as important as anyone else's."

## Utilizing Counterstatements

Now you are ready to go back and counter all of the negative statements you recorded on the worksheets for your various subpersonalities. Write down counterstatements in the right-hand column corresponding to each negative statement. Use extra sheets of paper if you need to.

Once you've completed writing out positive self-talk for each subpersonality in each situation, there are several ways you can work with your positive counterstatements:

- Read through your list of positive counterstatements slowly and carefully for a few minutes each day for at least two weeks. See if you can feel some conviction about their truth as you read them. This will help you integrate them more deeply into your consciousness.

- Make copies of your completed worksheets and post them in a conspicuous place. Take time once a day to carefully read through your positive counterstatements.

- Record your counterstatements, leaving about five seconds between each consecutive positive statement so that it has time to sink in. You can significantly enhance the effect of such a recording by giving yourself five to ten minutes to become very relaxed before listening to your counterstatements. You will be more receptive to them in a relaxed state. You may want to record the instructions for progressive muscle relaxation or one of the relaxing visualizations described in chapter 4 on the first ten to fifteen minutes of the recording.

- If you're having a problem with a particular phobia, you might want to work with positive counterstatements that are *specific just to that phobia*. For example, if you're afraid of speaking before groups, make a list of all your fears about what could happen, and develop positive statements to counter each fear. Then read through your list of counterstatements carefully each day for two weeks or make a short recording as described in the preceding item.

# Changing Self-Talk That Perpetuates Specific Fears and Phobias

Three factors tend to perpetuate fears and phobias: sensitization, avoidance, and negative, distorted self-talk. Chapter 7 focused on the first two conditions. A phobia develops when you become sensitized to a particular situation, object, or event—in other words, when anxiety becomes conditioned or associated with that situation, object, or event. If panic suddenly arises while you happen to be driving on the freeway or while you're home alone, you may start feeling anxious every time you're in either of these situations. Becoming *sensitized* means that the mere presence of—or even thoughts about—a situation may be enough to trigger anxiety automatically.

After sensitization occurs, you may start to *avoid* the situation. Repeated avoidance is very rewarding, because it saves you from having to feel any anxiety. Avoidance is the most powerful way to hold on to a phobia, because it prevents you from ever learning that you can handle the situation.

The third factor that perpetuates fears and phobias is distorted self-talk. The more *worry* and *anticipatory anxiety* you experience about something you fear, the more likely you are to be involved in unconstructive self-talk connected with that fear. You may also have negative *images* about what could happen if you had to face what you fear or about your worst fears coming true. Both negative self-talk and negative images serve to perpetuate your fears, guaranteeing that you remain afraid. They also undermine your confidence that you can ever get over your fear. Without negative self-talk and negative images, you would be much more likely to overcome your avoidance and confront your fear.

Fears come in many forms, but the nature of fearful self-talk is always the same. Whether you are afraid of crossing bridges, speaking up in a social situation, the sensation of a rapid heartbeat, the possibility of serious illness, or your children getting into trouble, the types of distorted thinking that perpetuate these fears are the same. *There are three basic distortions*:

**Note:** While this discussion primarily pertains to self-talk that perpetuates phobias, it can also be applied to self-talk that maintains excessive worry. See chapter 10, Overcoming Worry, for further guidelines on working with unconstructive self-talk that perpetuates worry.

1. *Overestimating a negative outcome.* Overestimating the odds of something bad happening is one type of distortion. Most of the time, your worries consist of "what-if" statements that overestimate a particular negative outcome. For example, "What if I panic and lose complete control of myself?" "What if they see me panic and think I'm weird?" "What if I flunk the exam and have to drop out of school?"

2. *Catastrophizing.* The second distortion is thinking that if a negative outcome did occur, it would be catastrophic, overwhelming, and unmanageable. Catastrophic thoughts contain such statements as "I couldn't handle it," "I'd be overwhelmed," "I'd never live it down," or "They'll never forgive me."

3. *Underestimating your ability to cope.* The third distortion is not recognizing or acknowledging your ability to cope if a negative outcome did, in fact, occur. This underestimation of your ability to cope is usually implicit in your catastrophic thoughts.

If you take any fear and examine the negative thinking that contributes to maintaining that fear, you'll probably find these three distortions. To the extent that you can overcome them with more reality-based thinking, the fear will tend to drop away. In essence, you can define fear as *the unreasonable overestimation of some threat, coupled with an underestimation of your ability to cope.*

Here are some examples of how the different types of distortions operate with various fears. In each example, the three types of distorted thoughts are identified. The distortions are then challenged in each case and modified with more appropriate, reality-based counterstatements.

## Example 1: Fear of Having a Panic Attack While Driving on a Freeway

### Overestimating Thoughts

"What if I can't handle the car? What if my attention wanders and I lose control of the car? What if I cause an accident and kill someone?"

### Catastrophic Thoughts

"I couldn't handle it if I lost control of the car. It would be a totally unmanageable situation—the end of the world—if I caused an accident." (Note: An image of a horrendous accident can accompany and amplify the force of a catastrophic thought.)

### Underestimating Your Ability to Cope

"I couldn't cope if I lost control of the car, especially if I got into an accident. I'll die of embarrassment if other drivers notice how frightened I am." "What would I say to a policeman—that I'm phobic?" "I wouldn't be able to start driving again if I got stopped for a ticket." "I couldn't live with myself if I caused physical injury to another person—and I know I couldn't face life in a wheelchair."

## Refuting Distorted Thinking

It's possible to refute each of these types of distorted thinking with questions and counterstatements. Examples follow below:

### Overestimating Thoughts

With overestimating thoughts, the appropriate question is *"Viewing the situation objectively, what are the odds of the negative outcome actually happening?"*

In the case of the previous example, the question is "If I did panic while driving, what are the true odds that I would lose control of the car?"

You could use this counterstatement: "It's unlikely that having a panic attack would cause me to lose complete control. The moment I felt my anxiety coming on, I could pull over to the shoulder on the side of the road and stop. If there weren't any shoulders, I could slow way down in the right lane, perhaps to forty-five miles per hour, put my flashers on, and keep a grip on myself until I reached the nearest exit. Once I got off the highway, my panic would begin to subside."

## Catastrophic Thoughts

With catastrophizing, the relevant question to ask is *"If the worst did happen, is it actually true that I couldn't handle it?"* The idea is to go ahead and imagine the worst that could happen and then ask yourself whether *in reality* you could handle the consequences or not.

In the above example, you would raise the question, "If the worst did happen—if I did get into an accident, one that even caused injury—would I be totally unable to handle it?"

You could then use a counterstatement, such as "As bad as having an accident would be, in most cases I would be able to handle it if I weren't injured. It's common for people to function in an emergency situation and then handle their anxiety later. So, in all likelihood, I would keep functioning in the event of an accident as long as I wasn't injured."

"Even if I were injured, and unable to handle the situation, the police and paramedics would soon arrive on the scene and take charge. There is simply no way in which the situation could become completely unmanageable."

## Underestimating Your Ability to Cope

Countering the idea that you couldn't cope often takes place in the process of answering catastrophic thinking with a more objective appraisal. However, the process isn't complete until you actually *identify and list specific ways in which you could cope.* In the above example, some possible coping strategies could include the following:

- "If I did have a panic attack, I could cope by getting off the highway immediately or driving slowly to the nearest exit and getting off."

- "In the very unlikely case that I actually caused an accident, I would still cope. I would exchange names and addresses with other parties involved. If my car were undriveable, the police would likely drive me to a place where I could call to have the car towed. It would be a very unpleasant experience, to say the least. But, realistically, I would continue to function. I've functioned in emergencies in the past, and I could function in this case, if I weren't injured."

- "Even given the remote possibility that I were injured, I wouldn't 'go crazy' or 'totally lose it.' I would simply wait until the paramedics came and took charge of the situation."

## *Example 2: Fear of Panicking While Speaking Up in a Class or Meeting*

### Overestimating Thoughts

"What if I panicked while speaking? Wouldn't others think I was really weird or crazy?"

*Questioning:* "Realistically, how likely is it that I would panic while speaking? What are the odds, if I did panic, that people would be aware of what I was thinking or make any judgments about me at all?"

*Counterstatements:* "It is possible that I could start to panic while speaking. If I did, I could simply abbreviate what I wanted to say and sit back down. As people tend to be caught up in their own thoughts and fears, no one would likely notice my difficulty or judge that I'd cut my comments short."

"Even if people did see me panic—if they saw my face turn red or heard my voice trembling—the odds are very slim that they'd think I was weird or crazy. It's much more likely that they'd express concern."

## Catastrophic Thoughts

"If I panicked while speaking and people thought I was weird, that would be terrible. *I'd never live it down.*"

*Questioning:* "Suppose the unlikely happened and people really thought I was strange or weird because I panicked. How terrible would that be?"

*Counterstatements:* "It's not going to be the end of the world if some people think I'm strange or that something's wrong with me. They have no way of knowing what it's like to have panic attacks, so they couldn't really understand. Even if people don't understand, or if they misperceive me, that doesn't decrease one bit my value or worth as a human being. If I believe in myself, then it really doesn't matter what others think. Certainly if others knew what it was like to have a panic attack, they would likely be sympathetic."

## Underestimating Your Ability to Cope

"I couldn't cope if people thought I was strange."

*Questioning:* "Is it realistic to assume that I couldn't cope? Is it realistic to suppose I'd never live it down?"

*Counterstatements:* "Even if people thought I was strange or different because I panicked, I could explain to them that I sometimes have panic attacks in social situations. With all the publicity about anxiety disorders that's around these days, they would likely understand. Being totally honest is one way I could handle the situation. And no matter what happened, I would forget about it after a while. It's just not true that I would never live it down."

## *Example 3: Fear of Serious Illness*

### Overestimating Thoughts

"I have no energy and feel tired all the time. Maybe I have cancer and don't know it!"

*Questioning:* "What are the odds that symptoms of low energy and fatigue mean that I have cancer?"

*Counterstatements:* "Symptoms of fatigue and low energy can be indicative of all kinds of physical and psychological conditions, including a low-grade virus, anemia, adrenal exhaustion or hypothyroidism, depression, and food allergies, to name a few. There are many possible explanations of my condition, and I don't have any specific symptoms that would indicate cancer. So the odds of my fatigue and low energy indicating cancer are very low."

## Catastrophic Thoughts

"If I were diagnosed with cancer, that would be the end. I couldn't take it. I'd be better off ending things quickly and killing myself."

*Questioning:* "If the unlikely happened and I really were diagnosed with cancer, how terrible could that be? Would I actually go to pieces and just want to die?"

*Counterstatements:* "As bad as a cancer diagnosis would be, it's unlikely that I would totally go to pieces. After an initial difficult adjustment to the fact—which might take days to weeks—I would most likely begin to think about what I needed to do to deal with the situation. It would certainly be difficult, yet it wouldn't be a situation that I was less equipped to handle than anyone else."

## Underestimating Your Ability to Cope

"If I were given a diagnosis of cancer, I simply couldn't cope."

*Questioning:* "Realistically, is it actually true that I would have no way of coping with the situation?"

*Counterstatements:* "Of course I would cope. After an initial period of adjusting to the situation, my doctor and I would plan the most effective possible treatment strategies. I would join a local cancer support group and get lots of support from my friends and immediate family. I would try alternative methods, such as visualization and dietary changes, that could help. In short, I would try everything possible to attempt to heal the condition."

# Summary: Countering Negative Self-Talk

The above three examples illustrate how overestimating and catastrophic thoughts can be challenged and then countered by more realistic, less anxiety-provoking thinking. Now it's your turn. During the next two weeks, monitor the times when you feel anxious or panicky. Each time you do, use the following five steps to work with negative self-talk:

**Step 1:** If you're feeling anxious or upset, do something to relax, such as abdominal breathing, progressive muscle relaxation, or meditation. It's easier to notice your internal dialogue when you take time to slow down and relax.

**Step 2:** After you get somewhat relaxed, ask yourself, "What was I telling myself that made me anxious?" or "What was going through my mind?" Remember to separate thoughts from feelings. For example, "I felt terrified" describes a feeling, while "This panic will never end" is an overestimating thought that might have led you to feel terrified.

**Step 3:** Identify the three basic types of distortions among your anxious self-talk. Sort out *overestimating thoughts*, *catastrophic thoughts*, and *thoughts that underestimate your ability to cope.*

**Step 4:** When you've identified your anxious, distorted thoughts, challenge them with appropriate questions.

- *For overestimating thoughts:* "What are the realistic odds that this feared outcome would actually happen?"

- *For catastrophic thoughts:* "If the feared outcome actually did occur, how terrible would it be? Is it really true that I would go to pieces and lose my ability to cope?"

- *For thoughts underestimating your ability to cope:* "If the feared outcome did occur, what could I actually do to cope?"

**Step 5:** Write counterstatements to each of your anxious self-statements. These counterstatements should contain language and logic that reflect more balanced, realistic thinking.

Use the *Countering Self-Talk Worksheet* that follows to write down your anxious thoughts and corresponding counterstatements for any specific fear or phobia you choose to work with. In the section at the bottom, list ways in which you could cope if the negative (but unlikely) outcome you fear actually occurred.

It would be a good idea to make photocopies of the worksheet before you begin, or download copies of the electronic version available online, so that you can fill out a separate sheet for each specific fear or phobia you have. (For more information about the download, see the very end of this book.)

# Countering Self-Talk Worksheet

Specific Fear or Phobia _____

| Anxious Self-Talk | Counterstatements |
| --- | --- |
| **Overestimating thoughts (or images)**<br>"What if...?" | |
| **Catastrophic thoughts (or images)**<br>"If the worst happened, then..." | |

**Coping strategies:** List the ways in which you would cope if a negative (but unlikely) outcome did occur. Use the other side of the sheet if needed. Change "What if" to "What I would do if (one of the negative predictions) actually did come about."

# Other Types of Distorted Thinking (Cognitive Distortions)

Overestimating and catastrophizing, along with underestimating your ability to cope, are three of the most common types of distortions in thinking that contribute to most phobias and fears. There are other types of distortions, however, that can skew the ways in which you perceive and evaluate both yourself and innumerable situations in everyday life. A well-known school of therapy known as cognitive therapy (Beck 1979; Burns 1980, 2008) enumerates ten types of distorted ways of thinking found in people with a tendency to be depressed and/or anxious. These cognitive distortions contribute not only to depression and anxiety, but also to guilt, shame, self-criticism and/or cynicism that you might feel. Learning to identify and then counter these unhelpful modes of thinking with more realistic, constructive self-talk can go a long way toward helping you handle everyday stresses of life in a more balanced, objective fashion. This, in turn, will significantly reduce the amount of anxiety, depression, and other unpleasant emotional states you experience. As you change your thinking, you change the way your world appears.

**Note:** The ten main cognitive distortions are listed in the same order David Burns presents them in his well-known book, *Feeling Good*.

*All-or-nothing thinking.* A tendency to view a situation as "either/or"—all good or all bad—with no allowance for shades of gray or a middle ground in between.

*Overgeneralization.* Similar to the tendency to overestimate something undesirable: if something bad happens once, you tend to overgeneralize that it will happen again and again.

*Filtering (mental filter).* Selectively focusing on negative details of a situation while filtering out all of the positive aspects. You find somebody's statement to be cruel or insensitive, and you quickly jump to the conclusion that people in general are cruel and/or insensitive.

*Disqualifying the positive.* More extreme than filtering, disqualifying the positive means you completely discount something positive and quickly convert it into something negative. You take a positive occurrence and tell yourself, "That was a fluke. It doesn't count." Or when someone gives you a legitimate compliment, you discount it by saying to yourself, "They were just being nice," or telling the other person, "Oh, it was nothing, really."

*Jumping to conclusions.* Assuming what another person is thinking or feeling—or exactly why they act the way they do—before actually checking out with the person what they are actually thinking or feeling, or the basis for their actions. David Burns, in his book *Feeling Good* (2008), often refers to this cognitive distortion as the "fortune-telling error," as if you had the capacity to read somebody's mind before even asking them what they were thinking or feeling.

*Magnification.* A tendency to "blow up" (magnify) your own or someone else's minor limitations, or conversely, minimize your or someone's strengths. For example, you make a minor mistake at work and conclude, "This is horrible" and "I could lose my job." Or you take a positive job review and minimize it, telling yourself, "This doesn't mean anything" and "The manager probably gives everyone this type of review."

*Emotional reasoning.* The fallacy that if something feels a certain way, then it must actually be true. You mistake feelings for reality. For example, if you feel stupid or boring in some situation, you conclude you must actually *be* stupid or boring.

*Should thinking.* Self-talk, including terms such as "should," "have to," or "must," that is commonly associated with a tendency to be perfectionistic. There is little or no room for mistakes. For more information about "should thinking," see the section "Perfectionism" in chapter 11, Personality Styles That Perpetuate Anxiety.

*Labeling.* A more extreme form of overgeneralization. If you make a simple mistake, you attach a label to yourself, such as "I'm a loser." Conversely, if you find you're upset by someone else's behavior, you apply a label to them, such as "loser," 'idiot," or even some obscene label.

*Personalization.* An excessive tendency to take another person's words or actions highly personally. Or you arbitrarily conclude that something that went wrong was entirely your fault, when, objectively, there is no basis for concluding whether you or the other person was at fault.

In his later work, Burns also mentions the following two types of cognitive distortions, bringing the total to twelve.

*Control fallacy.* The mistaken notion that you should have complete control over a situation that doesn't allow for total control.

*Blaming.* Holding someone else responsible for your own self-induced emotional pain. Alternatively, you may blame yourself for something, even when it's clearly out of your control.

As mentioned, the above list of cognitive distortions is highly abbreviated. For much more detailed information on identifying, understanding, and working with cognitive distortions, see the book *Cognitive Therapy and the Emotional Disorders* by Aaron Beck or *Feeling Good* by David Burns (see "Further Reading" at the end of this chapter). For quick reference, do a Google search of the term "cognitive distortions." You will find several websites that describe Beck and Burns's original ten cognitive distortions (the utilization of which came to be called "cognitive therapy") and other websites that propose still other types of distorted thinking.

# Summary: Guidelines for Identifying and Countering Self-Talk

Negative self-talk is nothing more than an accumulation of self-limiting mental habits. You can begin to break these habits by noticing occasions when you engage in unconstructive dialogues with yourself and then countering them, preferably in writing, with more positive, rational statements. It took repetition over many years to internalize your habits of negative self-talk; it will likewise take repetition and practice to learn more constructive and helpful ways of thinking.

Follow the steps below:

1. ***Notice.*** "Catch yourself in the act" of engaging in negative self-talk. Be aware of situations that are likely to be precipitated or aggravated by negative self-talk:

- *Any occasion when you're feeling anxious, including the onset of a panic attack* (watch for the Worrier and its tendency for overestimating and catastrophizing)

- *When you anticipate having to face a difficult task or a phobic situation* (again, the Worrier, overestimating, and catastrophizing can play a large role)

- *Occasions when you've made some kind of mistake and feel critical of yourself* (watch for the Critic and overuse of "should statements")

- *Occasions when you're feeling depressed or discouraged* (watch for the Victim, overestimating, catastrophizing, and underestimating your ability to cope)

- *Situations where you're angry at yourself or others* (watch for the Critic, the Perfectionist, and the words "should" or "must")

- *Situations where you feel guilty, ashamed, or embarrassed* (watch especially for the Perfectionist and the words "should" or "must")

2. ***Stop.*** Ask yourself any or all of the following questions:

    "What am I telling myself that is making me feel this way?"

    "Do I really want to do this to myself?"

    "Do I really want to stay upset?"

    If the answer to the last two questions is no, proceed to step 3.

    Realize that sometimes your answers may actually be yes. You may actually wish to continue to be upset rather than change your underlying self-talk. Often this is because you're having strong feelings that you haven't allowed yourself to fully express. It's common to stay anxious, angry, or depressed for a period of time when there are strong feelings that you haven't fully acknowledged—let alone expressed.

    If you're feeling too upset to easily undertake the task of identifying and countering self-talk, give yourself the opportunity to acknowledge and express your feelings. If there's no one available to share them with, try writing them down in a journal. When you've calmed down and are ready to relax, proceed with the steps below. (See chapter 13 for more guidelines and strategies regarding your feelings.)

    Another reason you may maintain your anxiety is because you perceive a strong need to "keep everything under control." Often you're overestimating some danger or preparing for an imagined catastrophe—and so staying tense and vigilant is the way in which you give yourself a sense of control. Your vigilance is validated by the feeling of control it gives you. Unfortunately, in the process you can make yourself more and more tense, until you reach a point where your mind seems to race out of control and you dwell on danger and catastrophe almost to the exclusion of anything else. This, in turn, leads to more anxiety and tension. The only way out of this vicious circle is to let go and relax. The next step, relaxation, is crucial for you to be able to slow down your mind and sort out patterns of negative self-talk.

3.  ***Relax.*** Disrupt your train of negative thoughts by taking some deep abdominal breaths or using relaxing visualizations. The point is to *let go, slow yourself down,* and *relax.* Negative self-talk is so rapid, automatic, and subtle that it can escape detection if you're feeling tense, speeded up, and unable to slow down. You'll find it difficult to recognize and undo such self-talk by merely thinking about it: it's very helpful to physically relax first. In extreme cases, it may take as long as fifteen to twenty minutes of relaxation, using breathing, progressive muscle relaxation, or meditation, to slow yourself down enough so that you can identify what you've been telling yourself. If you're not excessively wound up, you can probably do this step in a minute or two.

4.  ***Write down*** the negative self-talk or inner dialogue that led you to feel anxious, upset, or depressed. It's often difficult to decipher what you're telling yourself by merely reflecting on it. The act of writing things down will help clarify what specific statements you actually made to yourself. Use the *Subpersonality Worksheet(s)* or the *Countering Self-Talk Worksheet* to write down your unhelpful self-talk.

    This step may take some practice to learn. *It's important in identifying self-talk to be able to disentangle thoughts from feelings.* One way to do this is to write down just the feelings first and then uncover the thoughts that led to them. As a general rule, feeling statements contain words expressing emotions, such as "scared," "hurt," and "sad," while self-talk statements do not contain such words. For example, the statement "I feel stupid and irresponsible" is one in which thoughts and feelings are entangled. It can be broken down into a particular feeling ("I feel upset" or "I feel disappointed") and the thoughts (or self-talk) that logically produce such feelings ("I'm stupid" or "I'm irresponsible").

    To give another example, the statement "I'm too scared to undertake this" mixes a feeling of fear with one or more thoughts. It can be broken down into the feeling ("I'm scared"), which arises from the negative self-statement ("This is unmanageable" or "I can't undertake this"). You can ask yourself first, "What was I feeling?" and then ask, "What thoughts were going through my mind to cause me to feel the way I did?"

    Always keep in mind that *self-talk consists of thoughts, not feelings.* Most of the time these thoughts are judgments or appraisals of a situation or of yourself. The feelings are emotional reactions that *result* from these judgments and appraisals.

5.  ***Identify the type*** of negative self-talk you engaged in. (Is it from the Worrier, the Critic, the Victim, or the Perfectionist?) In what way does it include overestimating, catastrophizing, or underestimating your ability to cope? Also, after taking some time to familiarize yourself with them, you may want to look for any *cognitive distortions* that were present. Cognitive distortions are the basis of what was originally called "cognitive therapy" (which preceded the more modern-day "cognitive behavioral therapy"). You can do a Google search of the term "cognitive distortions" to learn more about distortions in thinking such as overgeneralizing, all-or-nothing thinking, or emotional reasoning (only a list of these distortions was provided in this chapter for reasons of space). After doing this for a while, you'll become aware of the particular types of negative inner dialogue (as well particular types of cognitive distortions) you're especially prone to use. With practice, you'll identify them more quickly as they come up.

6.  *Counter*—that is, answer or dispute—your negative self-talk with positive, rational, self-supportive statements. Answer each negative statement you've written by *writing down* an opposing, positive statement. These counterstatements should be worded so that they avoid negatives and are in the present tense and first person. They should also be *believable* and *feel good* to you (in other words, you should feel comfortable with them).

In many cases, you'll find it helpful to question and refute your negative statements with the Socratic questions enumerated earlier in this chapter.

In other instances, you may imagine a positive counterstatement immediately, without going through a process of rational questioning. This is fine, so long as you have some degree of belief in your counterstatement.

## Disrupting Negative Self-Talk: Short Form

Using worksheets such as the *Subpersonality Worksheets* and the *Countering Self-Talk Worksheet* will go a long way to help you overcome long-established mental habits that produce anxiety, depression, and low self-esteem. In many situations, however, you may have neither the time nor the opportunity to write down negative self-talk and positive counterstatements. Follow the three steps below whenever you wish to quickly *disrupt* a negative train of thought "on the spot."

1.  *Notice that you are engaging in negative self-talk.* The best time to catch yourself involved in negative inner dialogue is when you are feeling anxious, depressed, self-critical, or upset in general.

2.  *Stop.* Ask yourself any or all of the following questions:

    *"What am I telling myself that is making me feel this way?"*

    *"Do I really want to do this to myself?"*

    *"Do I really want to stay upset?"*

3.  *Relax and engage in some other activity.* In order to break a train of negative self-talk, you need to switch gears. This can be accomplished by slowing yourself down with deep, abdominal breathing *or* by finding some other activity in which you can immerse yourself. Often doing something *physical* (such as exercise, dancing, or household chores) will have the greatest power to supplant negative thinking because it moves you out of your head and into your body. Other coping tactics include engaging in conversation, reading, hobbies and games, relaxation recordings, and music. The purpose of this section is to suggest a quick, convenient method for disrupting negative self-talk "on the spot." It is *not* intended as a substitute for working out and writing down counterstatements that challenge specific negative self-talk you have identified. Only by using the latter approach and practicing over a period of a few weeks can you begin to effectively change your life-long habits of negative thinking that arise from the subpersonalities and cognitive errors described in this chapter.

# Summary of Things to Do

1.  Reread the section "Some Basic Points About Self-Talk" to reinforce your understanding of the automatic nature of self-talk and its role in maintaining both phobias and panic attacks.

2.  Familiarize yourself with the four subpersonalities that contribute to much of your negative self-talk: the Worrier, the Critic, the Victim, and the Perfectionist. Determine their role in your daily life by completing the worksheet for each subpersonality. Then take the time to counter the negative self-talk of each subpersonality (for relevant areas in your life, such as work, relationships, or specific phobias) with *positive counterstatements*. Write down and read over your lists of positive counterstatements on a regular basis for at least one, if not several, weeks. Or, you can record them on your smartphone so that you can listen to them first thing in the morning or while going to sleep at night. It is best to listen to them while you're relaxed, but not sleepy.

3.  Make a list of all your phobias and other specific fears, then rank them from the most to least bothersome. Complete the *Countering Self-Talk Worksheet* for each of your most difficult phobias, fears, or topics of worry. For each one, write down any overestimating or catastrophic thoughts that keep the fear going. Then refute these negative thoughts with more reasonable and positive counterstatements. Finally, write down ways in which you would cope if what you feared were actually to come about. (Remember to duplicate the worksheet so you have as many copies as you need to address all of your phobias.)

4.  Use the "short form" of disrupting negative self-talk when you want to quickly divert yourself from a train of negative thinking. Remember, this is not a substitute for doing the exercises in 2 and 3 above.

# Further Reading

Barlow, David, and Michelle Craske. *Mastery of Your Anxiety and Panic: Workbook.* 4th ed. New York: Oxford University Press, 2006.

Beck, Aaron T. *Cognitive Therapy and the Emotional Disorders.* New York: Meridian, 1979.

———, and Gary Emery. *Anxiety Disorders and Phobias: A Cognitive Perspective.* 20th anniversary ed. New York: Basic Books, 2005. (This book is primarily intended for helping professionals.)

Burns, David. *Feeling Good.* New York: HarperCollins, 1980. (The classic popular book on cognitive distortions.)

———. *Feeling Good.* New York: HarperCollins, 2008. (A revised and updated version of the classic book.)

Helmstetter, Shad. *What to Say When You Talk to Yourself.* Updated ed. New York: Gallery Books, 2017. (This book is timely and easy to read.)

McKay, Matthew, Martha Davis, and Patrick Fanning. *Thoughts & Feelings: Taking Control of Your Moods & Your Life.* 4th ed. Oakland, CA: New Harbinger Publications, 2011.

———, and Patrick Fanning. *Self-Esteem.* 4th ed. Oakland, CA: New Harbinger Publications, 2016.

Wilson, Reid. *Don't Panic: Taking Control of Anxiety Attacks.* 3rd ed. New York: HarperPerennial, 2009.

# 9

# Mistaken Beliefs

By now you may have asked, "Where does negative self-talk come from?" In most cases, it's possible to trace negative thinking back to deeper-lying beliefs or assumptions about ourselves, others, and life in general. These basic assumptions have been variously called "scripts," "core beliefs," "life decisions," "fallacious beliefs," or "mistaken beliefs." While growing up, we learned them from our parents, teachers, and peers, as well as from the larger society around us. These beliefs are typically so basic to our thinking that we do not recognize them as *beliefs* at all—we just take them for granted and assume them to reflect reality. Examples of mistaken beliefs that you might hold are "I'm powerless," "Life is a struggle," or "I should always look good and act nice, no matter how I feel." There is nothing new about the idea of mistaken beliefs—they are a part of what people have in mind when they refer to your "attitude" or "outlook."

Mistaken beliefs are at the root of much of the anxiety you experience. As discussed in the preceding chapter, you talk yourself into much of your anxiety by anticipating the worst (what-if thinking), putting yourself down (self-critical thinking), and pushing yourself to meet unreasonable demands and expectations (perfectionist thinking). Underlying these destructive patterns of self-talk are some basic false assumptions about yourself and "the way life is."

You could save yourself quite a bit of worrying, for example, if you let go of the basic assumption, "I must worry about a problem before there's any chance it will go away." Similarly, you would feel more confident and secure if you discarded the mistaken belief "I'm a failure unless I succeed" or "I'm nothing unless others love and approve of me." Once again, life would be less stressful and tense if you would let go of the belief "I must do it perfectly or it's not worth bothering to try." You can go a long way toward creating a less anxious way of life by working on changing the basic assumptions that tend to perpetuate anxiety.

Mistaken beliefs often keep you from achieving your most important goals in life. You might ask yourself right now, "What is it that I really want out of life? What would I attempt to do if I knew I could not fail?" Take a few minutes to seriously reflect on this and write your answer in the space below. (Use a separate sheet of paper if you need more room.)

Now, if you don't yet have what you want, ask yourself the simple question, "Why not?" List what reasons you can come up with in the space below or write them on another sheet of paper.

In the process of doing the above exercise, you may have discovered certain beliefs or assumptions that have been holding you back. Are these assumptions truly valid? Examples of assumptions that people hold themselves back with might include "I can't afford to have what I want," "I don't have the time to go back to school and study the subject that interests me," or "I don't have the talent to succeed." At a more unconscious level, you might even feel "I don't deserve to have what I truly want." None of these ideas necessarily reflects the true nature of reality—they all involve assumptions that might well turn out to be false if actually tested. Often you don't realize how such assumptions are affecting your behavior until someone else points it out to you.

Mistaken beliefs often set limits on your self-esteem and self-worth. Many such beliefs involve the idea that your self-worth depends on something outside yourself, such as social status, wealth, material possessions, the love of another person, or social approval in general. If you don't have these things, somehow you believe that you are not worth much. The belief that "Success is everything" or "My worth depends on what I accomplish" places the basis of your self-esteem outside of you. So does the belief "I'm nothing unless I'm loved (or approved of)."

The truth that takes some people a long time to realize is that self-worth is *inherent*. You have an essential value, worth, and dignity just by virtue of the fact that you're a human being. You have many qualities and talents, regardless of your outer accomplishments or the approval of others. Without thinking, we respect the inherent value of dogs and cats as animals. So, too, human beings have inherent value *just as they are*, apart from what they accomplish, what they possess, or whose approval they enjoy. As you grow in self-esteem, you can *learn* to respect and believe in yourself apart from what you have accomplished and without relying on others for your good feelings (or making others reliant on you).

## Examples of Mistaken Beliefs

There are innumerable mistaken beliefs. You have your own collection as a result of what you learned from your parents, teachers, and peers during childhood and adolescence. Sometimes you take on a false belief directly from your parents, such as when you are told, "Big boys don't cry" or "Nice girls don't get angry." At other times, you develop an attitude about yourself as a result of being frequently criticized (thus "I'm worthless"), ignored (thus "My needs don't matter"), or rejected (thus "I'm unlovable") over many years. The unfortunate thing is that you may live out these mistaken attitudes to the point where you act in ways—and get others to treat you in ways—that confirm them. Like computers, people can be "preprogrammed," and the mistaken beliefs of childhood can become self-fulfilling prophecies.

Below are some examples of fairly common mistaken beliefs that tend to influence many people. Following each are counterstatements that replace the negative belief with a positive one, much in the way negative self-talk was countered by positive self-statements in the preceding chapter. Positive statements that can be used to counter mistaken beliefs are often known as *affirmations*.

- I'm powerless. I'm a victim of outside circumstances.

  *I'm responsible and in control of my life. Circumstances are what they are, but I can determine my attitude toward them.*

- Life is a struggle. Something must be wrong if life seems too easy, pleasurable, or fun.

  *Life is full and pleasurable. It's okay for me to relax and have fun. Life is an adventure—and I'm learning to accept both the ups and the downs.*

- If I take a risk, I'll fail. If I fail, others will reject me.

  *It's okay for me to take risks. It's okay to fail—I can learn a lot from every mistake. It's okay for me to be a success.*

- I'm unimportant. My feelings and needs are unimportant.

  *I am a valuable and unique person. I deserve to have my feelings and needs taken care of as much as anyone else.*

- I always should look good and act nice, no matter how I feel.

  *It's okay simply to be myself.*

- If I worry enough, this problem should get better or go away.

  *Worrying has no effect on solving problems; taking action does.*

- I can't cope with difficult or scary situations.

  *I can learn to handle any scary situation if I approach it slowly, in small enough steps.*

- The outside world is dangerous. There is safety only in what is known and familiar.

  *I can learn to become more comfortable with the world outside. I look forward to new opportunities for learning and growth that the outside world can offer.*

Just *recognizing* your own particular mistaken beliefs is the first and most important step toward letting go of them. The second step is to develop a positive affirmation to counter each mistaken belief and continue to impress it on your mind until you are "deprogrammed."

What follows is a questionnaire that will help you identify some of your own mistaken beliefs. Rate each statement on a 1 to 4 scale, according to how much you think it influences your feelings and behavior. Then go back and check off the beliefs you rated 3 or 4.

# Mistaken Beliefs Questionnaire

How much does each of these unconstructive beliefs influence your feelings and behavior? Take your time to reflect about each belief.

1 = Not at all      3 = Strongly/frequently
2 = Somewhat/sometimes      4 = Very strongly

Place the appropriate number after each statement:

1. I feel powerless or helpless.

2. Often I feel like a victim of outside circumstances.

3. I don't have the money to do what I really want.

4. There is seldom enough time to do what I want.

5. Life is very difficult—it's a struggle.

6. If things are going well, watch out!

7. I feel unworthy. I feel that I'm not good enough.

8. Often I feel that I don't deserve to be successful or happy.

9. Often I feel a sense of defeat and resignation, a sense of "Why bother?"

10. My condition seems hopeless.

11. There is something fundamentally wrong with me.

12. I feel ashamed of my condition.

13. If I take risks to get better, I'm afraid I'll fail.

14. If I take risks to get better, I'm afraid I'll succeed.

15. If I recover fully, I might have to deal with realities I'd rather not face.

16. I feel like I'm nothing (or can't make it) unless I'm loved.

17. I can't stand being separated from others.

18. If a person I love doesn't love me in return, I feel like it's my fault.

19. It's very hard to be alone.

20. What others think of me is very important.

21. I feel personally threatened when criticized.

22. It's important to please others.

23. People won't like me if they see who I really am.

24. I need to keep up a front or others will see my weaknesses.

25. I have to achieve or produce something significant in order to feel okay about myself.

26. My accomplishments at work/school are extremely important.

27. Success is everything.

28. I have to be the best at what I do.

29. I have to be somebody—somebody outstanding.

30. To fail is terrible.

31. I can't rely on others for help.

32. I can't receive from others.

33. If I let someone get too close, I'm afraid of being controlled.

34. I can't tolerate being out of control.

35. I'm the only one who can solve my problems.

36. I should always be very generous and unselfish.

37. I should be the *perfect...* (Rate each below.)

    - employee    - professional

    - spouse      - parent

    - lover       - friend

    - student     - son/daughter

38. I should be able to endure any hardship.

39. I should be able to find a quick solution to every problem.

40. I should never be tired or fatigued.

41. I should always be efficient.

42. I should always be competent.

43. I should always be able to foresee everything.

44. I should never be angry or irritable. Or, I don't like (or am afraid of) anger.

45. I should always be pleasant or nice, no matter how I feel.

46. I often feel... (Rate each below.)

    - ugly            - inferior or defective

    - unintelligent   - guilty or ashamed

47. I'm just the way I am—I can't really change.

48. The world outside is a dangerous place.

49. Unless you worry about a problem, it just gets worse.

50. It's risky to trust people.

51. My problems will go away on their own with time.

52. I feel anxious about making mistakes.

53. I demand perfection of myself.

54. If I didn't have my safe person (or safe place), I'm afraid I couldn't cope.

55. If I stop worrying, I'm afraid something bad will happen.

56. I'm afraid to face the world out there on my own.

57. My self-worth isn't a given—it has to be earned.

You may have noticed that some of the beliefs on the questionnaire fall into specific groups, each of which reflects a very basic belief or attitude toward life.[1] Go back over your answers and see how you scored with respect to each of the groups of beliefs listed below.

Add up your scores for each of the following subgroups of beliefs. If your total score on the items in a particular subgroup exceeds the criterion value, then this is likely to be a problem area for you. It's important that you give this subgroup special attention when you begin to work with affirmations to start changing your mistaken beliefs.

| If your total score for questions 1, 2, 7, 9, 10, 11 is over 15: | You likely believe that you are powerless, have little or no control over outside circumstances, or are unable to do much that could help your situation. In sum, "I'm powerless" or "I can't do much about my life." |
|---|---|
| If your total score for questions 16, 17, 18, 19, 54, 56 is over 15: | You likely believe that your self-worth is dependent on the love of someone else. You feel that you need another's (or others') love to feel okay about yourself and to cope. In sum, "My worth and security are dependent on being loved." |
| If your total score for questions 20, 21, 22, 23, 24, 45 is over 15: | You likely believe that your self-worth is dependent on others' approval. Being pleasing and getting acceptance from others is very important for your sense of security and your sense of who you are. In sum, "My worth and security depend on the approval of others." |
| If your total score for questions 25, 26, 27, 28, 29, 30, 41, 42 is over 20: | You likely believe that your self-worth is dependent on external achievements, such as school or career performance, status, or wealth. In sum, "My worth is dependent on my performance or achievements." |
| If your total score for questions 31, 32, 33, 34, 35, 50 is over 15: | You likely believe that you can't trust, rely on, or receive help from others. You may have a tendency to keep a distance from people and avoid intimacy for fear of losing control. In sum, "If I trust or get too close, I'll lose control." |
| If your total score for questions 37, 38, 39, 40, 52, 53 is over 25: | You likely believe that you have to be perfect in some or many areas of life. You make excessive demands on yourself. There is no room for mistakes. In sum, "I have to be perfect" or "It's not okay to make mistakes." |

---

1   The idea for defining subgroups of beliefs was adapted from David Burns, MD, *Feeling Good*. See his book for further details on how to counter and work with mistaken beliefs.

# Countering Mistaken Beliefs

Now that you have an idea of those mistaken beliefs that have the greatest impact on you, how do you go about changing them? The first step is to ask yourself this question: *How strongly do I believe in them?* There are three possible ways to view a mistaken belief:

- You don't really believe it. The belief is simply a conditioned habit that you are ready to give up. You recognize the uselessness of the belief *and* you realize that it has no strong emotional hold on you. If that is the case, you are ready to develop a positive affirmation to counter the belief. You can proceed directly to the section "Guidelines for Constructing Affirmations" and follow the suggested steps for developing affirmations to counter a particular belief. You may also want to see the section "Examples of Affirmations" at the end of the chapter to get ideas for specific alternatives to any of the beliefs on the *Mistaken Beliefs Questionnaire*.

- You don't really subscribe to the belief on an intellectual level, but it still has an emotional grip on you and influences the way you act. You *don't want to believe* that "it's always important to be pleasing to others," for example, but you find that you continue to feel and act as if it were true. It's hard to "get the belief out of your system." If that is the case, it's important to subject the belief to questions 5 and 6 in the section "Six Questions for Challenging Mistaken Beliefs." Identify any belief you rated 3 or 4 that still affects you despite your intellectual doubts. Then use questions 5 and 6 to examine whether the belief is beneficial to your well-being and whether it developed out of your own choice or from your family history.

- You may really have faith in a particular belief. You're not convinced that it's inaccurate; you'll need some persuading before you'll consider giving it up. The idea of substituting a positive affirmation in place of an attitude you've long believed in seems superficial or naively optimistic. If that is the case, it's important to subject the belief to questions 1, 2, and 3 under "Six Questions for Challenging Mistaken Beliefs" listed below. These first three questions are taken from the Socratic questions described in chapter 8 and are especially useful for challenging a mistaken belief on a strictly logical level. If you discredit your belief on purely rational grounds, then proceed to questions 4, 5, and 6. These questions will enable you to see how the belief affects your personal well-being and to determine whether it's your own belief or was acquired— perhaps from your parents, or in some other way.

# Six Questions for Challenging Mistaken Beliefs

1. What is the evidence for this belief? Looking objectively at all of your life experience, what is the evidence that this is true?

2. Does this belief *invariably* or *always* hold true for you?

3.  Does this belief look at the whole picture? Does it take into account both positive and negative ramifications?

4.  Is this belief consistent with your personal values? To explore your values, consult the *Personal Values Inventory* in chapter 21, Personal Meaning.

5.  Does this belief promote your well-being and/or peace of mind?

6.  Did you choose this belief on your own or did it develop out of your experience of growing up in your family?

A few words need to be said about this last question. Many of your mistaken beliefs were likely acquired from your family while you were growing up. There are at least two ways this could happen. First, one or both of your parents may have held the belief and you simply learned it from them. For example, beliefs such as "The world outside is a dangerous place" or "It's risky to trust people" might have been attitudes held by your parents that you adopted wholesale, because no alternative views were presented to you as a child.

The other way you might have acquired a mistaken belief is as a *reaction to what happened* and/or *the way you were treated* as a child. For example, if your father died and then your mother went to work when you were five years old, you may have felt abandoned and developed the belief that "Being alone means being abandoned and unloved." Or if your parents expected you to achieve and criticized your mistakes and performance at school, your reaction would likely involve developing such beliefs as "My accomplishments are extremely important" and "It's not okay to make mistakes."

It's often helpful in the process of evaluating mistaken beliefs to see how they arose from unfortunate or dysfunctional circumstances during childhood. While such beliefs may have helped you survive as a child, *they have long lost their usefulness and only serve to create anxiety or stress for you now.* To investigate connections between your childhood and mistaken beliefs, refer to the section "Childhood Circumstances" in chapter 2, and complete the *Family Background Questionnaire* if you haven't done so already. You may also find it helpful to look at the section "Some Causes of Low Self-Esteem" in chapter 15 to get a clearer idea of the various types of dysfunctional childhood situations that can provide the basis for developing mistaken beliefs.

## Examples

The following examples illustrate the application of the above questions in challenging mistaken beliefs.

**Mistaken Belief:**    "I am powerless or helpless." (Note: When challenging beliefs from the *Mistaken Beliefs Questionnaire*, reword any belief beginning with the words "I feel..." to "I am..." This provides a more direct statement of the belief.)

*Questioning:*    1. "What is the evidence for this?"

2. "Is this *always* true for me?"

5. "Does this belief promote my well-being?"

*Counterarguments:*   1. "What is the evidence for this?"

"Though I often *feel* powerless or helpless, that doesn't necessarily mean that I *am* powerless or helpless." Recognize that the mistaken belief is an example of an attitude typically held by the Victim subpersonality described in chapter 8. It is also an example of the cognitive distortion "emotional reasoning," described in the section "Other Types of Distorted Thinking (Cognitive Distortions)" in chapter 8. "After all, I can work on mastering the strategies in this workbook and can consult a therapist specializing in anxiety disorders to help me overcome my condition. Also, I have the support of my family and friends who are backing me all the way. Thus, there is no strong evidence that I'm either powerless or helpless."

2. "Is this *always* true for me?"

"Some days I certainly *feel* powerless or helpless, but other days I feel more capable and optimistic. It's just not true that I *always* feel that way."

5. "Does this belief promote my well-being?"

"Believing that I'm powerless and helpless is destructive to developing confidence in myself and hope for recovery. Such a belief definitely does not promote my well-being or peace of mind."

*Affirmations:*   *I believe in myself.*

*I trust I have the capacity to overcome my problem with anxiety.*

**Mistaken Belief:**   "It's very important to please others."

*Questioning:*   2. "Is this *always* true for me?"

5. "Does this belief promote my well-being?"

6. "Did I choose this belief on my own, or did it develop from my childhood?"

*Counterarguments:*   2. "Is this *always* true for me?"

"Certainly there are some situations where it's helpful to come across in a pleasing manner. If I'm interviewing for a job, going out on a first date, comforting my friend, or hosting a party, I generally *want* to be pleasing. On the other hand, if I'm feeling exhausted or upset and need support from my partner or friends, it serves me better to ask them to be there for me rather than to have to deny my needs and keep up a pleasing front. In short, it's sometimes *more* important to attend to my own feelings."

5. "Does this belief promote my well-being?"

"In some situations, probably yes. I feel good about myself if I can be pleasant in situations where to come across as such might be appropriate. However, it doesn't serve me to try to be pleasing when I'm actually feeling upset or ill. I'll be more honest and in tune with myself to let people know what I'm feeling and ask for their support."

6. "Did I choose this belief on my own, or did it develop from my childhood?"

"My mother was ill and frequently complained during much of my childhood. I felt I always had to be on guard to protect her from my own problems. It seemed that I had to be pleasing to maintain her approval. No wonder I grew up to be such a people pleaser! I guess that I didn't freely choose this belief, but rather it was imposed on me by the circumstances of my childhood."

*Affirmations:*    *It's okay to not always be pleasing.*

*I can enjoy being pleasing at those times when I genuinely feel like it.*

**Mistaken Belief:**    "My accomplishments at work/school are very important."

*Questioning:*    2. "Is this belief *always* true?"

3. "Does this belief look at the whole picture?"

5. "Does this belief promote my well-being?"

6. "Did I choose this belief on my own, or did it develop from my childhood?"

*Counterarguments:*    2. "Is this belief *always* true?"

"No, in as much as other areas of my life (health, relationships, leisure time, creative pursuits) are also important. Accomplishing things at school or work is certainly important, but it's not *always important twenty-four hours a day, seven days a week.*"

3. "Does this belief look at the whole picture?"

"It's true that what I accomplish at school or work is important. I need to maintain a certain level of competence in school in order to earn the degree that will help me find a job." (Or "I need to maintain a certain level of performance at work to hold my job.") "But is it looking at the whole picture to regard my accomplishments as *supremely* important? If that were the case, they would be more important than my health, my peace of mind, my family, and everything else I value. Such an attitude would lead to an imbalanced and ultimately unhealthy lifestyle—a lifestyle where nothing else mattered except my success and accomplishments. Thus it's unreasonable to believe that my accomplishments are supremely important."

5. "Does this belief promote my well-being?"

"For reasons already mentioned, I recognize that an *exclusive* focus on accomplishments is unhealthy."

6. "Did I choose this belief on my own, or did it develop from my childhood?"

"My parents were both professionals who were successful in their careers and expected me to follow their example. I always had to do well in school to receive their approval and was criticized for any grade below an A. My attitude that achievement is so important came in large part from living with them—I didn't freely choose it."

*Affirmations:*      *My accomplishments are important and so are other things in my life.*

*I am learning how to balance work and play in my life.*

The above examples can serve as guidelines for challenging your own mistaken beliefs. If there is little evidence for a particular belief, if it is not always true, or if it doesn't promote your personal well-being, then it is most likely mistaken. If the belief was acquired out of dysfunctional family circumstances rather than freely chosen by you as an adult, it is equally likely to be mistaken. It is important to go through such a process of questioning if you feel at all attached to any particular belief.

Once you've completed the process of challenging all of those mistaken beliefs you rated 3 or 4, you're ready to develop positive affirmations to counter each one of them. The next section explains how to construct affirmations. Although it's preferable to develop your own affirmations, you can refer to the examples at the end of the chapter if you need help creating an affirmation for a particular mistaken belief.

After you've developed your affirmations, go back to the *Mistaken Beliefs Questionnaire* and write each affirmation in capital letters next to or under the particular mistaken belief it is intended to counter. (Refer to the examples of mistaken beliefs and affirmations earlier in this chapter.)

The process of countering mistaken beliefs with affirmations is very similar to that of countering negative self-talk with positive self-statements, which was described in chapter 8. The difference is that affirmations are very compact statements that you can easily rehearse (not unlike the coping statements for panic attacks listed in chapter 6). Writing affirmations repetitively on paper or listening to them repetitively on a recording can, with persistence, actually result in their supplanting unwanted mistaken beliefs in your mind. In the chapter on self-talk, the important process to master was "countering." By continually writing out counterstatements to negative self-talk, you eventually develop a *habit* of noticing and countering the anxiety-provoking thoughts you tell yourself. In this chapter, the important process is working with affirmations. This will actually change the core beliefs that underlie your negative self-talk.

## Guidelines for Constructing Affirmations

- An affirmation should be *short, simple, direct,* and usually in the *first person.* "I believe in myself" is preferable to "There are a lot of good qualities I have that I believe in."

- Keep affirmations in the *present tense* ("I am prosperous") or *present progressive tense* ("I am becoming prosperous"). Telling yourself that some change you desire will happen in the future always keeps it one step removed.

- Try to *avoid negatives.* Instead of saying, "I'm no longer afraid of public speaking," try "I'm free of fear about public speaking" or "I'm becoming fearless about public speaking." Similarly, instead of the negative statement "I'm not perfect," try "It's okay to be less than perfect" or "It's okay to make mistakes." Your unconscious mind is incapable of making the distinction between a positive and a negative statement. It can turn a negative statement, such as "I'm not afraid," into a positive statement that you don't want to affirm—that is, "I'm afraid."

- Start with a direct *declaration* of a positive change you want to make in your life ("I am making more time for myself every day"). If this feels a little too strong for you just yet, try changing it to "I am willing to make more time for myself." *Willingness* to change is the first step you need to take in order to actually make any substantial change in your life. A second alternative to a direct declaration is to affirm that you are *becoming* something or *learning* to do something. If you're not quite ready for a direct statement, such as "I'm strong, confident, and secure," you can affirm, "I am becoming strong, confident, and secure." Again, if you're not ready for "I face my fears willingly," try "I'm learning to face my fears."

- It's important that you have *some* belief in—or at least a willingness to believe in—your affirmations. It's by no means necessary, however, to believe in an affirmation 100 percent when you first start out. The whole point is to shift your beliefs and attitudes in favor of the affirmation.

## Ways to Work with Affirmations

Once you have made a list of affirmations, decide on a few that you would like to work with. In general, it's a good idea to work on only two or three at a time, unless you choose to make a recording containing all of them. Some of the more helpful ways you can utilize affirmations are listed below:

- *Write an affirmation repetitively,* about five or ten times every day, for a week or two. Each time you doubt your belief in the affirmation, write down your doubt on the reverse side of the paper. As you continue to write an affirmation over and over, giving yourself the opportunity to express any doubts, you'll find that your willingness to believe it increases. Here is an example:

| *Affirmation* | *Doubt* |
|---|---|
| "I'm learning to be fine by myself." | "Yes, for a few hours, but how will I ever manage for a whole day?" |
| "I'm learning to be fine by myself." | "What if I panic and no one is around?" |
| "I'm learning to be fine by myself." | "I'm not sure I'll be able to do this." |
| "I'm learning to be fine by myself." | |

Later, go back and counter your doubts one by one with positive statements. In the example above, the three doubts might be countered by the following three affirmations:

"Gradually, I can learn to extend the time I'm okay being alone to an entire day."

"If I panic while I'm alone, I can do abdominal breathing, go with the feeling, or call _____."

"If I break this down into small enough steps, I know I can do it."

- *Write your affirmation in giant letters* with a magic marker on a blank sheet of paper (the words should be visible from at least twenty feet away). Then attach the sheet to your bathroom mirror, your refrigerator, or some other conspicuous place in your home. Constantly seeing the affirmation day in and day out, whether or not you actively attend to it, will help to reinforce it in your mind.

- *Record a series of affirmations.* If you develop twenty or so affirmations to counter statements on the *Mistaken Beliefs Questionnaire*, you may wish to put all of them on a recording. You can either use your own voice or have someone else do the recording. Affirmations are best done in the first person because they are direct declarations about your personal beliefs, attitudes, or actions that you intend to do. Also, as you practice your list of affirmations, allow five to ten seconds between each successive affirmation so that it has time to sink in. Listening to the recording once a day for two or three weeks can lead to a major shift in your thinking and the way you feel about yourself. It's okay to play the recording at any time, even while cleaning the house or taking a shower. However, you can expedite the process by giving the recording your full attention in a very relaxed state when you've slowed yourself down enough to deeply feel each affirmation.

- *Take a single affirmation with you into meditation.* Repeating an affirmation slowly and with conviction while in a deep meditative state is a very powerful way of incorporating it into your consciousness. Meditation is a state in which you can experience yourself as a "whole being." Whatever you affirm or declare with your whole being will have the strongest tendency to come true.

# Increasing the Power of an Affirmation

There are two fundamental ways of reinforcing an affirmation or any new habit of thinking—*repetition* and *feeling*.

*Repetition*     It took repetition to "program" mistaken beliefs in your mind originally. Being told numerous times by your parents to "shut up" or "behave yourself" reinforced the fallacious belief "I'm unworthy" or "I'm unimportant." By the same token, repeated exposure to a positive affirmation can help instill it in your mind until it replaces the original, false belief.

*Feeling*     Saying affirmations with deep conviction and feeling is the *most* powerful method, in my opinion, for strengthening them. Getting a new belief *into your heart*—as well as into your head—will give it the greatest power and efficacy. A good way to do this is to attain a state of relaxation first (through progressive muscle relaxation or meditation) and then to say the affirmation slowly, with feeling and a sense of conviction. It has been said before that what you believe in with your whole heart becomes a part of you.

## Active Integration

You can also increase your conviction about an affirmation by keeping track of confirmations of it in real life. Select an affirmation you wish to work on and write it down on a note card. As you go through the day, write down on the other side of the card any event or situation, no matter how minor, that supports the affirmation. Keep this up for two or more weeks and see if you can compile a list of confirmations. For example, if you're working with the affirmation "I can recover by taking small risks at my own pace," then you might list all of your successes in reducing your anxiety and/or confronting phobic situations. Or if you're working with the statement "I'm learning that there is more to life than success in my career (or in school)," you can list all the occasions when you derived enjoyment from other activities to demonstrate the truth of your new belief.

Reinforcing an affirmation by noting real-life events that confirm it will go a long way toward strengthening your conviction of its truth.

# Examples of Affirmations

Below are examples of affirmations you can use to counter statements from the *Mistaken Beliefs Questionnaire*. Each numbered affirmation in this list corresponds to the same numbered mistaken belief in the *Mistaken Beliefs Questionnaire*. Use any that feel right to you, or use them as guidelines for making up your own.

1.   I'm responsible and in control of my life.

2.   Circumstances are what they are, but I can choose my attitude toward them.

3. I am becoming prosperous. I am creating the financial resources I need.

4. I am setting priorities and making time for what is important.

5. Life has its challenges and its satisfactions—I enjoy the adventure of life. Every challenge that comes along is an opportunity to learn and grow.

6. I accept the natural ups and downs of life.

7. I love and accept myself the way I am.

8. I deserve the good things in life as much as anyone else.

9. I am open to discovering new meaning in my life.

10. It's never too late to change. I am improving one step at a time.

11. I am innately healthy, strong, and capable of fully recovering. I am getting better every day.

12. I am committed to overcoming my condition. I am working on recovering from my condition.

13. I can recover by taking small risks at my own pace.

14. I am looking forward to the new freedom and opportunities I'll have when I've fully recovered.

15. Same as example 14.

16. I am learning to love myself.

17. I am learning to be comfortable by myself.

18. If someone doesn't return my love, I let it go and move on.

19. I am learning to be at peace with myself when alone. I am learning how to enjoy myself when alone.

20. I respect and believe in myself apart from others' opinions.

21. I can accept and learn from constructive criticism.

22. I'm learning to be myself around others. It's important to take care of my own needs.

23. It's okay to be myself around others. I'm willing to be myself around others.

24. Same as example 23.

25. I appreciate my achievements, and I'm much more than all of them put together.

26. I am learning how to balance work and play in my life.

27. I am learning that there is more to life than success. The greatest success is living well.

28. I'm a unique and capable person just as I am. I am satisfied doing the best I can.

29. Same as example 28.

30. It's okay to make mistakes. I'm willing to accept my mistakes and learn from them.

31. I'm willing to allow others to help me. I acknowledge my need for other people.

32. I am open to receiving support from others.

33. I am willing to take the risk of getting close to someone.

34. I am learning to relax and let go. I'm learning to accept those things I can't control.

35. I am willing to let others assist me in solving my problems.

36. When I love and care for myself, I am best able to be generous to others.

37. I'm doing the best I can as a _____. (*Optional:* I'm learning new ways to improve.)

38. It's okay to be upset when things go wrong.

39. I'm okay if I don't always have a quick answer to every problem.

40. It's okay to make time to rest and relax.

41. I'm doing the best I can, and I'm satisfied with that.

42. Same as example 41.

43. It's okay if I'm unable to always foresee everything.

44. It's okay to be angry sometimes. I am learning to accept and express my angry feelings appropriately.

45. I'm learning to be honest with others, even when I'm not feeling pleasant or nice.

46. I believe that I am an attractive, intelligent, and valuable person. I am learning to let go of guilt.

47. I believe that I can change. I am willing to change (or grow).

48. The world outside is a place to grow and have fun.

49. Worrying about a problem is the real problem. Doing something about it will make a difference for the better.

50. I am learning (or willing) to trust other people.

51. I'm making a commitment to myself to do what I can to overcome my problem with

   _____.

52. I'm learning that it's okay to make mistakes.

53. Nobody's perfect—and I'm learning (or willing) to go easier on myself.

54. I'm willing to become (or to learn to become) self-sufficient.

55. I'm learning to let go of worrying. I can replace worrying with constructive action.

56. I am learning, one step at a time, that I can deal with the outside world.

57. I'm inherently worthy as a person. I accept myself just the way I am.

The purpose of this chapter has been to increase your awareness about mistaken beliefs and help you identify some of your own. Countering negative self-talk and mistaken beliefs with positive thinking and affirmations can go a long way toward helping you lead a calmer, more balanced, and anxiety-free life. While the earlier chapters on relaxation and exercise were designed to help you overcome the physiological bases of anxiety, the intent of the last two chapters has been to give you tools to deal with that part of anxiety that is in your mind—what you say to yourself and what you believe. Chapter 13 will examine the important relationship between anxiety and feelings.

## Summary of Things to Do

1. Complete the *Mistaken Beliefs Questionnaire*, checking off those beliefs you rated 3 or 4. Note any subgroupings of beliefs where your total score exceeds the criterion value for that group. The theme for that subgroup deserves your special attention.

2. Reread the section "Countering Mistaken Beliefs" until you are thoroughly familiar with various ways to challenge them. Use the "Six Questions for Challenging Mistaken Beliefs" to call into question any belief that has an emotional hold on you or seems intellectually plausible.

3. After challenging your mistaken beliefs, develop affirmations to counter each one of them. Use the "Guidelines for Constructing Affirmations" to assist you, and refer to the section "Examples of Affirmations" at the end of the chapter for a list of examples. On the questionnaire, write each of your affirmations in capital letters underneath the particular mistaken belief you're countering.

4. Reread the section "Ways to Work with Affirmations" and decide which method of rehearsing affirmations you want to use—for example, writing them repetitively, listening to them on a recording, working with a partner, or taking one or two of your affirmations into meditation. Work with this method for two weeks to one month on a daily basis, and afterward whenever you feel the need.

# Further Reading

Bloch, Douglas. *Words That Heal: Affirmations and Meditations for Daily Living.* Portland, OR: Pallas Communications, 1998.

Burns, David. *Feeling Good: The New Mood Therapy.* New York: Harper, 2008.

Handly, Robert, and Pauline Neff. *Anxiety and Panic Attacks: Their Cause and Cure.* New York: Random House, 1987. (Popular book for phobics on how to utilize affirmations and visualization.)

McKay, Matthew, and Patrick Fanning. *Prisoners of Belief.* Oakland, CA: New Harbinger Publications, 1991.

# 10

# Overcoming Worry

Worry often can become a negative spiral that escalates. When you're caught in a spiral of worry, you tend to ruminate on every facet of a perceived danger until your worry eclipses all other thoughts and you feel trapped. Some indications that you are caught in a worry cycle include these:

- Repeatedly making negative predictions about the future

- Overestimating the odds of something threatening or dangerous happening

- Underestimating the odds of your being able to cope in the unlikely event that the source of your worry actually came true

- Trying to stop worrying by suppressing it or distracting yourself in order to flee from it

On a physiological level, unpleasant body symptoms of anxiety (such as sweating, shaking, tight muscles, rapid heartbeat, feeling light-headed or dizzy, among others) are your body's natural response to the experience of your mind spinning out of control.

Because escalating worry tends to dominate your attention, it takes a deliberate act of will to move away from it. This involves not so much an attempt to escape it by distraction, but a deliberate effort at *disrupting* the cycle of worried thoughts. Although deliberately disrupting your worry cycle may be difficult at first, with practice it gets easier.

Please see the section below, "Disrupting Worry," for a variety of methods that can empower you to move out of excessive worry. First, though, it's important to avoid beliefs and actions that only increase your worry.

## What Can Increase Your Worrying

Here are some things you might do, most likely unconsciously, to make your worry worse:

- You repeatedly attempt to talk yourself out of the worry.

- You overthink your worry and argue with yourself about why you shouldn't be worrying. The result simply puts more attention on your worry process.

- You try to suppress the worry. Attempting to suppress your worry almost always results in enlarging it. The old maxim "what you resist persists" applies in this instance.

- You try to obtain complete certainty in a situation that is inherently uncertain or ambiguous. For example, you worry you might panic when you take a flight or go to the dentist's office for a procedure. There is simply *no way to completely ensure* that you won't have an anxiety surge during one of these experiences. The more you seek *certainty about avoiding anxiety* in such a situation, the more you tend to worry about it in advance, a process referred to as *anticipatory anxiety*.

  What is more helpful is to put together a "repertoire" of coping strategies, such as using abdominal breathing, utilizing preferred coping statements, or even relying on a support person (in real life or by phone) to assist with better negotiating the situation. Then you approach the situation with relative degrees of *acceptance* rather than worrying that you could have excessive anxiety.

## Recognizing and Letting Go of Metacognitive Beliefs About Worry

Many people have underlying, hidden beliefs—or what are sometimes called *metacognitive beliefs*—about the nature of worry itself that can further aggravate their issues with excess worrying. Here are some of the most important of these "metabeliefs" about worry:

- *Your thoughts should be completely under your control.* In truth, it is impossible to completely control the stream of thoughts that come into your mind.

- *Worrying enough about something will make it less likely to come true.* In truth, there is an "optimal" amount of worry for any particular situation. If you have an upcoming exam or job interview, not to worry at all about it might lead you to underprepare and be less successful. However, if you overworry about it, your resulting anxiety may not only cause increased suffering but actually interfere with you making your best performance. A little worry can be a good thing; too much—the idea that only by worrying enough will you prevent a problem—can actually aggravate the problem.

- *Worrying about something too much might actually cause it to happen.* This is a common but irrational belief. Looking at things objectively, there is no correlation between the amount of time you spend worrying about something and the odds that your worry will come true. You can worry quite a bit about the threat of an earthquake or a tornado, but it is seismic conditions or the weather that affects the odds, not the amount of your worry.

- *Your excessive worry is an indication that something must be seriously wrong with you.* This is yet another faulty belief. Worrying a lot does not imply you have some physical illness (though having a serious illness might lead to worrying about it). Nor does excessive worrying imply you have a serious psychiatric disorder. One of the hallmarks of serious psychiatric disorders (such as schizophrenia or bipolar disorder) is that you are out of touch with reality. In worrying too much, you may exaggerate reality, but you are not distorting it.

Yes, there is a psychiatric name for an excessive tendency to worry: *generalized anxiety disorder* (GAD). However, GAD is by far one of the most common problems people can have; it affects nearly 5 percent of the population at any time. GAD is not a serious psychiatric illness. See the section "Generalized Anxiety Disorder" in chapter 1 of this book for more information.

- *If a thought keeps repeating itself in your mind, it must be important.* In truth, having a repeating thought in your mind is not much different from having a repeating song going through your mind. It is nothing more than a common aspect of worrying, which has a tendency to lead you into repetitive thoughts. The frequency with which a given thought—or song—recurs has nothing to do with its importance or significance.

## Disrupting Worry

As mentioned before, it takes a deliberate act of will to disrupt a repetitive worry cycle. Following the path of least resistance is likely to keep your mind spiraling until bodily anxiety symptoms begin to take hold (and, in turn, these body symptoms feed back to your mind and aggravate the repetitive mental aspect of worrying). Getting "out of your head and into your life" by doing or focusing on something outside yourself is an excellent way to disrupt the worry spiral.

In short, you need to redirect your focus away from the cerebral toward the practical. This is *not* a knee-jerk, reflexive distraction or escape from worry that may only tend to increase it. Instead, you need to become engaged in a project or an activity so that your concentration shifts away from your worries about a possible future danger. This might involve engaging in 1) a practical activity that is inherently enjoyable or 2) a practical strategy for completing some immediate task at hand (for example, driving far from home or making a speech).

The stance you take toward the activity you choose to disrupt your worry is critical. You're aiming for a stance of *acceptance*, in spite of whatever worry might be going on. Because you can't force worry to go away, it's entirely okay for worry to come up. You might respond to the recurrence of worry with a statement of acceptance like "Okay, there's the worry—it can just be here and run its course while I get on with my business." Your focus is directed toward the practical activity rather than wrestling with whatever worry might be coming up. Consider the following activities as ways to disrupt your worry.

### Do Physical Exercise

This can be your favorite exercise or sport, or just a household chore. If you don't want to have an exercise session, take a look around the house or office. What needs to be done? Do you have a project you've been putting off for a while? It can be as mundane as changing shelf paper or waxing the floor. Most people have an unwritten, long-term "to-do list" of projects around the house. Write down your own list and decide what you would like to do first.

## Talk to Someone

The modern world has sharply curtailed the amount of time we spend in conversation. Technology, the fast pace of contemporary life, and a general trend toward isolation have limited the time we devote not only to deep, meaningful conversations, but even to everyday, simple chatting. Conversation is a great way to shift your focus away from your worries. Generally, you want to talk about something other than your worries, unless you want to express your feelings about them.

## Do Twenty Minutes of Deep Relaxation

Your body is usually tense when you are stuck in worry. If you take time out of your schedule to practice a relaxation technique, you'll often find your mind will tend to let go of whatever you were stuck on. Longer periods of relaxation (fifteen to twenty minutes) work better than short periods. You can use abdominal breathing, progressive muscle relaxation, a guided visualization, or meditation, as described in chapters 4 and 19, to induce a state of deep relaxation.

## Listen to Evocative Music

Feelings like sadness and anger may underlie and drive obsessive worrying. Music has a powerful ability to release these feelings. Take a look at your music collection and find a song or a whole CD that unlocks emotions for you. Or you can stream your favorite music online. Many people find that, without consciously intending to, they've assembled an eclectic selection of music that they can choose from according to their mood. If this is true for you, take advantage of it to cut short a worry spiral.

## Experience Something Immediately Pleasurable

You cannot be worried and feel comfortable and pleasant at the same time. Fear and pleasure are incompatible experiences. Anything you find pleasurable—whether it be a good meal, a warm bath, a funny movie, a back rub, cuddling, sexual activity, or simply walking in a beautiful setting—can help move you away from worry and fearful thinking.

## Use Visual Distractions

Simply look at something that absorbs your attention. This can be TV, movies, video games, your computer, or non-screen activities such as uplifting reading, arts and crafts, or working with a coloring book.

### Express Your Creativity

It's difficult to worry when you're being creative. Try craft projects, playing an instrument, painting or drawing, gardening, or just rearranging your living room. If you have a hobby, spend some time working on it. Is there something you always wanted to try, like making jewelry or watercolor painting? This is an opportune time to begin new and rewarding activities.

### Find an Alternative Positive Obsession

You can swap your negative obsession for a positive one by working on something that requires focused, steady concentration. For example, work out a crossword or jigsaw puzzle. Or get into puzzle books.

### Repeat an Affirmation

A healthy ritual for moving away from worry can be to sit quietly and practice repeating a positive affirmation that has personal significance. Repeat the affirmation slowly and deliberately. When your mind gets distracted, bring it back to the affirmation. Keep this up for five to ten minutes, or until you're fully relaxed. If you're spiritually inclined, here are some possible affirmations:

- Let go and let God.

- I abide in Spirit (God).

- I release (or turn over) this negativity to God.

If you prefer a nonspiritual tack, try these:

- Let it go.

- These are just thoughts—they're fading away.

- I'm whole, relaxed, and free of worry.

Two lists of affirmations in this book might help you as you create your own list. One list can be found in the section "Examples of Affirmations" in chapter 9, Mistaken Beliefs. The other list can be found in appendix 4, Affirmations for Overcoming Anxiety.

## Defusion

*Defusion* is a series of techniques derived from a form of therapy called acceptance and commitment therapy, or ACT (Hayes, Strosahl, and Wilson 1999; Harris 2019; and Eifert and Forsyth 2005).

These techniques offer a method for *disentangling yourself from the ongoing stream of your thoughts*. Defusion techniques help introduce some distance or "space" between conditioned, automatic thoughts and your awareness of those thoughts. They increase your capacity to observe rather than be enmeshed in the thoughts. These techniques are especially helpful for dealing with worry.

When you are "fused" with your thoughts, you tend to believe them as if they were absolute truth, even if they refer to some future danger that hasn't even happened (and isn't likely to). For example, if your heart races when you're anxious, you may be fused with the idea that you are going to have a heart attack. You may absolutely believe this, even if the likelihood of it happening is remote.

Another type of fusion includes adherence to rigid rules about what you should or shouldn't feel or do. Such thinking includes the words "should," "must," or "have to." Common examples include "I shouldn't be feeling this way" and "I have to do this right, or it's not worth trying at all."

Yet another type of fusion is closely identified with the negative judgments of your "inner critic," the voice within that tends to put you down. In this case, you really believe negative self-judgments such as "I'm worthless," "I'm weak," "I'm a failure," or "I can't cope." Fusion with such self-critical statements can lead to depression and feelings of hopelessness.

The problem with fusion is that what you take to be absolutely true and real *are simply strings of words and images in your head.* These strings of words and images that your mind creates may have nothing to do with reality, and yet you may wholeheartedly believe them as if they were utterly true. Being enmeshed or "entangled" with such thoughts can lead to a lot of suffering. The way out is *to stop believing everything you think.*

In worrying, fearful thoughts tend to be linked together in a lengthy sequence. Each fearful worry tends to be linked to another, and, as the chain continues, your anxiety tends to increase. Defusion helps you take a step back from this chain. All defusion techniques are based on the basic principle of *learning to observe* your thoughts.

Defusion itself begins by simply asking yourself to step back and carefully notice what you're thinking. How do you do this? You might say to yourself:

- "Okay, so what is my mind telling me right now?"

- "What thoughts are going through my mind right now?"

- "Can I just notice what my mind is saying?"

- "What judgments am I making right now?"

Once you've identified several of your specific thoughts—perhaps even written them down—the next important question to ask is *whether they are helpful or not—whether they work for you or not.* In contrast with cognitive behavioral therapy, defusion is less concerned with the truth or falsity of a given thought than whether it's *workable*—whether it's helpful and leads to a richer, fuller, or more meaningful life (as opposed to leading to more stress and suffering). If you are fused with the thought "I'm fat," defusion is not concerned with whether this thought is true or not (unlike your counselor at the local Jenny Craig program); rather, it's concerned with whether the thought is helpful. In brief, defusion is concerned with loosening up unworkable thoughts, whether they are true or not. The whole point is to hold painful/critical/fearful thoughts less tightly so that they are less likely to run your life.

## Common Defusion Techniques

Here are some common defusion techniques you can use.

**Notice what your mind tells you.** Just notice what your mind is telling you right now. Recall this question: "Okay, what is my mind telling me right now?"

**Write as many thoughts down as possible.** Especially when you feel upset, take a few deep abdominal breaths until you feel relaxed, sit or lie down, notice your thoughts, and then write them down separately on index cards or write all of them on a piece of paper.

**Bracket a thought.** Take a thought that you notice and preface it with the phrase "I'm having the thought that…" For example, you could take the self-destructive thought "I'm a loser" and defuse it, or gain some distance from it, by saying to yourself, "I'm having the thought that 'I'm a loser.'"

**Imagine leaves on a stream.** Imagine that you're sitting on the bank of a gentle stream. Leaves have dropped into the stream and are floating by you. Now, for the next few minutes, take every thought that pops into your head, place it on a leaf, and let it flow by. Whether you like the thought or not, place it on a leaf and just let it flow by. Don't try to make the stream move faster or slower, just imagine it flowing at its own rate. If a leaf gets stuck, let it hang around. Don't force it to float away. If you start to feel bored or impatient, acknowledge *that* thought: "Here's a feeling of boredom" or "Here's a feeling of impatience." Then place that thought on a leaf, and let the leaf float by.

**Watch your thinking.** Relax, support your head, center yourself in your body, and engage in abdominal breathing for one or two minutes. Now shift your attention to your thoughts. Ask yourself: *Where* are they? Where do they seem located in space? Are they inside my head? Are they floating around in "mental space" in my mind? Are they someplace else?

**Notice the *form* your thoughts take.** Are they more like words, pictures, or sounds? Notice whether your thoughts are moving rapidly, slowing down, or practically still. If they are moving, at what speed and in what direction are they moving? Notice what is above and below your thoughts. Are there any gaps between them? How large are these gaps? From time to time, you may find you get caught up in your thoughts. This is perfectly natural and normal. When it happens, just gently acknowledge it, and go back to watching your thoughts.

**Imagine a computer screen.** Imagine your thoughts are moving across a computer screen from left to right. See them in the middle of the screen or as captions running across the bottom. Watch them as they appear on the left of the screen and move steadily across the screen from left to right. If the thoughts are moving too fast to read all of them, then just use phrases or short words in lieu of full thoughts. If the thoughts stall, just allow that to happen; be patient, and see what happens. Just keep watching the thoughts go by until you can get a sense of how one thought leads to the next one, and so on. If you feel inclined, try changing the font, color, or even the format of the words as they move by. You might even try animating the thoughts with images.

**Explore the "natural history" of a thought.** Ask yourself whether you can remember when you first had a particular thought (or worry). What was going on in your life when you first became aware of the thought? *Why* do you think your mind keeps bringing up this particular thought or worry? What is your mind trying to accomplish or protect you from by having the worry? How has this thought worked for you? Has it helped you feel more happy, safe, or secure? Has the thought led you to avoid anything that you might have otherwise enjoyed? Spend a few minutes continuing to explore a given thought or worry with such questions.

**Sing the thought.** For example, take the thought "I'm a loser" and sing it to the tune of "Happy Birthday." (This is one of the zanier defusion techniques, which may or may not appeal to you, but it works for many people.)

**Consider the thought's workability.** Ask yourself these questions: "If I go along with a particular thought, buy into it, and let it control me, where does that leave me?" "What do I get for buying into it?" "Does buying into this thought lead me to a better and more meaningful life?"

Defusion techniques like those above can be used at any time to disentangle yourself from worried thoughts. As mentioned earlier, defusion is an aspect of acceptance and commitment therapy (ACT). If you are interested in learning more about ACT, a good place to start is *ACT Made Simple* by Russ Harris.

# Worry Exposure

*Worry exposure* is a form of imagery exposure (see chapter 7) where you imagine in detail a worst-case scenario regarding a particular worry, say, for example, failing an exam or flubbing up a job interview or presentation. The purpose is to repeatedly imagine the worrisome situation until you get bored and eventually neutralize it. This means getting used to something by repeatedly facing it to the point where it "loses its charge" and no longer has any power to provoke anxiety.

## *Practicing Worry Exposure for All of Your Worries*

You may have one particular worry that bothers you the most, or you may have a variety of worries that you find troublesome.

To properly execute worry exposure, proceed with the following steps:

1.  On a sheet of paper, make a list of all of your worries. They may concern performance at school or work, personal relationships with significant others or friends, making mistakes, health, physical danger, and so on.

2.  Take your list of worries and write a second list that ranks them in order of severity (that is, how much they bother you)—from the least severe to the most severe. So, let's say you

have ten worries: the least severe one will be ranked #1 and the most severe one will be ranked #10.

3.   Pick the worry you wish to work on first, preferably one of the less bothersome ones, and write a *detailed script* of everything included in the worry, with an emphasis on making it a *worst-case scenario*. Write up your script not only in words but also in images, including sights, sounds, physical sensations, and even smells. List all the aspects of the situation from start to finish. Strive to include everything in the script *as if it were actually occurring,* as if it were really happening to you. For example, if your worry is about an upcoming job interview, write a script that includes the night before the interview and then the day of the interview itself—driving to the interview, waiting for the interview to begin, receiving questions that are difficult to answer, imagining that you stumble in attempting to answer, seeing your interviewer look impatient or even contemptuous, imagining the interviewer suddenly stopping the interview and in a loud voice asking you to leave, and then later receiving a two-sentence rejection letter in the mail. Or in the case of taking an exam, write a detailed scenario where you study for the exam, sit down and wait for the exam to be passed out, receive the exam, and realize with growing apprehension that you can only answer a few of the questions. You feel upset that you have to leave many questions blank, so you get up and leave early while everyone else is still taking the exam. Other examinees stare at you as you walk out. You wait to get your exam results, and then receive your results by mail, where you get a failing grade, which in turn affects your grade point average to such a degree that you fail the course.

4.   Now read through your complete script slowly, experiencing it word for word.

   **Important:** After reading your script, close your eyes and *visualize the scene* for about five to ten minutes. If it helps to set a timer, please do so.

   If you feel anxiety in response to visualizing your worry scenario, you have done a good job of writing it up. To repeat, in order to fully neutralize a worry scenario, you need to feel at least *some anxiety* when you initially expose yourself to it. Then you need to repeat your exposure to the scenario several times until it becomes so routine that it no longer has any power to evoke anxiety.

   Try not to let your attention be drawn to other scenarios. Stay with your worst-case scenario for up to five to ten minutes without escaping into some distraction. Be willing to make that kind of time commitment. When your mind starts to wander, focus again on your detailed worry scenario. Keep going through the scene *until any anxiety you experience starts to subside or even to the point where you get bored.*

5.   Repeat step 4 at least *two or three times* in succession for a particular worry on a given day. If your anxiety subsides after the second exposure, you can skip doing a third exposure to your worst-case scenario for that day. The total time for worry exposure could take you anywhere from ten up to thirty minutes if you spend significant time with a particular exposure. If you're anxious throughout the entire period the first time, that is okay. On a scale of 1 to 10, if you feel anxiety in the 4 to 7 range when you do your first exposure, you are doing well. Feeling anxiety sensations is quite necessary for you to be able to

eventually neutralize the worry situation and to learn that, in truth, it is typically harmless. If you feel little or no anxiety, and would rate your anxiety no more than a 1 or 2 on a 10-point scale, then move on to a more difficult worry on your list. On the other hand, if you feel *very high or even overwhelming anxiety* in the range of 8 to 10 on the scale, postpone exposure to that particular worry and find an easier worry on your list with which you to begin worry exposure. After successfully overcoming anxiety to less challenging worries on your list, you will find it easier to take on the most difficult worries.

6.  After you have finished your worry exposure session for the day, allow yourself to imagine an *alternative positive outcome* that is easier or works out better than your worst-case scenario. Be sure that you've visualized your worst-case worry scenario at least two or three times—or spent from ten up to as long as twenty minutes with it—before you imagine an alternative outcome that is easier. It's particularly helpful to utilize coping strategies such as abdominal breathing or coping statements in your alternative, positive scenario.

    For example, in the case visualizing a job interview, practice abdominal breathing (see chapter 4) in advance of your positive interview scenario and/or rehearse confidence-building coping statements (see chapter 6, "Coping Statements"). Then imagine the interview going well, with the interviewer smiling, asking simple questions that you can easily answer, and mentioning at the end of the interview that she or he thinks the company can find a place for you. In the case of the exam scenario, practice abdominal breathing before the positive exam scenario to placate your anxiety. Then imagine that you find the questions on the exam easy to answer, you breeze through all of the questions, and you even leave early, feeling confident you have done well on the exam.

    Whatever level of anxiety you may have initially felt while visualizing your worst-case worry scenario, that anxiety should be significantly reduced by the time you follow up with alternative "success scenarios."

7.  Practice worry exposure with two or three exposures to your worst-case scenario on a given day, and, if you still feel some anxiety after the first day, then for up to three days every week. Eventually, sooner or later, you will find that the worry loses its power to evoke anxiety. Be sure to start with a worry that leads to just "midrange" anxiety (rather than very low or very high anxiety). After you have practiced worry exposure for a particular worry enough times *so that it no longer causes anxiety (or only nominal anxiety),* you are done with exposure for that worry. Congratulations! You have learned to overcome that worry, although you may want to occasionally return to running through your worry scenario as a kind of "booster session" to build on your success.

8.  Go to the next most difficult worry on your list. Repeat steps 3 to 7 for that particular worry, creating a detailed scenario and then exposing yourself to it in your imagination.

**Note:** The difference between exposure to actual phobias, as described in chapter 7, is that it involves exposures done in *real life*. Worry exposure is a process of normalizing your most challenging worries, whose locus is in your mind, with the long-term goal of being able to entertain any and all of your worries without anxiety.

The purpose of worry exposure is to get to the point where a worry no longer causes anxiety or has a distressing impact on you. After doing worry exposure, when a worry comes up spontaneously, you naturally feel that you have already run through the worry so many times in the exposure process that it's lost its potency. With sufficient exposure practice, you can learn that almost all worries (apart from those that have some realistic basis, such as, perhaps, passing the bar exam or having a high-profile interview) are either harmless or highly improbable.

## Postpone Your Worry

Rather than trying to stop worry or obsessive thoughts altogether, you may opt to try postponing them for a bit. This strategy can be especially helpful when your attempt to stop worry abruptly—as in the disruption techniques mentioned at the beginning of the chapter—feels difficult to achieve.

In a sense, you pay some credence to your worries or obsessive thoughts by telling them that *you will only ignore them for a few minutes, but then you will get back to them later*. In that way, you avoid a fight with the part of your mind that seems compelled to keep worrying.

When you first try this technique, try postponing worry only for a short time, perhaps one or two minutes. Then, at the end of the allotted time, try postponing the worry again for a short time, perhaps three to five minutes. When that period of time is up, set another specified time to postpone your worried thoughts even longer. The trick is to keep postponing worry for as long as you can. Often you will be able to postpone a particular worry long enough that your mind moves on to something else—because you have postponed it so long, the worry just loses its strength. For example, suppose you're trying to get work done and a worry about how you're going to pay all of your expenses keeps entering your mind. Don't try to push the worry away. *Accept* the worry without trying to fight with it, but tell yourself you'll postpone thinking about it for five minutes. After five minutes is up, tell yourself that you're going to postpone thinking about your worry for another five minutes. Continue attempting to postpone it until your mind moves on to something else.

When you first try out this technique, work with short periods of postponement, such as a few minutes. After you gain proficiency with it, try postponing for longer periods—for up to an hour or even a few hours during a day. If, after postponing worry two or three times, you feel you just can't postpone it any longer, give yourself five or ten minutes of *worry time*—that is, deliberately focus on your worry, reviewing the worrisome thoughts and any accompanying images in your mind for a short, predesignated period of time, such as five to ten minutes. At the end of the time, try to postpone the worry again. If you're having difficulty with resuming postponement, then utilize either the disruption or defusion techniques described earlier in this chapter.

Postponing worry is a skill that you can improve on with practice. As with the other worry-disruption techniques, gaining skill with worry postponement will increase your confidence in your ability to handle all kinds of worries as well as recurring obsessive thoughts.

# Plan Effective Action to Deal with Your Worries

Worrying about getting through a job interview, making a speech, or taking a long flight can be more stressful than the actual experience. That's because your body's fight-or-flight system makes no distinction between your fantasies about the situation and the situation itself. Worrying about an imagined threat causes your muscles to tighten and your stomach to churn just as much as when you're faced with a real threat. When you feel stuck in a particular worry, a useful strategy is to develop a plan of action to deal with the worry. The simple process of developing such a plan will help redirect your mind away from the worry. It will also help replace any sense of victimization you might be feeling with a more optimistic, hopeful attitude.

## Exercise: Make a Plan to Deal with Your Worry

Think about what worries you the most. Is it money? A particular relationship? Your kids? Your health? Your problem with anxiety itself? An upcoming public speaking situation? Among your worries, which one has highest priority for you to take action on right now? If you are ready and willing to take action, follow the sequence of steps below, adapted with permission from *The Worry Control Workbook* by Mary Ellen Copeland.

Write down the particular situation that is worrying you below:

1. Make a list of possible things you can do to deal with and improve the situation. Write them down, even if they seem overwhelming or impossible to you right now. Ask family and friends for ideas as well. Don't judge any possible options at this point—simply write them down.

2. Consider each idea. Which ones are not possible? Which ones are doable but difficult to implement? Put a question mark after these. Which ones could you do in the next week or perhaps the next month? Put a check after these.

3. Make a contract with yourself to do all the things you checked off. Set specific dates by which you will complete them. When you have completed the checked items, go on to the more difficult things. Make a similar contract with yourself to do them and complete them by specific dates.

4. Are there any other items that originally looked impossible that you might be able to do now? If so, make a contract with yourself to do these, too—again completing them by specific dates.

5. Once you've fulfilled all of your contracts, ask yourself how the situation has changed. Has your worry been satisfactorily resolved? If the situation has not been resolved, go through this process again.

If you continue to have problems with a particular worry, perhaps you have some self-limiting thought patterns or beliefs that are getting in your way. To understand and modify your personal thought patterns or belief system, see chapter 8, Self-Talk, and chapter 9, Mistaken Beliefs.

## Summary of Things to Do

1. Notice how your mind creates worry by repetitively making negative predictions about the future, overestimating the odds of a threat, underestimating the odds of your ability to cope in the unlikely event the threat actually happens, or trying to fight or suppress worry.

2. Be aware of the ways you might actually increase your worrying, such as attempting to talk yourself out of it, striving to obtain certainty in a situation that is inherently uncertain, or holding "metacognitive beliefs" about worry—such as the more you worry, the less likely the object of your worry will happen; overworrying will bring on the very thing you worry about; or excessive worry is an indication that something is seriously wrong with you.

3. Use disruption techniques to redirect your mind away from worry. Disruption is not the same as distraction, which is an attempt to escape from your worrying. Disruption techniques proactively help you "get out of your mind and into your life" by engaging in practical activities such as physical exercise, abdominal breathing, talking to someone, or engaging in some creative activity.

4. Use defusion techniques to "defuse" from your thoughts. Defusion provides a series of strategies to increase your capacity to stand back and *witness your worried thoughts and images* rather than being so enmeshed in them. All common defusion techniques are variations on the same theme: they empower you to *observe* your conscious stream of inner experience.

5. Use worry exposure to mentally neutralize your most challenging worries. In worry exposure, you write a script containing detailed thoughts and images to create a "worst-case scenario" of a particular worry (such as worrying about an upcoming exam or a job interview). Then both read through your detailed script as well as imagine it in your mind a number of times. If moderate anxiety comes up while running through the script, it means that worry exposure is working. Continue rehearsing the script in your mind until your anxiety eventually subsides. This can occur in one day doing several exposures to a given worry scenario, or it could take up to a few days of repetitive exposures. By doing this, you learn that the original worry is overrated or highly improbable. At that point, the worry has lost its power to evoke anxiety.

6. Postponing your worry is another quick trick to disrupt a worry. The moment the worry comes up, postpone thinking about it for a minute. If the worry comes back again, slightly lengthen the time you postpone it to two or three minutes. The idea is to keep postponing

the onset of the worry enough times that you finally move away from it and get involved in a more productive activity.

7.   Plan effective action to deal with your worry. When you are worried about something that has a practical solution, brainstorm effective steps you can take to deal with the situation and then systematically carry out those steps. The final section of this chapter provides a step-by-step process for taking action on those worries that can be resolved through real-life action.

## Further Reading

Bourne, Edmund. *Coping with Anxiety*. Rev. 2nd ed. Oakland, CA: New Harbinger Publications, 2016. (See especially chapter 9.)

Copeland, Mary Ellen. *The Worry Control Workbook*. Oakland, CA: New Harbinger Publications, 2000.

Eifert, G., and J. P. Forsyth. *Acceptance and Commitment Therapy for Anxiety Disorders*. Oakland, CA: New Harbinger Publications, 2005.

Harris, Russ. *ACT Made Simple*. 2nd ed. Oakland, CA: New Harbinger Publications, 2019.

Hayes, Steven, K. D. Strosahl, and K. G. Wilson. *Acceptance and Commitment Therapy: An Experiential Approach to Behavior Therapy*. New York: Guilford Press, 1999.

McKay, Matthew, Michelle Skeen, and Patrick Fanning. *The CBT Anxiety Solution Workbook: A Breakthrough Treatment for Overcoming Fear, Worry, and Panic*. Oakland, CA: New Harbinger Publications, 2017. (See especially chapter 8.)

# 11

# Personality Styles That Perpetuate Anxiety

People who are prone to anxiety disorders tend to share certain personality traits. Some of these traits are positive—such as creativity, intuitive ability, emotional sensitivity, empathy, and amiability. Such traits as these endear anxiety-prone people to their friends and relatives. Other common traits tend to aggravate anxiety and interfere with the self-confidence of people with anxiety disorders. This chapter focuses on four of these traits, all of which need to be addressed at some point in the process of recovery.

- Perfectionism

- Excessive need for approval

- Tendency to ignore physical and psychological signs of stress

- Excessive need for control

You may not possess all four of these traits. But if panic, phobias, or generalized anxiety have been part of your life for any length of time, you may identify with at least one or more of them.

## Origins of Anxiety-Provoking Traits

What's the origin of these traits that perpetuate anxiety? Such traits as creativity and emotional sensitivity may well be part of the hereditary component of anxiety disorders. On the other hand, perfectionism and excessive need for approval or control *often* have their origin in childhood experiences. There are various ways in which you can acquire such traits. If your parents have these traits, you may learn them directly by following their example. If your mother and father are high achievers and demand perfection of themselves, you may have internalized their values and behave in a similar way. Alternatively, such traits may develop out of your *response* to the ways in which you were treated by one or both of your parents. If, for example, you were frequently criticized or reprimanded, you may have decided early on that nothing you could do was good enough. As a result, you strive to do everything perfectly. Or you might constantly seek reassurance and approval. In the process, you may have also learned to repress your feelings and ignore signs of stress.

If you would like to obtain more insight about how you developed any of the traits considered in this chapter, you can start by referring to chapter 2, Major Causes of Anxiety Disorders, and the *Family Background Questionnaire,* which you will also find in chapter 2. Reflecting on your answers to the questions will help you better understand your past.

Below you'll find guidelines to help you identify, work with, and change each of the four traits that perpetuate anxiety: perfectionism, excessive need for approval, the tendency to ignore physical and psychological signs of stress, and the excessive need for control.[1]

# Perfectionism

Perfectionism has two aspects. First, you have a tendency to have expectations about yourself, others, and life that are unrealistically high. When anything falls short, you become disappointed and/or critical. Second, you tend to be overconcerned with small flaws and mistakes in yourself or your accomplishments. In focusing on what's wrong, you tend to discount and ignore what's right.

Perfectionism is a common cause of low self-esteem. It is critical of every effort and convinces you that nothing is ever good enough. It can also cause you to drive yourself to the point of chronic stress, exhaustion, and burnout. Every time perfectionism counsels you that you "should," "have to," or "must," you tend to push yourself forward out of anxiety, rather than from natural desire and inclination. The more perfectionistic you are, the more often you're likely to feel anxious.

Overcoming perfectionism requires a fundamental shift in your attitude toward yourself and how you approach life in general. The following seven guidelines are intended as a starting point for making such a shift.

### Let Go of the Idea That Your Worth Is Determined by Your Achievements or Accomplishments

Outer accomplishment may be how society measures a person's "worth" or social status. But are you going to allow society to have the last word on your value as a person? Work on reinforcing the idea that your worth is a given. People ascribe inherent worth to pets and plants just by virtue of their existence. You as a human being have the same inherent worth just because you're here. Be willing to recognize and affirm that you're lovable and acceptable as you are, apart from your outer accomplishments. When self-reflective people are near death, there are *often* only two things that seem to have been important to them about their lives: learning how to love others and growing in wisdom. If you need to measure yourself against any standard, try these rather than society's definitions of value.

### Recognize and Overcome Perfectionistic Thinking Styles

Perfectionism is expressed in the way you talk to yourself. "Should/must thinking," "all-or-nothing thinking," and "overgeneralization" characterize a perfectionist attitude. Below are

---

1 Outlines of the sections on perfectionism and the excessive need for approval in this chapter were adapted with permission from chapters 6 and 8 of *Anxiety, Phobias, and Panic: A Step-by-Step Program for Regaining Control of Your Life* by Reneau Z. Peurifoy, MA, MFCC. See this useful book for more detailed discussions of these issues.

examples of self-statements associated with each thinking style and corresponding, more realistic counterstatements.

| Thinking Style | Counterstatements |
|---|---|
| *Should/Must Thinking* | |
| "I should be able to do this right." | "I'll do the best I can" |
| "I must not make mistakes." | "It's okay to make mistakes." |
| *All-or-Nothing Thinking* | |
| "This is all wrong." | "This is not *all* wrong. There are some parts of it that are okay and some that need attention." |
| "I just can't do it at all." | "If I break this down into small enough steps, I can do it." |
| *Overgeneralization* | |
| "I *always* foul things up." | "It's simply untrue that I *always* foul things up. In this particular case, I'll go back and make the necessary corrections." |
| "I'll *never* be able to do this." | "If I take small steps and keep making an effort, over time I'll accomplish what I set out to do." |

Spend at least a week noticing all the instances when you get involved in should/must thinking, all-or-nothing thinking, or overgeneralization. Keep a notebook with you so that you can write down thoughts as they occur to you. Examine what you're telling yourself at times when you feel particularly anxious or stressed. Pay special attention to your use of the words "should," "must," "have to," "always," "never," "all," or "none." After you've spent a week writing down your perfectionist self-statements, compose counterstatements for each one. In subsequent weeks, read over your list of counterstatements frequently to encourage yourself to develop a less perfectionistic approach to life. See chapter 8 for further information on how to develop and work with counterstatements.

## Stop Magnifying the Importance of Small Errors

One of the most problematic aspects of perfectionism is its mandate to focus on small flaws or errors. Perfectionists are prone to come down very hard on themselves for a single, minute mistake that has few or no immediate consequences, let alone any long-term effects. When you really think about it, how important is a mistake you make today going to be one month from now? Or one year from now? In a majority of cases, the mistake will be forgotten within a short period of time. There is no real learning without mistakes or setbacks. No great success was ever attained without many failures and mistakes along the way.

## Focus on Positives

In dwelling on small errors or mistakes, perfectionists tend to discount their positive accomplishments. They selectively ignore anything positive they've done. A way to counter this tendency is to take inventory near the end of each day or week of positive things you've accomplished. Think about the ways, small or large, you've been helpful or pleasant to people during the day. Think of any small steps you've taken toward achieving your goals. What other things got done? What insights did you have?

Pay attention to whether you disqualify something positive with a "but"—for example, "I had a good practice session, but I became anxious near the end." Learn to leave off the "but" in the assessments of your attitudes and behavior.

## Work on Goals That Are Realistic

Are your goals realistically attainable, or have you set them too high? Would you expect of anyone else the goals you set for yourself? Sometimes it's difficult to recognize the overly lofty nature of certain goals. It can be helpful to do a "reality check" with a friend or counselor to determine whether any given goal is realistically attainable or even reasonable to strive for. Are you expecting too much of yourself and the world? You may need to adjust some of your goals a bit to be in line with the limiting factors of time, energy, and resources. If your determination of self-worth truly comes from within rather than from what you achieve, you will be able to do this. Acceptance of personal limitations *is* an ultimate act of self-love.

## Cultivate More Pleasure and Recreation in Your Life

Perfectionism has a tendency to make people rigid and self-denying. Your own human needs get sacrificed in favor of the pursuit of external goals. Ultimately, this tendency can lead to a stifling of vitality and creativity. Pleasure—finding the enjoyment in life—reverses this trend.

There is a wise saying attributed to a Native American chief: "The first thing people say after their death is—'Why was I so serious?'" Are you taking yourself too seriously and not allowing yourself time for fun, recreation, play, and rest? How can you make more time for leisure and pleasure? You can change by taking time every day to do at least one thing you enjoy.

## Develop a Process Orientation

If you engage in sports, do you play to win or just to enjoy the activity of playing? In your life in general, are you "playing to win"—channeling your energies into excelling at all costs—or are you enjoying the process of living day by day as you go along?

Most people find, especially as they get older, that to get the most enjoyment out of life, it works best to place value on the *process* of doing things—not just on the product or accomplishment. Popular expressions of this idea include "The journey is more important than the destination" and "Stop and smell the roses."

# Excessive Need for Approval

All human beings need approval. Yet for many people struggling with anxiety and phobias, the need for approval can be excessive. Being overly concerned with approval often arises from an inner sense of being flawed or unworthy. This leads to the mistaken belief that you are unacceptable just the way you are ("If people really saw who I am, they wouldn't accept me"). Individuals with an excessive need for approval are always looking for validation from other people. In trying to be generally pleasing, they may conform so well to others' expectations that they often ignore their own needs and feelings. Frequently, they have a difficult time setting boundaries or saying no.

The long-term consequence of always accommodating and pleasing others at the expense of yourself is that you end up with a lot of withheld frustration and resentment over not having taken care of your own basic needs. Withheld frustration and resentment may form the unconscious foundation for a lot of chronic anxiety and tension.

There are many ways to get over *feeling* excessively needy for approval. The following guidelines can help you start.

## *Develop a Realistic View of Other People's Approval*

When people don't express approval toward you—or even act rudely or critically—how do you receive it? Do you tend to take it personally, to see it as further evidence of your own ineptness or lack of worth? Below are some common attitudes characteristic of people who place excessive emphasis on always being liked. These might be called "people-pleasing" attitudes. Following each is an alternative view which represents, in most cases, a more realistic outlook.

*Common Attitude:*     "If someone isn't friendly to me, it's because I did something wrong."

*Alternative View:*     "People may be unable to express warmth or acceptance toward me for reasons having nothing to do with me. For example, their own problems, frustrations, or fatigue may get in the way of their being friendly and accepting."

*Common Attitude:*     "Others' criticism only serves to underscore the fact that I really am unworthy."

*Alternative View:*     "People who find fault with me may be projecting their own faults, which they can't admit to having, onto me. It's a human tendency to project unconscious flaws onto others."

*Common Attitude:*     "I think I'm a nice person. Shouldn't everyone like me?"

*Alternative View:*     "There will always be some people who just won't like me—no matter what I do. The process by which people are attracted to or repelled by others is often irrational."

*Common Attitude:*    "Others' approval and acceptance of me is very important."

*Alternative View:*    "It's not necessary to receive the approval of everyone I meet in order to live a happy and meaningful life—especially if I believe in and respect myself."

The next time you feel put off or rejected, take a moment to calm down and think about whether the person acting negatively is reacting to something you did or might simply be upset about something that has little or nothing to do with you. Ask yourself whether you might be taking the other person's inconsiderate remarks or behavior too personally.

## Deal with Criticism in an Objective Fashion

An excessive need for approval is often accompanied by an inability to handle criticism. You can learn to change your attitude toward criticism, ignoring those critical remarks that are unfounded and accepting constructive criticism as a positive learning experience.

The following three guidelines may be helpful:

**Evaluate the source of the criticism.** If you find yourself criticized, it's important to ask *who* is making the criticism. Is this person qualified to criticize you? Does he or she know enough about you, your skills, or the subject involved to make a reasonable assessment? Does this person have a bias that would make it impossible for him or her to be objective? (The more emotionally charged the relationship, the more likely this is to be true.) Is this person speaking emotionally or rationally? You can often soothe the sting of criticism by exploring the answers to these questions.

**Ask for details.** This is especially important if you receive a blanket criticism, such as "That was a lousy job" or "I don't think you know what you're doing." Don't accept a global judgment. Ask the person offering the criticism to indicate specific behaviors or issues that seem to fall short. You can ask that person's point of view about what actions you might take to improve your performance or correct the situation.

**Decide whether the criticism has some validity.** You've evaluated the source of criticism and also, in the case of a global criticism, asked for details. The next question to ask is whether the criticism has some merit. Usually when a criticism has some truth to it, it has a little more sting— you may feel somewhat pained or disturbed by it. If a criticism has no validity, you're likely to have little emotional reaction to it at all: you may dismiss it as irrelevant, absurd, or uninformed.

The best way to handle criticism that rings true is to view it as important feedback that can help you learn something about yourself. Also, be sure to remind yourself that the criticism is—or should be—directed toward only one aspect of your behavior, not toward you as a total person. Here are some good affirmations to help cultivate a positive response:

- This criticism is a good opportunity to learn something.

- This criticism concerns only a few of my actions, not my entire being.

- Although this criticism feels uncomfortable, it doesn't mean that I'm totally rejected or disapproved of.

## *Recognize and Let Go of Codependency*

Check off any of the following statements that generally reflect your beliefs:

☐   If someone important to me expects me to do something, I should do it.

☐   I should not be irritable or unpleasant.

☐   I shouldn't do anything to make others angry at me.

☐   I should keep people I love happy.

☐   It's usually my fault if someone I care about is upset with me.

☐   My self-esteem comes from helping others solve their problems.

☐   I tend to overextend myself in taking care of others.

☐   If necessary, I'll put my own values or needs aside in order to preserve my relationship with my significant other.

☐   Giving is the most important way I have to feel good about myself.

☐   Fear of someone else's anger has a lot of influence on what I say or do.

If you checked three or more statements, codependency may likely to be one of the issues you need to deal with.

*Codependency* can be defined as the tendency to put others' needs before your own. You accommodate others to such a degree that you tend to discount or ignore your own feelings, desires, and basic needs. Your self-esteem depends largely on how well you please, take care of, and/or solve problems for someone else (or many others).

The consequence of maintaining a codependent approach to life is a lot of resentment, frustration, and unmet personal needs. When these feelings and needs remain unconscious, they often resurface as anxiety—especially *chronic, generalized anxiety*. The long-term effects of codependency are stress, fatigue, burnout, and possibly even serious physical illness.

Recovering from codependency in essence involves learning to love and take care of yourself. It means giving at least equal time to your own needs alongside the needs of others. It means setting limits on how much you will do or tolerate, and learning to say no when appropriate. The following list of affirmations will encourage you to develop a more self-nurturing attitude that can move you beyond codependency (see chapter 9, Mistaken Beliefs, for suggestions on how to work with affirmations):

•   I'm learning to take better care of myself.

•   I recognize that my own needs are important.

•   It's good for me to take time for myself.

•   I'm finding a balance between my own needs and my concern for others.

•   If I take good care of myself, I'll have more to offer others.

- It's okay to ask for what I want from others.

- I'm learning to accept myself just the way I am.

- It's okay to say no to others' demands when I need to.

- I don't have to be perfect to be accepted and loved.

- I can change myself, but I accept that I can't make another person change.

- I'm letting go of taking responsibility for other people's problems.

- I respect others enough to know that they can take responsibility for themselves.

- I'm letting go of guilt when I can't fulfill others' expectations.

- Compassion toward others is loving; feeling guilty about their feelings or reactions accomplishes nothing.

- I am learning to love myself more every day.

In order to work with your own codependency issues, you may want to read some of the classic books on the subject, such as *Codependent No More* by Melody Beattie, *Facing Codependence* by Pia Mellody, and *Women Who Love Too Much* by Robin Norwood. Also consider attending a local meeting of Codependents Anonymous, which offers a 12-step approach to overcoming codependent attitudes.

The three guidelines cited earlier in this section are only a start in the direction of learning to be less concerned with others' approval. The chapters on assertiveness and self-esteem in this book will also help you learn to rely on yourself rather than others for a sense of your inherent worth and acceptability.

## Tendency to Ignore Physical and Psychological Signs of Stress

People with anxiety disorders are often out of touch with their bodies. If you are anxious or pre-occupied with worrying, you may, as the expression goes, be "living in your head"—not feeling strongly connected with the rest of your body, below your neck. Try checking in with yourself at various times though the day, particularly at times when you are not looking at a screen or focused on a mental task. Do you feel as if most of your energy—your "center of gravity"—is situated from your neck up? Or do you feel more solidly connected with the rest of your body, in touch with your chest, stomach, arms, and legs? To increase a sense of connection with your full body, almost any form of exercise will help. See chapter 5, Physical Exercise, for more information on exercise.

To the extent that you are out of touch with your body, you may ignore—often unconsciously—an entire range of physical symptoms that arise when you're under stress. Examples of physical symptoms that may signify stress are fatigue, headaches, nervous stomach, tight muscles, cold hands, and diarrhea, to mention a few. Unfortunately, when you're unaware that you're under stress, you're likely to keep pushing yourself without taking time out or slowing down. You may keep going until you reach a state of exhaustion or illness.

Many individuals with anxiety disorders have a long history of pushing themselves very hard and continually overextending themselves—trying to fit too much into too little time. Driven by perfectionist standards, they keep striving to do more and be more for everyone. Often they may go for months at a time—even years—without noticing, or simply ignoring, that they are under high levels of stress.

One possible outcome of chronic, cumulative stress is that the neuroendocrine regulatory systems in the brain begin to malfunction, and you develop panic attacks, generalized anxiety, depression, mood swings, or some combination of these three (see chapter 2). You might also develop ulcers, hypertension, headaches, or other psychosomatic illnesses under conditions of prolonged or chronic stress. If it is your neurotransmitter systems that happen to be vulnerable, the effects of chronic stress are likely to show up in the form of an anxiety or mood disorder. Although these disorders cause significant distress in themselves, *they are, in fact, warning signs.* The body has built-in mechanisms for preventing its self-destruction. Developing panic disorder or depression may be viewed as a way in which your body forces you to slow down and alter your lifestyle before you push yourself into serious illness.

One of the themes of this workbook is that your recovery from anxiety disorders depends in great measure on your ability to manage and cope with stress. This, in turn, requires that you learn to *recognize* your own symptoms of stress and then *do* something about them—to relieve your symptoms through deep relaxation, exercise, downtime, supportive social interaction, recreation, and so on—so that stress does not become cumulative.

Stress can manifest itself not only in the form of physical symptoms but as emotional and psychological symptoms as well. The psychological symptoms are a *direct* indication that your nervous system (and possibly endocrine system) is being overtaxed. Not just anxiety and depression, but also forgetfulness, feeling "overloaded," mood swings, difficulty concentrating, boredom, excessive worrying, and spells of excessive guilt are all examples of psychological symptoms of stress.

The *Checklist for Symptoms of Stress* that follows is designed to help you increase your awareness of both physical and psychological symptoms of stress. You may want to make a number of copies of the checklist, or download the digital version available online (see the very end of this book for details) and complete it periodically to get a reading of your own stress level.

The *Life Events Survey* in chapter 2 measured your level of cumulative stress over a period of one or two years. The *Checklist for Symptoms of Stress* (below) will enable you to determine the stress load on your body and psyche over the past few weeks or month. Take some time to complete the checklist now.

Handling stress involves two steps. The first is to *recognize and identify* your own symptoms of stress. The second is to *decide not to ignore* them. If you would truly like to find relief from anxiety disorders, you need to *do* something to reduce and better manage your stress. Some of the stress management strategies described in this workbook include deep relaxation, regular exercise, downtime and time management, cultivating constructive self-talk and attitudes, expressing feelings, learning assertiveness, self-nurturing skills, and good nutrition.

Many other strategies for coping with stress are available. You will find them described in books on stress management such as *Guide to Stress Reduction*, 2nd ed., by John Mason and *The Relaxation & Stress Reduction Workbook*, 7th ed., by Martha Davis, Elizabeth Eshelman, and Matthew McKay. A list of twenty-four positive coping skills for dealing with stress follows the *Checklist for Symptoms of Stress*.

# Checklist for Symptoms of Stress

*Instructions:* Check each item that describes a symptom you have experienced to any significant degree during the last month, then total the number of items checked.

## Physical Symptoms

☐ Headaches (migraine or tension)

☐ Backaches

☐ Tight muscles

☐ Neck and shoulder pain

☐ Jaw tension

☐ Muscle cramps, spasms

☐ Nervous stomach

☐ Other pain

☐ Nausea

☐ Insomnia (sleeping poorly)

☐ Fatigue, lack of energy

☐ Cold hands and/or feet

☐ Tightness or pressure in the head

☐ High blood pressure

☐ Diarrhea

☐ Skin condition (e.g., rash)

☐ Allergies

☐ Teeth grinding

☐ Digestive upsets (cramps, bloating)

☐ Stomach pain or ulcer

☐ Constipation

☐ Hypoglycemia

☐ Appetite change

☐ Colds

☐ Profuse perspiration

☐ Heart beats rapidly or pounds, even at rest

## Psychological Symptoms

☐ Anxiety

☐ Depression

☐ Confusion or "spaciness"

☐ Irrational fears

☐ Compulsive behavior

☐ Forgetfulness

☐ Feeling "overloaded" or "overwhelmed"

☐ Hyperactivity—feeling you can't slow down

☐ Mood swings

☐ Loneliness

☐ Problems with relationships

☐ Dissatisfied/unhappy with work

☐ Difficulty concentrating

☐ Frequent irritability

☐ Restlessness

☐ Frequent boredom

☐ Frequent worrying or obsessing

☐ Frequent guilt

☐ Temper flare-ups

☐ Crying spells

☐ Nightmares

☐ Apathy

☐ Sexual problems

☐ Weight change

☐ Overeating

☐ When nervous, use of alcohol, cigarettes, or recreational drugs

*Evaluate your stress level as follows:*

| Number of Items Checked | Stress Level |
| --- | --- |
| 0–7 | *Low* |
| 8–14 | *Moderate* |
| 15–21 | *High* |
| 22+ | *Very High* |

## 24 Positive Coping Strategies for Stress

**Physical and Lifestyle Strategies**
(see chapters 4 and 5)

1. Abdominal breathing and relaxation

2. Low-stress diet

3. Regular exercise

4. Downtime (including "mental health days")

5. Mini-breaks (5- to 10-minute periods to relax during the day)

6. Time management (appropriate pacing)

7. Practice guidelines for improving sleep (see chapter 17)

8. Choosing a nontoxic environment

9. Material security

**Emotional Strategies**
(see chapters 13, 14, and 15)

10. Social support and relatedness

11. Self-nurturing

12. Good communication skills

13. Being more assertive

14. Recreational activities ("playtime")

15. Emotional release

16. Sense of humor—ability to see things in perspective

**Cognitive Strategies**
(see chapters 8 and 9)

17. Constructive thinking—ability to counter negative thinking

18. Helpful diversion tactics—the ability to disrupt and move beyond negative preoccupations (see appendixes 2, 3, and 4)

19. Task-oriented (versus reactive) approach to problems

20. Acceptance (ability to accept/cope with setbacks)

21. Tolerance for ambiguity—ability to "live in the question" rather than seeking immediate closure

**Philosophical/Spiritual Strategies**
(see chapter 21)

22. Consistent goals or purposes to work toward

23. Positive philosophy of life

24. Religious/spiritual life and commitment

# Excessive Need for Control

The excessive need for control makes you want to have everything in life be predictable. It's a kind of vigilance that requires all the bases to be covered—the opposite of letting go and trusting in the process of life.

Often an excessive need for control has its origins in a traumatic personal history. After living through experiences in which you felt frightened, vulnerable, or violated and powerless, it's easy to grow up feeling defensive and vigilant. You may go through life this way, ready to put up your defenses in response to any situation that seems to challenge your sense of security (whether it actually does or not). Survivors of severe trauma often develop highly controlled and/or controlling personalities, or else they may have been so distressed that they decided to give up, feeling depressed and discouraged about maintaining any control of their lives (the latter outcome has been referred to as "learned helplessness").

Overcoming the excessive need for control takes time and persistence. Key strategies that have been helpful to many people are described in the sections below.

## *Acceptance*

Acceptance entails learning to live more comfortably with the unpredictability of life—with the unexpected changes that occur daily on a small scale and, less often, on a large scale. It's inevitable that you'll encounter changes in your environment, in the way others choose to behave, and in your own physical health that you are simply unable to predict or control. You may have resources to cope with these changes, but you are not always going to be prepared for them. There will be times when your personal life situation may seem relatively chaotic, disordered, or out of control. Developing acceptance means acquiring a willingness to take life as it comes. Rather than fearing and struggling with those occasions when circumstances don't obey your expectations, you can learn to go with the change. Popular expressions for this are "go with the flow" and "take things in stride." In a word, acceptance implies *nonresistance*.

There are numerous ways in which to cultivate greater acceptance. Certainly letting go of perfectionism, as described earlier in this chapter, will provide a good start. A willingness to let go of unrealistic expectations can save you a lot of disappointment. Relaxation is also an important key. The more relaxed you remain, the less likely you are to be fearful and defensive when circumstances suddenly change and don't go your way. When you're relaxed, you slow down, and it's easier to go with rather than balk against the unexpected.

Finally, a sense of humor toward life can be very helpful. Humor enables you to step back from those times when everything appears to be in disarray and to get some perspective. If you can remain relaxed and laugh a little at situations that appear out of control, your response begins to change from "Oh my God!" to "Oh well—that's just the way it goes." Acceptance ensures that you will be able to cope better and sooner. You are likely to say, "Now what do I need to do?" a lot sooner after "Oh well…" than after "Oh my God!"

Affirmations that can help you develop acceptance include:

- "I'm learning to take life as it comes."

- "It's okay to let go and trust that things will work out."

- "I can relax and tolerate a little disorder and ambiguity."

- "I'm learning not to take myself or life so seriously."

## Cultivating Patience

People who have an overcontrolled approach to life's problems want to have them all figured out by tomorrow. Yet it's often true that difficult situations cannot be worked out immediately. All the pieces that contribute to a solution come together gradually over a period of time. Developing patience means allowing yourself to tolerate temporary muddles and ambiguity while you wait for all the necessary steps of the solution to unfold. As you develop patience, you learn to let go and wait for a resolution or an answer to emerge.

## Trusting That Most Problems Eventually Work Out

Developing trust goes along with cultivating patience. You may not see the solution to a particular difficulty easily or quickly. But if you always need to see in advance how something is going to work out, you can end up making yourself very anxious. There is an old saying, "Life is a river—you can't always see what's coming around the bend." Developing trust means believing that just about everything *eventually does work out.* Either you find a solution, or, if the problem can't be changed externally, you learn to alter your attitude toward it so that coping becomes easier. When you look back over the problems you've encountered in your life, you'll find that in most if not all cases, the problem eventually worked itself out.

## Developing a Spiritual Approach to Life

Developing a spiritual approach to life can mean many things (for further discussion of this topic, see chapter 21, Personal Meaning). In essence, it means believing in a Higher Power, Force, or Intelligence that transcends the world as you ordinarily perceive and know it. Very often it also implies having a personal relationship—in your inner experience—with that Power, Force, or Intelligence.

Developing your spirituality offers at least two ways in which to reduce an excessive need for control. First, it gives you the option to "turn over" or "let go" of any problem that seems insoluble, overwhelming, or just plain worrisome to the care of your Higher Power. This possibility is expressed in the third step of all 12-step programs: "[We] made a decision to turn our will and our lives over to the care of a Higher Power as we understood that Power." This does *not* mean that you relinquish responsibility for handling the problems that come up in life. It does mean that you have trust in a higher resource ("higher" in the sense of being beyond your own capabilities) that can be of support and assistance when you've reached the point where a problem appears insoluble, despite your best efforts. Faith in such a resource enables you to let go of the idea that you have to fully control everything. Some of my clients find that they can approach a phobic situation more easily by "turning over" their worry and anxiety to a Higher Power.

The second way in which developing your spirituality can reduce your need for control is in nurturing your belief that *there is a larger purpose in life beyond the overt appearance of what happens from day to day.* If you believe that there is no spiritual foundation to reality, then the unpredictable and unforeseen events of life can seem random and capricious. You can feel distressed because there is no explanation for why this bad event happened or that apparently unfair situation occurred. Most forms of spirituality offer the alternative view that the universe is not random. Events that may appear meaningless and brutal from a human perspective have some meaning or purpose in a broader scheme of things.

A popular phrase that expresses this idea is "Everything happens for some purpose." Often hindsight provides us with clearer vision. When you reflect deeply on some of the unforeseen mishaps in your life, you may see in retrospect how they served you—either in an obvious way or simply in promoting your growth and development as a human being.

The four traits described in this chapter—perfectionism, excessive need for approval, tendency to ignore physical and psychological signs of stress, and excessive need for control—are shared by many people who deal with anxiety on a day-to-day basis. By this point you've hopefully become more aware of which of these traits might be a problem for you. Actually changing traits such as perfectionism or the excessive need for control will take time and commitment on your part. Part of the process involves changing particular mistaken beliefs you may hold, as was described in chapter 9, Mistaken Beliefs. Ultimately, though, you may need to reevaluate and shift certain basic values and priorities in your life.

## Summary of Things to Do

1.  What are you willing to do today—and each day—to relax your quest for perfection? Can you let go of some of the demands you put on yourself in order to make time for your anxiety recovery program—or simply for rest and relaxation? Each day, find something you would ordinarily do that doesn't *have to* get done (such as work or household chores) and defer it to another day.

2.  If excessive need for approval is an important issue, be sure to spend extra time with the chapters on assertiveness and self-esteem in this book. It's important to work on developing 1) greater self-respect, 2) an ability to nurture yourself, 3) knowledge of your basic rights, and 4) a willingness to ask for what you want. If you suspect that codependency is an issue for you, consult the references on that subject below, or attend a Codependents Anonymous meeting, if available in your area.

3.  Complete the *Checklist for Symptoms of Stress* to get an idea of your level of stress over the past month. If stress is a real problem, focus on the chapters on relaxation, exercise, and nutrition in this book to get started with a program of stress management. Working on mistaken beliefs (chapter 9) and perfectionism (from this chapter) are also important. Consult the references on the subject of stress reduction below.

4. Learning to let go of the excessive need for control can be a challenge for people who are prone to anxiety. Cultivating a sense of humor and an ability to laugh at life's limitations is one way to get started. You tend to loosen up as you learn how to laugh and have more fun with your life. Another way to proceed, if you feel so inclined, is to develop your spirituality and trust in a Higher Power (see chapter 21).

5. Finally, the author's book *Beyond Anxiety & Phobia*, contains an entire chapter on strategies for letting go of control. That book also discusses how to deal with other personality traits prevalent in people who struggle with anxiety (and depression), such as insecurity and overdependency, the fear of abandonment, overcautiousness, and the fear of illness or injury. *Beyond Anxiety & Phobia* has its own chapter on personality traits that can foster anxiety, entitled Address Your Personality Issues.

# Further Reading

Beattie, Melody. *Codependent No More.* 25th anniversary ed. Center City, MN: Hazelden, 1992.

Bourne, Edmund. *Beyond Anxiety & Phobia.* Oakland, CA: New Harbinger Publications, 2001.

Davis, Martha, Elizabeth Robbins Eshelman, and Matthew McKay. *The Relaxation & Stress Reduction Workbook.* 7th ed. Oakland, CA: New Harbinger Publications, 2019.

Mason, John. *Guide to Stress Reduction.* Rev. ed. Berkeley, CA: Celestial Arts, 2001.

Mellody, Pia. *Facing Codependence.* San Francisco: HarperSanFrancisco, 2003.

Norwood, Robin. *Women Who Love Too Much.* New York: Pocket Books, 2008.

Peurifoy, Reneau. *Anxiety, Phobias, and Panic: A Step-by-Step Program for Regaining Control of Your Life.* Rev. ed. New York: Warner Books, 2005.

# 12

# Ten Common Specific Phobias

A *specific phobia* involves a *fear of one particular type of object or situation*—for example, flying, a type of animal, or going to the dentist. You tend to avoid the situation altogether or else endure it with dread. The fear is of the situation itself, not of having a panic attack. If you avoid a situation primarily out of fear of having a panic attack, you are more likely to be dealing with agoraphobia (see chapter 1). Yet panic can occur if you unexpectedly find yourself confronted with a specific phobic situation you've routinely avoided.

Specific phobias affect many people. More than half of the population in the United States has some degree of performance anxiety, and fear of flying affects approximately 20 percent of the population. To be diagnosed with a specific phobia, however, not only do you have a strong fear and avoidance of a specific situation, but your phobia also interferes significantly with your occupational and/or social functioning. Using this stronger criterion, about 10 percent of the population has a diagnosable specific phobia that causes impairment at some time in their life.

There are many types of specific phobias, and phobia lists enumerate more than a hundred types with exotic names. This chapter provides descriptions of ten common types of specific phobias, along with proposed causes and common approaches to their treatment. Resources such as books and audio programs relevant to a particular type of phobia are mentioned, when available. Although the list of common phobias described here is by no means complete, the cognitive behavioral principles and treatment strategies described can be applied to any type of phobia.

The phobias described include the following:

- Performance anxiety

- Fear of flying

- Claustrophobia

- Fear of disease (hypochondria)

- Dental phobia

- Blood/injection phobia

- Fear of vomiting (emetophobia)

- Fear of heights (acrophobia)

- Animal and insect phobias

- Fear of death

Even if you are not dealing with any of the specific phobias described above, reading through the chapter will provide some insight into the variety of causes as well as the most common effective treatments for phobias of all kinds. For an in-depth description of the details and mechanics of facing phobias in general, see chapter 7.

# Performance Anxiety

The fear of performing or speaking in front of an audience is the most common phobia, affecting up to 60 percent of the population worldwide at some time in their life. In the context of fear of public speaking, it's sometimes referred to as *glossophobia*. Performance anxiety in general can involve any one or all of the following components:

- Fear of being judged as awkward or inadequate when speaking in front of others

- Fear of underperforming or making a mistake, as in a musical recital or sports performance

- Fear of having your anxiety be outwardly visible to others, as in sweating, stammering, or blushing

- Fear of failure and/or rejection, as in a job interview or an oral examination

- Anxiety over uncertainty about how you will do when you have to perform

Performance anxiety often has a strong anticipatory aspect, with considerable worry in advance of the performance or speaking presentation. The anxiety usually increases as the time of the performance approaches. For many, the anxiety goes away as soon as they actually start speaking, singing, or performing. Others, however, continue to have distracting symptoms during the performance, such as pounding heart, hand tremors, sweating, nausea, or dry mouth. In the worst case, the anxiety becomes severe enough to interfere with the performance and/or disrupt speech.

Performance anxiety affects all kinds of people whether they are novices or professionals. Singer Barbra Streisand, for example, spent twenty-seven years avoiding any performance before a live audience.

## Causes

The long-term cause of performance anxiety may be a single traumatic experience with speaking before a group or doing a musical recital as a child. Or you may simply be prone to social anxiety and shyness from early childhood. You consistently avoid speaking or performing in front of others. A more general tendency to avoid groups and social situations is not performance anxiety but *social phobia* or *social anxiety disorder* (see chapter 1 for more information). Performance anxiety is a distinct problem from social phobia; however, it affects large numbers of people who otherwise do not avoid or fear participating in groups.

The immediate cause of performance anxiety often lies in deep-seated core beliefs and images where you may think or picture yourself losing control or being incompetent in front of others. You may imagine that you will make dreadful mistakes, believe that your performance has to be perfect to be acceptable, or exaggerate the importance or status of the people you will speak to. These self-defeating thoughts can be very stubborn and persistent, leading to long-term avoidance of any situation where you might have the opportunity to perform or speak before others.

## Treatment

Cognitive behavioral treatment of performance anxiety consists of identifying self-defeating core beliefs (and images) and gradually internalizing more constructive beliefs, such as:

- You really do have the ability to perform well in front of others.

- It's possible to embrace or "flow with" anxiety when it comes up rather than resist it.

- It's human and okay to make mistakes.

- Others will approve of you if you are "just yourself."

- You will likely not appear anxious to others, even if you feel anxious inside.

- People are not scrutinizing you to see if you flub the speech or performance.

- By focusing on the message you want to convey, you can deflect attention away from anxiety.

- With practice and adequate rehearsal, you can assure a good performance.

The replacement of dysfunctional beliefs is then followed by a hierarchy of exposures to progressively more challenging performance opportunities. For example, in the case of public speaking, you might start by speaking to one or two friends, then speak to a larger group of friends, and finally speak before a small group of strangers, and ultimately before a large group of strangers. Also, the number and perhaps status of the people you speak to could gradually be increased. Some people prefer to do performance anxiety exposures without proceeding in an incremental order of difficulty. They opt to do the exposures in a random order of varying difficulty. For them, the total time to complete exposure to performance anxiety can be much shorter. The risk of having to endure high levels of anxiety, on the other hand, may be higher.

An important facet of treatment includes learning to refocus away from excessive concern about yourself and your appearance and instead think about how what you do might benefit, help, or entertain the people in your audience. Refocusing on how you can help or benefit people can make a big difference. The more you can think about how you might be contributing to your audience, the less you focus on your own internal thoughts and feelings.

Other practical tips often mentioned in programs on public speaking include these:

- Spend plenty of time rehearsing your speech or performance in advance (ideally in front of a friend) to build confidence.

- Take a walk to release nervous energy an hour or two before your performance, and make sure you don't perform on an empty stomach. (Keep your blood sugar level up.)

- Have a glass of water available next to the podium so you have something to do should your mind get distracted by anxious thoughts or body symptoms.

- If you're afraid of your audience, imagine them as babies with bonnets or in their underwear to remind yourself they are just people.

- If it's part of your philosophy, say a prayer and turn your performance over to your higher power or deity.

## Medication

Many performers use beta-blocker medications such as *propranolol* or *metoprolol* in advance of a performance to reduce body symptoms such as sweating, shaky hands, or pounding heart. These medications can be quite effective. Less common but sometimes useful are tranquilizers before the performance or sedatives the night before (to ensure sleep). While the latter can be helpful in reducing anxiety or aiding sleep, they have the downside of sometimes flattening access to your feelings and inner spontaneity. Too high a dose can also interfere with mental clarity.

## Resources

The books and CDs of Janet Esposito are highly recommended for dealing with performance anxiety. Her first book, *In the Spotlight*, provides an excellent general introduction, while her later book, *Getting Over Stage Fright*, provides specific affirmations and practices to help reframe your approach and attitude toward performing in front of others. You may want to do a Google search on performance anxiety to look at many different websites on the topic.

# Fear of Flying

Fear of flying is the second most common phobia (after fear of public speaking). About 8 percent of the US population avoids flying altogether or achieves it only with difficulty. A larger percentage of the population dislikes flying and is inclined only to do so when necessary, such as for business or to attend an important family event. Sometimes fear of flying can interfere with a person's life in major ways—he or she might avoid desirable jobs that require flying or going on vacations to visit family and friends.

Frequently, the fear of flying overlaps with other phobias, particularly *claustrophobia*—the fear of being enclosed with no ability to exit for a set period of time. Fear of heights (*acrophobia*) may also play a role. For some, the main fear is of a plane crash, despite the realistic odds of a crash being less than one in ten million. Other fears can include a fear of encountering air turbulence, a fear of hijackers, or just a general fear of relinquishing control—putting one's life in the hands of the pilots.

Flying phobia can involve avoiding flights altogether or flying only with the aid of sedation from alcohol and/or prescription tranquilizers. Fearful fliers are often afraid they will have a full-blown panic attack while flying, and this may be based on a previous bad experience.

## Causes

The most frequent cause of flying phobia is a traumatic experience with flying, either related to another phobia (such as heights or feeling enclosed) or as a result of encountering severe air turbulence, getting sick (vomiting) while in flight, and/or having a bad panic attack. Once you start to avoid flying, the longer you avoid it, the more formidable the idea of ever flying again seems to become.

Occasionally, witnessing scenes of an air crash on TV will be enough to initiate a phobia in certain individuals. Also, having a negative experience *after* the flight, such as flying to a meeting only to be told you are fired, could be traumatic enough to instigate a strong negative association with flying.

## Treatment

Education and cognitive behavioral therapy are the mainstays of effective treatment for flying phobia. Education includes information on how planes fly and all of the multiple precautions that are taken to ensure safety. The fact that planes are designed to withstand several times the amount of air turbulence they would ever encounter is helpful in diminishing fears that come up around the prospect of a bumpy ride due to turbulence. Understanding that certain abrupt noises, such as putting the landing gear down, are just a routine part of the flight can help those who jump at any unexpected sound. Finally, just knowing that the statistical odds of any single commercial plane crashing are less than one in ten million—much more favorable odds than being killed or badly injured in an auto crash—helps many people.

Cognitive behavioral therapy consists of teaching people panic-control strategies (see chapter 6) and then working to shift catastrophic thoughts based on the individual's specific fears. A hierarchy of progressive exposures to flying is set up, beginning with a trip to the airport and culminating with an actual flight, usually no more than one hour in duration. Sometimes therapists who specialize in flying phobia have an arrangement with an airline to allow their clients to enter and sit on a grounded plane a few days in advance of making an actual flight—an important intermediate exposure. On the day of the actual first flight, the therapist may accompany the client or have a support person accompany them.

Having constructive ways to divert your attention is often helpful in facilitating a less anxious initial flight. A therapist or support person can continuously talk to you both before and during the flight to divert your attention away from fearful thoughts and body symptoms. You may also take a "tool kit" on board the flight, with favorite forms of diversion, such as magazines, a CD player with guided visualizations, or puzzle books. Many air carriers offer movies to help divert attention away from the flight itself.

Medication may be an additional treatment intervention in some cases. Tranquilizers such as Xanax or Ativan, or beta blockers such as propranolol or metoprolol, may be used to help both the subjective experience of anxiety as well as physical body symptoms prior to and during the flight. Many people uneasy with flying self-medicate with alcohol both before and during the flight. One problem with this is that alcohol has a stronger effect in a pressurized cabin (due to lower oxygen levels), so one or two drinks may produce high levels of intoxication for some people.

Additional guidelines for fearful fliers:

- Educate yourself about how planes operate. For example, it's helpful to know that even if an engine fails, the plane can continue to fly. The SOAR program, mentioned in the "Resources" section below, provides detailed education about flying.

- If feeling confined is an issue, be sure to choose an aisle seat (also advisable if height above the ground is an issue).

- Give yourself plenty of time the day you make your initial flight—don't end up rushing.

- Have a support person go with you and talk to you during the flight.

- If possible, make your initial flight no more than one hour long each way.

- Have a "tool kit" of things that can divert your attention while on board the plane.

- Use prescription medication only if you feel you need to have an extra safety margin against anxiety. Avoid all caffeine the day you fly.

### Resources

There are several special programs and websites that have a wealth of information (as well as paid programs) for flying phobia. Captain Tom Bunn offers the well-known *SOAR program* for fear of flying (see fearofflying.com). Reid Wilson, PhD, offers a popular program called *Achieving Comfortable Flight* (see anxieties.com). Many books on fear of flying are available through amazon.com.

# Claustrophobia

Most people know that *claustrophobia* refers to a fear of being closed in and having no escape. It can take a variety of forms, including fear of small and/or crowded rooms such as restaurants or movie theaters, fear of being stuck in traffic, fear of tunnels, fear of subways, fear of being stuck waiting in line, or fear of sitting in a chair while receiving a procedure. It can overlap with other phobias. Many people who fear flying are really afraid of the forced confinement of being on board the plane for a set period of time. Or a fear of elevators may have a strong claustrophobic component. One of the best-known forms of claustrophobia occurs in the course of being confined in the small, tunnel-like chamber of an MRI scanner. This can be a significant problem if you need such a procedure.

For a certain proportion of claustrophobics, there is a second stage of the problem. The fear of confinement, if not relieved, leads to a fear of suffocation, of not getting enough air. Either the fear of confinement, or confinement combined with the fear of suffocation, can lead to panic attacks. Panic attacks include the usual array of symptoms, such as sweating, shaking, and heart palpitations. With claustrophobia, you may also feel that the walls are closing in on you and you may experience a desperate urge to escape.

Claustrophobia can generalize to a whole range of situations. You may come to avoid crowds in general, or you may always sit near the door of any room containing other people in order to have easy access out. Traveling may be very difficult for some claustrophobics, since any form of traveling, whether by plane, train, or car, requires a sustained period of confinement.

## Causes

There is no clear consensus on what causes claustrophobia. The most common explanation is a traumatic experience in childhood where you were frightened while being confined in some way. However, there are plenty of people with claustrophobia who cannot recall any such experience. Some degree of resistance to confinement is common for all animals and humans, but claustrophobia appears to be a very exaggerated form of this reaction.

## Treatment

As with other phobias, cognitive behavioral therapy is used effectively to treat claustrophobia. In the cognitive component, the therapist would help you identify and challenge catastrophic beliefs, such as the false idea that being confined to a crowded room or a crowded plane is potentially threatening or dangerous. You would work on strengthening the belief that there are many advantages to being able to travel over avoiding travel simply because of your fear of confinement. After working on shifting your fearful beliefs, you would undergo a custom-made hierarchy of exposures progressing from simple to more difficult types of confinement situations that bother you. For example, in the case of tunnels, you would progress from short to longer ones, likely having a support person go with you at first. In the case of public transportation (buses or trains), you would progress from short trips with a support person eventually to longer trips alone. An exposure *hierarchy* typically involves confronting a progression of incrementally more difficult situations related to the specific phobia, but in some cases certain people seem to do fine with a random order of difficulty among various exposures to confinement (see chapter 7 for further information).

*Virtual reality* has also been used effectively to treat claustrophobia. Researchers found that virtual reality—re-creating a three-dimensional video experience of an MRI procedure—reduced anxiety when subjects subsequently went through the real procedure (Garcia-Palacios et al. 2007).

Medications, including tranquilizers and beta blockers, are sometimes used to treat claustrophobia in instances where the situation you are afraid of occurs infrequently, such as making a flight.

## Resources

Entire books on the topic of claustrophobia are available on amazon.com.

# Fear of Disease (Hypochondria)

*Hypochondria* is defined as excessive worry about having a serious disease, even after medical reassurance. Often a particular body symptom, such as gastric discomfort, intermittent headaches, or heart palpitations, is taken to be evidence of a life-threatening disease. Having a bad headache might be taken as evidence of a brain tumor, or a chronic cough as evidence for cancer. Forgetting where you put something might be taken as an indication of Alzheimer's disease.

Some people continuously seek out various doctors and have repeated exams to confirm whether they have the dreaded disease, while others avoid doctors altogether out of fear that their worst-case scenario will turn out to be true.

Hypochondria is often thought of as an *OC* (obsessive-compulsive) *spectrum disorder* because it frequently involves intrusive fears followed by compulsive checking, such as feeling for lumps or continually retaking one's blood pressure. (See chapter 1 of this book for more information about OC spectrum disorders.) In other cases, it is more like a phobia, consisting of excessive sensitivity and avoidance around anything that reminds you of, for example, cancer. One difference between OCD and hypochondria is that OCD sufferers tend to fear and obsess about getting a disease, while hypochondriacs fear they already have a disease and interpret minor symptoms as evidence of the disease.

About 4 to 6 percent of the population who already have a medical issue demonstrate hypochondria at some time in their lives. The percentage is lower for people who have not had any history of significant medical issues. Men and women are about equally affected by hypochondria.

## Causes

Many different kinds of factors can lead to hypochondria. It may develop through unconscious identification after the death or serious illness of a close family member. Suddenly you begin to fear that you have developed the same or a similar disease. Even approaching the age at which a loved one's premature death occurred may be enough to trigger worry about oneself.

Predicted pandemics, such as a worldwide flu outbreak, lead some people to become obsessed with becoming ill. Even seeing a special on TV about a particular illness may be enough to trigger serious worry about that disease.

Family studies of hypochondria find little evidence of a genetic predisposition. However, having a first-degree relative with OCD increases the likelihood that you might develop obsessive preoccupation with a particular disease.

## Treatment

Cognitive behavioral therapy is the first-line treatment for hypochondria. The cognitive component focuses on identifying and countering false beliefs that lead you to overestimate the threat posed by your symptoms. The odds of actually having a life-threatening disease are usually very low, much lower than your estimated risk. The behavioral part focuses on stopping the quest for continual reassurance from doctors and others. Also, you would work on stopping continuous monitoring of your body for evidence of the problem, which only reinforces your fear. Excessive research about the disease on the Internet would also be discontinued. Being frequently exposed to symptoms that evoke worry about disease—without engaging in body monitoring, reassurance seeking, or Internet research—is an approach very similar to exposure and response prevention utilized in the treatment of OCD.

Another approach used with hypochondria is imaginal exposure. Here you would write out your worst-case scenario of having the dreaded disease (such as cancer or AIDS) in vivid detail. Your script could be audiorecorded, and you would listen to the recording repeatedly until you neutralized the fears and worries it evokes. While this can be an uncomfortable process at first, it ultimately reduces the frequency and intensity of intrusive worries about the disease.

Mindfulness-based therapy may be used to treat hypochondria just as it is in the case of OCD. The goal of mindfulness-based therapy (such as acceptance and commitment therapy) is to develop the ability to more willingly experience uncomfortable thoughts, feelings, and sensations without struggling with or trying to control them. This may naturally lead you to engage in less worry-based behavior such as doctor visits, body monitoring, or reassurance seeking.

Finally, as with OCD, SSRI (selective serotonin reuptake inhibitor) medications can be helpful in reducing anxiety (and depression) around excessive concern about having a disease.

### Resources

Many good books on health anxiety are available. See, for example, *Overcoming Health Anxiety* by Katherine Owens and Martin Antony.

# Dental Phobia

Dental phobia can involve fear and avoidance of dentistry in general, or a more specific fear about having a particular dental procedure. In some cases, it appears that the problem is not a phobia at all but symptoms of post-traumatic stress disorder in response to a previous, traumatic dental experience.

More than half of adults in America experience some anxiety about going to the dentist, though a much smaller number are phobic to the point of avoiding dentists altogether unless they have an acute, painful dental emergency. Obviously, this can create very serious problems for dental health, resulting in much more serious and intrusive procedures down the road when you have not had regular cleanings and routine dental maintenance over the years.

Women and young children report a higher incidence of dental phobia than men. The more invasive the procedure (for example, oral surgery), the greater the likelihood of dental phobia or at least considerable anticipatory dental anxiety.

### Causes

There are multiple ways you can develop a fear of going to the dentist. The most common is actually having had a painful or traumatic dental experience. A second factor is the personality of the dentist. Even in the absence of painful experiences, many people develop fears simply as the result of working with a dentist they found cold, impersonal, or uncaring.

Other causes can include hearing about someone else's bad experience or a generalization of fear from doctor phobia—that is, you can be afraid of receiving any procedure in an antiseptic clinic administered by a health professional.

Often a dental phobia can overlap with the fear of confinement (being in a chair you can't leave for a period of time) or a fear of loss of control (relinquishing complete control to the dentist, especially in the cases where you are sedated or put to sleep for the procedure). Sometimes there is a fear of surrendering to the effects of the anesthetic.

## Treatment

As with other phobias, the first-line treatment for dental phobia is cognitive behavioral therapy. This would include three components:

- Learn panic-control techniques as described in chapter 6 of this book (for example, abdominal breathing and the use of specific coping statements).

- Identify and challenge catastrophic fears about the phobic situation—the tendency both to overestimate the danger or threat of the situation and to underestimate your ability to cope, as described in chapter 8. See, in particular, the section in that chapter "Changing Self-Talk That Perpetuates Specific Fears and Phobias."

- Undergo gradual exposure to the phobic situation. A hierarchy of exposures would be set up in regard to the dentist's office, then the treatment room, and, finally, a specific procedure, such as receiving an injection before a filling. In the latter case, you might first see the lidocaine syringe, then handle it, then witness the dentist giving a "placebo" injection to himself, then finally receive the injection while in an induced state of relaxation.

There is one crucial variable beyond cognitive behavioral therapy that is critical for successful treatment: the personality and style of the dentist in caring for his or her patients.

Most dental phobics will attest to the fact that the most important factor in helping them overcome their fear was the bedside or "chairside" manner of the dentist. Is she or he warm, caring, attentive, reassuring, and willing to explain things simply and clearly? Such personal qualities go a long way to mitigate anxiety. Other things that can be done to make the overall dental environment easier for dental phobics include dispensing with traditional antiseptic smells, having the staff wear nonclinical clothes, and playing relaxing music in the background.

Specialized clinics that claim to offer fear-free dentistry exist in many major metropolitan areas. It's helpful to ask friends if they have found a dentist with whom they feel an easy and comfortable rapport.

Medications are commonly used to manage anxiety about dental procedures. Nitrous oxide (or "laughing gas") may be used to help you relax, though some people are afraid of the mask that needs to be worn to administer the gas. Benzodiazepine tranquilizers such as Xanax or Valium may be administered orally or intravenously ahead of the procedure. While such medications help you relax, you remain conscious and able to communicate with the dentist. In general, if you are prone to dental anxiety, ask your dentist about using a dental anesthetic that does not contain epinephrine.

Some general tips helpful for dental phobics:

- When trying out a new dentist, meet in advance of any procedure to get a feel for him or her personally as well as to scope out how you feel about the office setting.

- Take a supportive friend along when you go to the dentist, but don't let your friend speak for you. Instead, be sure you communicate directly to the dentist.

- For any new procedure, have the dentist explain and demonstrate the procedure in some detail before actually performing it.

- Have a predetermined hand signal you can use to let the dentist know when you need to take a break or in case you need more local anesthetic.

- Expect that you can find a dentist who is caring, responsive to your needs, willing to explain everything, and able to provide lots of positive reinforcement. If the dentist is not someone you can trust and feel comfortable with, look for someone else.

### Resources

For further helpful information on dealing with dental phobias, do a Google search for "help for dental phobia," where you will find a large number of sites on the topic.

## Blood/Injection Phobia

Fear of blood, fear of injuries associated with blood, and fear of injections or blood draws often go together. The prevalence of these fears in the adult population is about 4 percent. A complete phobia of injections can have very serious health consequences, if you refuse to receive blood tests or potentially life-saving medication that needs to be administered by injection or IV. About 25 percent of people with blood/injection phobias jeopardize their health by avoiding visits to doctors altogether (Thompson 1999).

Of all anxiety disorders, blood/injection phobia has the strongest degree of family association. Up to 60 percent of people with this type of phobia have a family member with the same or related problem, whereas the incidence in the general population, as mentioned, is about 4 percent. While extensive research on this question has not been done, one study found the heritability of blood/injection phobia to be 59 percent (LeBeau et al. 2010). An unusual characteristic of blood/injection phobias, distinguishing them from all other phobias, is that they often involve a fainting response. When confronted with the sight of blood (your own or another's) or the prospect of receiving an injection, there is a twofold response. The first phase is a normal anxiety response with increased heart rate, increased blood pressure, and other panic-like symptoms. This is followed by a sudden drop in blood pressure, slowing down of heart rate (called *bradycardia*), and reduced blood flow to the brain, which may result in fainting or prefainting reactions such as dizziness, sweatiness, tunnel vision, or nausea. These symptoms are due to a phenomenon called a "vasovagal response." It appears that the vagus nerve, the tenth of your twelve cranial nerves, stimulates your parasympathetic nervous system to overcompensate for the initial sympathetic nervous system arousal associated with high anxiety. (For more information about the parasympathetic and sympathetic nervous systems, see the section "The Physiology of Panic" in chapter 2.) About 75 percent of people with blood/injection phobias tend to have prefainting symptoms or actually faint, allowing them to escape from the feared stimulus.

## Causes

Causes of blood/injection phobia are yet to be fully understood. There is some evidence suggesting this class of phobias has a hereditary basis, as mentioned above. However, many people with blood/injury phobias cite a traumatic cause in childhood as their perceived source of the problem. Blood/injury phobia may develop in childhood in response to a frightening experience at the doctor's office.

## Treatment

Cognitive behavioral therapy, emphasizing exposure therapy, works well for blood/ injection phobias. However, because of the fainting response, an additional technique called "applied tension" is included. Upon the first sensation of possibly fainting, you are instructed to tense your feet, legs, arms, and shoulders quickly all at once. Then you release them and tense them again. This raises blood pressure and blocks the fainting response. Even more important, it gives you confidence that you have a coping strategy you can use to overcome fainting. With this confidence, it's much easier to negotiate exposure.

It takes some resourcefulness to come up with effective exposures for this type of phobia. A possible hierarchy of exposures for blood phobia would include:

1. Read an article about bleeding.

2. Look at photos of blood.

3. Look at photos of injuries involving blood.

4. Watch videos or movies involving blood and injuries.

5. Hold a jar or test tube containing blood.

6. Visit a blood bank.

7. Witness a veterinary surgery (if this can be arranged).

For injection phobia, a possible exposure hierarchy might include:

1. Look at photos of people receiving a shot.

2.  Look at videos of people receiving a shot.

3.  Visit a doctor's office and watch someone get a shot.

4.  Visit a doctor's office and watch someone receive a blood draw.

5.  Handle syringes.

6.  Have a health professional touch a syringe needle to your skin without penetration.

7.  Receive a shot in the arm.

8.  Receive a blood draw.

As with other phobias, it is best to start the hierarchy at whatever step causes mild anxiety, and repeat any more difficult steps more than once if they cause excessive anxiety. For some people, doing exposures in a random order of difficulty instead of a progressive order may expedite the process. A support person going with you to a medical setting at first can be quite helpful. Medication (a tranquilizer) can be used to help negotiate a particularly difficult step, but it's generally not recommended if you are prone to fainting. In order to gain confidence that you won't faint, applied tension should be used the moment you feel light-headed. As described above, this includes suddenly tensing your feet, legs, arms, and shoulders together at once. Hold them tight for at least five seconds. Then release all your muscles, followed by tensing them and relaxing them again. In some cases where fainting is a difficult problem, the exposures may be done first lying down, then sitting up, and finally standing.

In medical and particularly dental settings, a variety of anesthetics may be used to reduce the fear of being injected. These usually include some kind of numbing gel applied to the gum followed by a very gradual injection of anesthetic. Often you aren't even aware of the needle at all. Most competent dentists are proficient in administering painless injections.

### Resources

As with all specific phobias, a variety of useful websites may be found by doing a Google search for "blood/injury phobia."

## Fear of Vomiting (Emetophobia)

Fear of vomiting, sometimes called *emetophobia*, is surprisingly prevalent. It can take various forms, including the fear of vomiting itself, a fear of doing so in public, a fear of seeing vomit, or a fear of seeing someone else throw up.

Emetophobia can develop in childhood or adulthood and last for years without treatment. Sometimes it accompanies other fears, such as the fear of eating, or other disorders, such as eating disorders (anorexia and/or bulimia) or obsessive-compulsive disorder.

Most people with emetophobia rarely actually vomit and may not have done so since childhood. Yet when the fear is severe, your life can be restricted in many ways. You may avoid long car trips or only go places where you know a restroom is easily available. You may only want to drive when you can be the driver or even only when you are able to drive alone. Or you may be afraid to be around babies or sick people who you believe have an increased risk of throwing up. Frequently, you are hypervigilant around any gastrointestinal symptoms. In this phobia, nausea is just about the worst thing that can happen to you. You are afraid you might vomit, which aggravates more nausea, which in turn increases the urge to vomit, and around the cycle goes until you may panic.

Sometimes the fear of vomiting becomes associated with a fear of eating. You may strongly restrict what you eat or undereat to avoid the possibility of feeling full (as the feeling of being full could potentially precede vomiting). In rare cases, emetophobia can be associated with anorexia.

## Causes

A general fear of losing control can often be found in the background of people who are fearful of vomiting. For some, the phobia begins with a particularly bad instance of vomiting in childhood, or seeing vomiting in a loved one who is very ill. The more traumatic the initial experience was, the more likely a phobia may develop. In other cases, no traumatic past incident can be found, and the fear seems to center more around losing control of yourself.

## Treatment

If you are emetophobic, the first thing to find out is what it is you are truly afraid of. Is it vomiting itself, or is it a fear of rejection if others were to see you vomit? Or does it have to do more generally with losing control of your body? It's important to identify and work through the core fear or fears.

Next, it's important to make a list of all the situations you avoid because of your fear. For example, you might avoid long car trips, taking a boat cruise, eating certain foods that you think could make you sick, being around babies and young children, or going on amusement park rides. List all of the situations you avoid in order of difficulty and then gradually take the risk to face and enter each one of them. Working with a progression of exposures will help you reclaim your life as well as reduce the fear of vomiting itself.

Finally, exposure to the vomiting itself will help you overcome your fear. One way to do exposure is to write down a series of vomiting scenarios, starting off easy and progressing up to the worst-case vomiting scenario you can imagine (for example, you describe in graphic detail vomiting all over yourself and others while being in the presence of work associates who disapprove). Read through your written vomiting scenarios repeatedly, or, better yet, have someone read them to you over and over several times, until the scenes lose their ability to evoke much anxiety. You can also record your series of vomiting scenarios on your smartphone and play them back.

Another way to do exposure (not exclusive of the first) is to look at a series of vomiting scenes, progressing from color photos of vomiting to videos and movies that have graphic vomit scenes. Ultimately, you should progress to a live vomiting situation—for example, a nursery where babies are having lunch and spit up on themselves. If you are bold, you can progress to self-induced vomiting, though emetophobic experts are mixed on whether this is helpful.

By doing one or both types of exposure, you will become more used to vomiting and shift your core beliefs away from vomiting being something horrific to it merely being a normal bodily function.

Medications are generally not used for emetophobia (except sometimes in helping you enter a previously avoided situation). If acid reflux is a part of emetophobia, medications for that problem can be helpful. Many emetophobics tend to avoid antianxiety medications for fear they will cause vomiting. Natural remedies for nausea, such as ginger tea or 7Up, may be helpful in reducing long-lasting symptoms of nausea that exacerbate anxiety.

### Resources

Many excellent websites on emetophobia are available online.

## Fear of Heights

The fear of heights, or *acrophobia*, is another very common phobia. Frequently, it combines with other phobias, such as the fear of flying, fear of riding elevators, or a fear of driving over a high bridge. The most frequent form of the fear is being high up in a building. About 5 percent of the adult population suffers from acrophobia, and the condition affects more women than men.

Sometimes the fear of heights is confused with vertigo. *Vertigo* is a sensation of spinning usually caused by a medical condition, and it rarely occurs with acrophobia. A more common reaction to heights is dizziness and difficulty trusting your own sense of balance. Frequently, you may grab on to something to steady yourself, and, if that doesn't help, you may panic.

People with acrophobia should avoid construction work at heights or climbing tall ladders. Unfortunately, this is one phobia where panic might, in some circumstances, lead to a dangerous fall.

Acrophobia can result in severe restrictions on your life if it causes you, for example, to avoid taking a job offer that would involve being high up in a building or visiting a close relative in the hospital who is on a high floor.

### Causes

A certain amount of acrophobia is instinctive in all animals. It has an evolutionary advantage in preventing falls. However, a true phobia of heights is typically learned and is an exaggeration of the normal, adaptive fear response to heights. It may develop as the result of an actual fall or the memory of an incident where you were very afraid of falling as a child. People prone to having problems with balance may be more susceptible to developing a fear of heights, but the research on this is inconclusive.

## Treatment

Cognitive behavioral therapy is effective in overcoming the fear of heights. The acrophobic is first taught panic-control strategies (see chapter 6) and then undergoes a hierarchy of exposures to situations that involve increasing heights. This can be done by going up successive floors in a building and looking out a window or even walking onto balconies. As with other phobias, having a support person accompany you when you first attempt exposure can be very helpful. Here is an example of a hierarchy of exposures for the fear of heights:

1.  Go to the second story of a building and look out a window for ten to sixty seconds. Have a support person go with you if you wish.

2.  Look out of a second-story window for two to five minutes. Look straight out and then down. Have a support person go with you at first, if you wish, then do it alone.

3.  Go to the third floor of a building and look out a window for ten to sixty seconds. Take someone with you, if you wish.

4.  Repeat the previous step for two or three minutes. Look straight ahead and then down.

5.  Repeat the previous two steps with phone access to your support person, then do them again alone.

6.  Continue the process you did with the preceding steps for progressively higher floors in a taller building. Beyond the fourth floor, take an elevator to higher floors.

7.  Continue advancing to higher floors until you reach your desired goal (ideally, the highest floor of the tallest building in the area where you live).

8.  If possible, go out on a balcony or an observation deck at your goal height (you may want to try balconies on lower floors first).

**Note:** The above exposure hierarchy pertains only to dealing with tall buildings, which may or may not be close to where you live. Acrophobia may also involve a fear of high, steep roads or high bridges. In either case, you may want to write out detailed scenarios where you visualize undertaking a high road or bridge first, then confront the height in real life, perhaps first with a support person and ultimately alone. For acrophobia that comes up during flying, see the section of this chapter on fear of flying.

Virtual exposure has also been used effectively with the fear of heights. This involves re-creating a hierarchy of height scenarios in virtual reality using special equipment. Clinics that can afford the equipment prefer this option because it allows therapists to treat more people in a more efficient and timely manner.

## Resources

Several good books on the fear of heights are available on amazon.com.

# Animal and Insect Phobias

Phobias of specific types of animals or insects abound. The fear can be of snakes, bats, mice or rats, dogs, cats, certain birds, frogs, spiders, bees, or cockroaches, to name some of the most common examples. People with this type of phobia avoid not only a particular animal/insect but also areas where they believe they might be exposed to the feared creature. Evidence of the presence of the feared animal/insect, such as seeing a spiderweb, hearing a dog bark, or being near a zoo, is enough to evoke strong fear. Sometimes merely seeing a picture of the creature will lead to a panic attack.

In childhood, some of these fears are so common that they are considered normal. Only when they significantly disrupt your life and/or cause you significant distress—as a child or an adult—do they qualify as a full-blown phobia. In general, animal and insect phobias tend to be more common in women than men, especially in regard to snakes, mice, spiders, and cockroaches.

## Causes

It has been proposed that certain animal or insect phobias, such as fears of snakes or large animals, are innate in all mammals because they confer an evolutionary advantage in promoting survival. In many cases, though, the cause of the phobia appears to be a previous traumatic experience, such as being bitten by a dog, scratched by a cat, or stung by a wasp. It's also possible for children to acquire fears of animals or insects from their parents. Simply observing a parent express fear at the sight of a mouse or a spider may instill the same fear in the child. There have also been instances where simply watching a horror film that featured a particular animal or insect was sufficient to cause a phobia.

## Treatment

Overcoming animal and insect phobias is straightforward and usually involves a hierarchy of exposures to the feared creature. As with exposure to any other type of phobia, it's important to set up a series of exposures in increasing order of difficulty. You may want to do your exposure series incrementally, progressing from photos and videos to eventual approach and ultimately possible contact with the living creature (for example, in the case of phobias of harmless garden snakes or frogs). Some people prefer doing the exposures in a random order of difficulty, which may be more anxiety-provoking but expedites the process of overcoming the phobia. A generic exposure hierarchy, applicable to any animal/insect phobia, might run something like this:

1. Draw a picture of the animal/insect.

2. Look at black-and-white photos of the animal/insect.

3. View color photos of the animal/insect.

4. Watch a video featuring the animal/insect.

5. Handle a toy version of the animal/insect.

6. Look at the animal/insect from a distance (this could involve a trip to a pet store or zoo).

7. Move progressively closer to the live animal/insect.

8. Watch someone touch or hold the animal/insect.

9. Touch or hold the animal/insect in a cage and, ultimately, directly (if it is safe to do so).

**Note:** The last two steps may require a visit to a pet store, nature center, or zoo. In cases where it's not possible to touch the creature (bears, for example), sustained close observation at a zoo would be the final step in the exposure hierarchy.

As with all exposure therapy, working through the various steps of the exposure hierarchy requires commitment, perseverance, and a willingness to tolerate varying degrees of anxiety. If anxiety becomes extreme, it can be useful to have a support person accompany you through the early phases of exposure. Sometimes medication, such as a beta blocker or a benzodiazepine, may be helpful to facilitate getting through a particularly challenging step, but the medication eventually needs to be relinquished. See chapter 7 for the distinction between "coping exposure" and "full exposure." In beginning a hierarchy of exposures, it's common to start off with whatever step evokes mild to moderate anxiety, skipping any early steps that do not elicit anxiety at all. Repeat any step that causes very high anxiety more than once if you need to until your anxiety diminishes to a tolerable level.

In working through exposure to animals or insects, it's also important to think about what it is about the animal or insect that you find particularly frightening. In the case of a dog, for example, is it the barking, the appearance, the size, the way the dog moves, or mainly the idea of being attacked? If you have a phobia of spiders (*arachnophobia*), is it the appearance of the spider, the way it moves, or the size of the spider that triggers your fear? Once you pinpoint what specific characteristics of the creature bother you the most, then it's important to focus on those characteristics as you progress through your exposure. Once you've become less conditioned to the most bothersome characteristics by repeated exposure, you are more likely to remain free of the phobia indefinitely.

### Resources

To explore further information on the nature and treatment of animal as well as insect/spider phobias, you might want to consult some of the books on these topics available on amazon.com. You may find the book *Overcoming Animal and Insect Phobias* by Martin Antony and Randi McCabe to be helpful.

## Fear of Death

The fear of death, sometimes referred to as *thanatophobia*, can involve any one or several of a variety of distinct fears. Here are some of the most common types:

- Fear of nonexistence, a permanent end to life

- Fear of the unknown—not knowing what will happen after death

- Fear of a negative afterlife based on religious beliefs, such as the ideas of hell or purgatory

- Fear of sickness, pain, and suffering associated with death

- Fear of the death of a loved one to whom you are closely attached

- Fear of what will happen to loved ones in your family after your death

- Fear of dead things, such as a corpse, or things associated with death, such as coffins, funeral homes, and cemeteries (this type of fear is referred to as *necrophobia*)

Sometimes the basic fear is simply one of losing control. Dying is out of your control, and you may attempt to hold death at bay through frequent visits to doctors and ritualistic health practices (an instance where the fear of death overlaps with hypochondria). Approximately 20 percent of Americans express some degree of fear of death.

## Causes

Causes of the fear of death vary depending on which of the above fears is dominant. Existentialist philosophy maintains that the fear of nonexistence is innate to the human condition and shared by all human beings at a deep level. Some have even gone so far as to claim that the fear of death (in the sense of permanent nonexistence) is the "core" or underlying fear behind all fears. There is certainly at least some truth to the existentialist point of view. All of us, at one point or another, have had anxiety about our eventual demise.

Other fears of death center around religious beliefs about punishment and hell in the afterlife. Counselors who deem these beliefs to be fictitious need to be sensitive in working with clients who take them quite seriously.

The fear of pain and suffering associated with death may arise from a traumatic experience of witnessing a loved one go through a protracted process of dying. Often the death of a loved one may lead to an increased fear of one's own death as well as a fear of sights and objects associated with death.

Anxiety about death naturally increases with aging and often in association with illnesses that occur with aging. Increased death anxiety as a result of minor body symptoms is analogous to hypochondria and, if the fears and thoughts about death are consistent and intrusive, may be considered an OC spectrum disorder.

## Treatment

Treatment of thanatophobia, of course, depends on the specific nature of your particular fear. Working with the fear of nonexistence may require some deep philosophical reflection on the meaning of life and the recognition that probably the best way to deal with death is to live life as well as you can. It's also important to realize that none of us is unique in this regard; everyone has to deal with death.

Some people respond favorably to reading literature that provides evidence for the survival of consciousness following death. An extensive literature on near-death experiences, and numerous individual accounts of what people "saw" during such experiences, provides compelling evidence for many that death is not a permanent end to existence.

Among books that describe visions of the "other side" by people who have had near-death experiences, the following are a good place to start: *Life After Life* by Raymond Moody, *Evidence of the Afterlife* by Jeffrey Long, or *Proof of Heaven* by Eben Alexander. Fear of the death of a loved one can be difficult, but may be seen as a "spiritual call" to develop inner strength and the capacity to stand on your own even in the absence of someone dear. Some people are heartened by the belief that, after their death, they will be reunited with loved ones who "went before," a possibility that is clearly indicated by the literature on near-death experiences.

Finally, if your fear of death started with a traumatic experience of witnessing a friend or family member's death, it may be helpful to try hypnotherapy or eye movement desensitization and reprocessing (EMDR) to work through and reconfigure traumatic memories. (For more information, do a Google search of EMDR.)

### Resources

As with all of the phobias listed in this chapter, a search on amazon.com for "overcoming the fear of death" will bring up a number of helpful books on the topic.

## Summary of Things to Do

1. Read about any specific phobia in this chapter that affects you. You may wish to work with a therapist or a supportive friend in actually undertaking a detailed exposure plan to overcome your fear. A Google search of any of the phobias described in this chapter will yield websites that offer further information, advice, and various treatment options. A search on amazon.com using the term "fear of _____" will bring up books on how to overcome the specific phobia in many cases.

2. Even if you struggle with phobias that are not described in this chapter (such as thunderstorms or seasickness, for example), reading the treatment sections for all of the various phobia types may give you some new insights on how to work through whatever phobia(s) you do have. Also see chapter 7 for further information on the details of facing a phobia in general. There are hundreds of different types of phobias, but the basic principles for facing and overcoming them are the same.

# Further Reading

Alexander, Eben. *Proof of Heaven*. New York: Simon & Schuster, 2012.

Antony, Martin M., and Randi E. McCabe. *Overcoming Animal & Insect Phobias*. Oakland, CA: New Harbinger Publications, 2005.

Bourne, Edmund J. *Overcoming Specific Phobia: Therapist Protocol and Client Manual* (two-book set). Oakland, CA: New Harbinger Publications, 1998.

Brown, Duane. *Flying Without Fear*. 2nd ed. Oakland, CA: New Harbinger Publications, 2009.

Esposito, Janet. *Getting Over Stage Fright*. St. Louis, MO: Love Your Life Publishing, 2009.

———. *In the Spotlight: Overcoming Your Fear of Public Speaking and Performing*. Bridgewater, CT: In the Spotlight, 2000.

Garcia-Palacios, A., H. Hoffman, T. Richards, E. Seibel, and S. Sharar. 2007. "Use of Virtual Reality Distraction to Reduce Claustrophobia Symptoms During a Mock Magnetic Resonance Imaging Brain Scan: A Case Report." *CyberPsychology and Behavior* 10(3): 485–88.

LeBeau, Richard, Daniel Glenn, Betty Liao, Hans-Ulrich Wittchen, Katja Beesdo-Baum, Thomas Ollendick, and Michelle G. Craske. 2010. "Specific Phobia: A Review of DSM-IV Specific Phobia and Preliminary Recommendations for *DSM-5*." *Depression & Anxiety* 27(2): 148–67.

Long, Jeffrey. *Evidence of the Afterlife: The Science of Near-Death Experiences*. New York: HarperCollins, 2010.

Moody, Raymond. *Life After Life: The Bestselling Original Investigation That Revealed "Near-Death Experiences."* New York: HarperOne, 2015.

Thompson, Alandra. 1999. "Cognitive Behavioral Treatment of Blood-Injury-Injection Phobia: A Case Study." *Behavior Change* 36: 182–90.

Weisinger, Hendrie, and J. P. Pawliw-Fry. *Performing Under Pressure*. New York: Crown Books, 2015.

# 13

# Dealing with Feelings

As you progress in your recovery, you may notice unaccustomed emotions and feelings beginning to surface. This is particularly true if you're beginning to confront your phobias. It's entirely normal to experience feelings more intensely when you begin to face situations you've been avoiding for a long time. If this is happening to you, you're on the right track.

Many people who are phobic and prone to anxiety tend to have difficulty with feelings. You may have a problem just knowing *what* you're feeling. Or you may be able to identify your feelings but unable to express them. When feelings begin to come up in the course of facing phobias or dealing with panic, there is often a tendency to withhold them, which only aggravates your stress and anxiety. The purposes of this chapter are 1) to help you increase your awareness of feelings and 2) to give you some tools and strategies for identifying and expressing them more readily.

## Some Facts About Feelings

- Feelings, unlike thoughts, involve a *total body reaction*. They are mediated both by a part of your brain called the limbic system and by the involuntary, autonomic nervous system in your body. When you're emotionally excited, you "feel it all over" and experience bodily reactions such as increased heart rate, quickened respiration, perspiration, and even shaking or trembling. (Note the similarity to panic, which is another type of intense emotional state.)

- Feelings do not come out of the blue but are *influenced by your thoughts and perceptions*. They arise from the way you perceive or interpret outer events and/or the way you react to your own inner thought processes or "self--talk" (see chapter 8), imagery, or memories. If you can't identify a stimulus for a particular emotional reaction (for example, a spontaneous panic attack), that stimulus may be unconscious. Feelings are also affected by stress. When you're under stress, your body is already in a state of physiological arousal similar to that which accompanies an emotion. Since you're already primed to have emotional reactions, it may not take much to set you off. The particular type of emotion you happen to experience will depend on your view of external events and what you tell yourself about them.

- Feelings can be divided into two groups—*simple* and *complex*. There is much controversy and disagreement about how to do this—and even whether it can be done—

but for our purposes here, a distinction will be made between *basic emotions* such as anger, grief, sadness, fear, love, excitement, or joy, and more *complex feelings* such as eagerness, relief, disappointment, or impatience. Complex feelings may involve a combination of more basic emotions and are also shaped by thoughts and imagery. Many of the feelings on *The Feeling List* presented later in this chapter are complex. Complex feelings can last a long time and are more tied to thought processes, while basic emotions tend to be short-lived, more reactive, and more tied to involuntary physical reactions mediated by your autonomic nervous system. Fear or panic is a basic emotion, while free-floating anxiety (anxiety without an object) is an example of a more complex feeling.

- Feelings are what give you *energy*. If you're in touch with your feelings and can express them, you'll feel more energetic. If you're out of touch with your feelings or unable to give them expression, you may feel lethargic, numb, tired, or depressed. As you'll see shortly, blocked or withheld feelings can lead to anxiety.

- Feelings often come in *mixtures* rather than in pure form. Sometimes you may experience a simple, basic emotion such as fear, sadness, or rage. More often, though, you'll find that you feel two or more emotions at the same time. For example, it's common to feel anger and fear at the same time when you're threatened. Or you may feel anger, guilt, and love all at the same time in response to arguing with your partner, parent, or close friend. The common expression *sorting out feelings* reflects the fact that you can feel several things at once.

- Feelings can be *contagious*. If you're close to someone who is crying, you may start to feel sad or even cry yourself. Or you may pick up on another's excitement or enthusiasm. Phobic and anxiety-prone individuals are often particularly susceptible to taking on the feelings of people around them. The more you learn to be in touch with and comfortable with your own feelings, the less prone you'll be to "catch" those of others.

- Feelings are *not* right or wrong. As reactions, feelings simply *exist*. Fear, joy, guilt, and anger are not in and of themselves valid or invalid—you just happen to have these feelings and usually will feel better if you can express them. The *perceptions* or *judgments* you made that *led* to your feelings, however, may be right or wrong, valid or invalid. Be careful not to judge yourself or anyone else as wrong for simply having a feeling, whatever that feeling may be.

- Strong feelings are often clues to unmet needs. Perhaps you're feeling anxious because you're afraid of what other people will think of you if you show signs of panic. The need for acceptance underlies your fear. Or you're feeling angry because your partner broke an important agreement you had. The need behind your anger is for respect and consideration. Often, by looking for the need behind your feelings, you give your feelings a new and deeper perspective. When you've gained more insight into your needs, you can begin to address how to go about meeting them.

- Feelings are often subject to *suppression*. Sometimes you may actively control or "hold in" your feelings. For example, you're still upset from an argument with your spouse and then you have to talk to a colleague at work. You deliberately and consciously hold back your feelings, because you know that it would be inappropriate for them to carry over into your work situation. On other occasions, you may start to experience feelings that are unpleasant and decide that you don't want to deal with them. Instead of deliberately suppressing them, you just get busy and put your mind on something else—in essence, you ignore them. Over time, the practice of continually suppressing your feelings can lead to increased difficulty in expressing or even identifying them. When the process of suppression begins in childhood, you may grow up being out of touch with your feelings and going through life experiencing a certain numbness or "emptiness."

## Why Phobic and Anxiety-Prone People Have a Tendency to Suppress Their Feelings

People with anxiety disorders tend to withhold their feelings. There are several reasons for this.

First, many such people tend to have a very strong need for control and/or a fear of losing control (see the section "Excessive Need for Control" in chapter 11). It's difficult to surrender to the partial loss of control involved in the full experience of your feelings. When feelings have been chronically denied for a long time, they can loom very large and overwhelmingly when they first begin to surface. You can even experience irrational fears of "going crazy" or "coming apart" when you give in to the full force of these long-withheld feelings. Note that these are the very same fears that occur during a panic attack. In fact, in some cases *panic itself may be a signal that suppressed feelings are trying to emerge.* Instead of dealing with feelings that seem overwhelming, you panic instead. It's important to learn that feelings only *seem* overwhelming or scary at the point when they first begin to surface. This scariness goes away as soon as you allow yourself to accept and *feel* them. It's simply not possible to "go crazy" by fully feeling your emotions. In fact, "craziness"—or severe emotional disturbance—is more likely to develop as an outcome of not experiencing your feelings.

A second reason why phobic people have difficulty expressing their feelings is because often they grew up in families with overly critical parents who set unrealistically high or perfectionist standards. In such a situation, a child doesn't feel free to express her or his natural impulses and feelings. Parental approval is so essential to us as children that we will always suppress our natural reactions and feelings if they are in conflict with parental expectations. As adults, many of us continue to make that choice. Anger is typically the most common feeling to be withheld because it was frequently not tolerated in childhood or its expression was punished. To the child, anger becomes truly dangerous if its expression threatens the continued approval and affection of their parents, on whom that child is completely dependent for survival. More will be said about anger later in this chapter.

# Identifying, Expressing, and Communicating Feelings

Because phobic people, by their very nature, tend to be emotionally reactive and have feelings, it is especially important for them to learn to express rather than withhold what they feel. Actually, a three-stage process is involved here.

Perhaps you have so withheld your emotions that much of the time you don't even know *what* you're feeling. An important first step is to learn how to *identify* your feelings. Once this awareness and ability to identify feelings have both developed, the second step is learning to *express* them. This typically involves being willing to share your feelings with another person. Alternatively, you may choose to "write out" your feelings in a journal, or physically discharge them (for example, by crying or venting anger into a pillow).

Once you've given some expression to your feelings, you're ready for the third and final step: *communicating* them to whomever you perceive to have contributed to "triggering" these particular emotions. For the purposes of this chapter, "communicating" a feeling means to let someone know that your feeling involves something he or she said or did.

The good news is that identifying, expressing, and communicating your feelings is something that can be learned—and something that can be improved upon with practice. It does take some time and perseverance, however, if you've been accustomed to withholding or ignoring feelings for much of your life.

To sum up, your ability to gain awareness of and express your feelings is an *essential* part of the process of recovering from anxiety disorders. It is just as important as relaxation, exposure, and the cognitive skills discussed in previous chapters.

# Identifying Your Feelings

How can you identify what you're feeling? It will help to follow these three steps:

1.  Recognize the symptoms of suppressed feelings.

2.  Tune in to your body.

3.  Identify the exact feeling.

## *Recognize the Symptoms of Suppressed Feelings*

Held-in feelings frequently make themselves known through several types of bodily and psychological symptoms:

*Free-floating anxiety.* Anxiety arises from many sources. Sometimes it's simply fear in the face of uncertainty. Sometimes it's the result of anticipating a negative outcome ("what-if" thinking). If anxiety doesn't seem to relate to any specific situation—if it's only a vague, undefined uneasiness—this may be because it arises from strong but unexpressed feelings. Every feeling carries a charge of energy. When we hold that energy in and do not give it expression, it may create a state of tension or vague anxiety. The next time you hold in your anger toward someone, notice whether you feel anxious afterward. Holding in enthusiasm or excitement about something can also produce anxiety.

*Depression.* In his well-known book *The Road Less Traveled*, M. Scott Peck defines depression as "stuck feelings." Often we may feel depressed when we're holding in unexpressed grief or sadness over some loss. Letting out tears and crying often helps us feel better—we effectively mourn the loss. Depression can also result from holding in anger. Gestalt psychologists were the first to point out that depression can mask anger turned in against the self. If you find yourself feeling depressed without any obvious recent loss, it may help to ask yourself what you're angry about. This is an especially good question if you find that you're attacking and criticizing yourself.

*Psychosomatic symptoms.* Common psychosomatic symptoms such as headaches, acid reflux, high blood pressure, and asthma are often the end result of chronically withheld feelings. While psychosomatic symptoms can arise from any type of chronic stress, the holding in of feelings over many years is a form of stress that is especially likely to take its toll on your body. Learning to identify and express strong feelings can lead to a reduction or even a remission of many types of psychosomatic symptoms.

*Muscle tension.* Stiff, tight muscles are a common symptom of chronically withheld feelings. You tend to tighten certain groups of muscles when you suppress and hold in what you feel. Different feelings may be held in by tightening different muscle groups. Anger or frustration may be suppressed by tightening the back of your neck and shoulders. Grief and sadness can be held in by tightening muscles in the abdomen or chest and around the eyes. Fear can be held in through tightening up in the stomach/diaphragm area.

These correlations between areas of the body and suppression of specific feelings should not be viewed as absolute. Anger, for example, can be held in by tightening many different muscle groups from the eyes to the pelvis. The point is that tight muscles and physical tension in any region may be a sign of chronically bottled-up feelings. This relationship between suppressed feelings and muscular tension has been explored in great depth by the school of therapy known as *bioenergetics*.

Any of the above four symptoms may indicate that you've been withholding strong feelings. Once you've recognized this, the next step is to tune in to exactly what it is you're feeling.

## Tune in to Your Body

Staying in your head, preoccupied with daily worries and concerns, tends to keep you out of touch with your feelings. To switch gears and gain access to your feelings, it's necessary to shift your focus from your head to your body. Again, feelings tend to be held in the body. Our use of language reflects this in expressions such as "heartbroken," "pain in the neck," and "gut-level feeling." By making time to tune in to your body, you can learn to get in touch with and identify your feelings. Many people have found the following steps to be useful. (They are based on a process called "experiential focusing" developed by Eugene Gendlin—see the reading list at the end of this chapter.)

1. Physically relax. It's difficult to know what you're feeling if your body is tense and your mind is racing. Spend five to ten minutes doing progressive muscle relaxation, meditation, or some other relaxation technique to slow yourself down.

2. Ask yourself, "What am I feeling right now?" or alternatively, "What is my main problem or concern right now?"

3. Tune in to that place in your body where you feel emotional sensations such as anger, fear, or sadness. Often this will be in the area of your heart or your gut (stomach/diaphragm), although it may be other areas higher or lower in the body. This is your "inner place of feelings."

4. Wait and listen carefully to whatever you can sense or pick up on in your place of feelings. *Don't try to analyze or judge* what's there. Be an observer and allow yourself to sense any feelings or moods that are waiting to surface. Simply *wait* until something emerges. What emerges has been described as a "felt sense" (Gendlin 2007).

5. If you draw a blank on steps 3 and 4 or are still stuck in your head (that is, your thoughts are racing), go back to step 1 and start over again. Most likely you need more time to relax. A few minutes of slow, deep breathing will often help increase your awareness of your feelings.

6. Once you've obtained a general sense of what you're feeling, it may help you to make it seem more concrete by answering the following questions:

   - *Where in my body is this feeling?*
   - *What is the shape of this feeling?*
   - *What is the size of this feeling?*
   - *If this feeling had a color, what would it be?*

If, after taking the time to relax and tune in to what you're feeling, you still have only a vague sense of what's there, it may be useful to look at a list of "feeling words" to help you identify the exact feeling you're experiencing.

## Identify the Exact Feeling: The Feeling List

The list of feeling words that follow may help you identify exactly what you're feeling. Use the list anytime you have a vague sense of some feeling but are unsure of exactly what it might be: read down the list until a particular feeling word stands out and then check to see if it matches your inner experience.

# The Feeling List

## Positive Feelings

| | |
|---|---|
| Accepted | Grateful |
| Affectionate | Great |
| Alive | Happy |
| Amused | Hopeful |
| Beautiful | Joyful |
| Brave | Lovable |
| Calm | Loved |
| Capable | Loving |
| Caring | Loyal |
| Cheerful | Passionate |
| Cherished | Peaceful |
| Comfortable | Playful |
| Competent | Pleased |
| Concerned | Proud |
| Confident | Quiet |
| Content | Relaxed |
| Courageous | Relieved |
| Curious | Respected |
| Delighted | Safe |
| Desirable | Satisfied |
| Eager | Secure |
| Energized | Self-reliant |
| Excited | Sexy |
| Forgiving | Silly |
| Friendly | Special |
| Fulfilled | Strong |
| Generous | Supportive |
| Glad | Sympathetic |
| Good | Tender |

## Negative Feelings

| | |
|---|---|
| Afraid | Hostile |
| Angry | Humiliated |
| Anxious | Hurt |
| Apprehensive | Ignored |
| Ashamed | Impatient |
| Awkward | Inadequate |
| Bitter | Incompetent |
| Bored | Indecisive |
| Confused | Inferior |
| Contemptuous | Inhibited |
| Defeated | Insecure |
| Dejected | Irritated |
| Dependent | Isolated |
| Depressed | Jealous |
| Despairing | Lonely |
| Desperate | Melancholy |
| Devastated | Miserable |
| Disappointed | Misunderstood |
| Discouraged | Muddled |
| Disgusted | Needy |
| Distrustful | Outraged |
| Embarrassed | Overwhelmed |
| Exasperated | Panicky |
| Fearful | Tired |
| Foolish | Touchy |
| Frantic | Trapped |
| Frustrated | Troubled |
| Furious | Unappreciated |
| Guilty | Unattractive |
| Hateful | Uncertain |
| Helpless | Uncomfortable |
| Hopeless | Uneasy |
| Horrified | Unfulfilled |

# Expressing Feelings

Once you're able to identify what you're feeling, it's important to express it, particularly if you feel strongly. *Expressing* feelings, here, is defined as "letting them out" by 1) sharing them with someone else, 2) writing them out, or 3) physically discharging them (such as by hitting a plastic bat against your bed or crying into a pillow). Expressing your feelings does *not* mean "dumping" or directing them toward someone you perceive to be responsible for how you feel. The skill of letting people know how you feel about them (or better, their behavior) is discussed later, in the section "Communicating Your Feelings to Someone."

Feelings can be compared to charges of energy that need physical release or discharge from your body. When unexpressed, they tend to become stuck in your body in the form of tension, anxiety, or other symptoms previously described. Your physical health, as well as your sense of well-being, depends on your willingness to acknowledge and express feelings at or close to the time they occur. Here are some useful ways of expressing your feelings.

## Talk It Out

Probably the best way to express feelings is to share them with a supportive friend, mate, or counselor. Sharing means not just talking *about* your feelings but actually letting them out. It's important that you have a high level of trust toward the person you share with in order to open up and fully disclose your true feelings. Also, it's important that the person *listen carefully*—in other words, he or she does not offer advice, opinions, or suggestions while you're sharing. Your ability to share fully will in part be determined by your partner's willingness to do nothing more than just listen without interrupting until you are finished.

## Write It Out

If your feelings are running high and there's no one immediately available to talk to, take a pen and paper and write out what you feel. You may wish to keep a "feeling journal" in which you enter your strong feelings from time to time (see *Exercise 2: The Feeling Journal*, at the end of this chapter). Weeks later it may be very instructive to go back and read through the journal to get an idea of broad patterns or themes running through your life. Whether you keep a journal or not, the act of writing out your feelings will often suffice as an outlet until you have the opportunity to talk them out.

## Discharging Sadness

You might want to ask yourself the following questions:

- Do you ever cry?

- Under what circumstances do you cry?

- Do you cry because someone hurt you? Because you feel lonely? Because you're scared?

- Do you cry for no apparent reason?

- Do you cry only when alone, or do you permit someone else to see you crying?

Sometimes you may have a feeling of being on the verge of tears. You feel like you would like to cry but are having difficulty "getting it out." At this point, you may find that a particular artistic prompt will help. Evocative pieces of music that have personal significance can often help to elicit tears. Watching an emotional movie, reading poetry or literature, or even certain television programs may also bring an initially vague sense of sadness to the surface.

## Discharging Anger

Often you may feel angry or frustrated but are reluctant to express it for fear of hurting others. It's quite possible, and often healthy, however, to discharge your anger in ways that are not destructive—ways that do not involve "dumping" your anger on someone else. *Going through the physical motions associated with aggression* may bring anger to the surface. The target of these actions, however, always needs to be an inanimate object. All of the following have been helpful to many people in releasing angry feelings:

- Hitting a large pillow with both fists

- Screaming into a pillow

- Hitting a punching bag

- Yelling within the confines of a car

- Chopping wood

- Hitting a life-size inflatable doll

- Hitting an old tennis racket or a plastic baseball bat against a bed

- Having a vigorous physical workout

It's not recommended that you engage in any of the above (with the exception of physical exercise) on a daily basis. There is evidence, reported by Carol Tavris in her book *Anger: The Misunderstood Emotion*, that excessive expression of anger only tends to produce more anger. The popular term "rageaholic" describes the type of person who has become addicted to anger through *excessive* expression of it. On the other hand, many phobic and anxiety-prone people have a tendency to withhold or deny angry feelings under most circumstances. Anger may be such a difficult emotion for you that some additional comments are warranted.

# Dealing with Anger

Of all the different emotions that can give rise to anxiety, anger is the most common and pervasive one. Anger comprises a continuum of emotions ranging from rage at one extreme to impatience and irritation at the other. Frustration is perhaps the most common form of anger that most of us experience.

A proneness to phobias and obsessive-compulsive behavior is often associated with withheld anger. *Your preoccupation with phobias, obsessions, and compulsions may increase during those times when you're feeling most frustrated, thwarted, and otherwise angry with your situation in life.* Often, however, you are entirely (or almost entirely) unaware of these angry or frustrated feelings.

Why should people suffering from phobias and other anxiety disorders be predisposed to deny or withhold anger? There are several reasons:

- Individuals who are prone to phobias and anxiety tend to be "people pleasers." They want to think of themselves—and appear to others—as pleasant and nice. That leaves less room for experiencing, let alone expressing, anger.

- Such people, especially if they suffer from agoraphobia, are often unusually dependent on relationships with significant others. Outward expressions of anger are taboo because they might threaten to alienate the very person on whom the agoraphobic feels dependent for survival.

- People who are prone to anxiety have a high need for control. But anger, when full-blown, is probably the least rational and least controllable of our feelings. Giving in to anger, with the attendant loss of control, is very frightening if you are someone who always feels the need to "keep a grip" on yourself.

The consequences of withholding anger over time have been discussed in the previous section detailing the symptoms of suppressed feelings. Generalized anxiety can be a sign of suppressed anger. So can depression or psychosomatic symptoms such as acid reflux, neck and upper back tension, or tension headaches. Some additional signs of withheld anger include these:

- *An increase in phobic concerns*, such as a tendency to avoid new situations without any obvious reason

- *An increase in obsessive thoughts* and/or compulsive behaviors

- *Self-defeating behaviors*, such as excessive self-criticism, maximizing what's wrong with your life while discounting the good, complaining about problems without taking any action, passive-aggressive behavior such as procrastination or always being late, blaming others, or worrying about the future instead of enjoying the present

## Some Guidelines for Learning to Deal with Anger

Once you've become aware of the signs and symptoms of suppressed anger, what can you do to better deal with these feelings? The following guidelines may be helpful:

1. *Be willing to let go of the standard of always having to be nice or pleasing in all situations.* Expand your self-concept so that you can allow yourself to express irritation or anger in situations when to do so might be appropriate. Examples would include occasions when

someone keeps responding to you with snide remarks or subtle put-downs—or a situation where someone breaks an important agreement he or she made with you. Remember that expressing your anger does *not* mean dumping it on someone else, but rather sharing with someone (preferably *not* the person you feel anger toward) that you're feeling angry. You need to do this with feeling, rather than merely talking in a detached manner about your anger. Expressing your anger might alternatively mean to write out or physically "exercise out" your angry feelings. When you're ready to tell people you're angry with them or their behavior, there are specific skills you can learn to communicate your feelings without hurting or belittling the other person. See the section below, "Communicating Your Feelings to Someone," for guidelines about communicating anger or other feelings.

2. *Work on overcoming "what-ifs" about what might happen if you let your anger out.* Usually these what-ifs are exaggerated and unreasonable—for example, "What if I go berserk or crazy?" or "What if I do something terrible?" Remember that anger withheld for a long time may *seem* ominous at first. Its intensity may startle you during the first few moments you give it vent, but it is not going to cause you to "fall apart," "go crazy," or "do something destructive." The intensity of your angry feelings will diminish quickly as soon as you allow yourself to experience them. This is especially so if you express your anger in a benign way. If your anger is intense, try discharging it onto inanimate objects or on paper in the ways previously described, instead of "dumping" it onto someone you'd like to blame for your feelings.

3. *Work on overcoming fears about alienating people you care about when you allow your anger to show.* Being able to *appropriately communicate* angry feelings to significant others is, in fact, an indication that you do care about them. If you didn't care, you would be more likely to withdraw from them and withhold your true feelings. While overexpression of anger can be destructive to others or yourself, not ever communicating angry feelings to someone you love may convey either indifference or a kind of phony, "holier-than-thou" equanimity.

4. *Learn to communicate angry feelings assertively rather than aggressively.* It is quite possible to convey your anger or frustration toward other people in a way that respects their dignity—in a way that doesn't blame or put them down. One way is to begin what you say in the first person, speaking about how you yourself feel rather than blaming the other person with some kind statement: "You…"—in other words, "I feel angry when you break your agreements" instead of "You make me so mad when you break your agreements." "I-statements" maintain respect for the other person; "you-statements" put people on the defensive and assign them the blame for your feelings. Other people don't *make* you angry. Rather, you react angrily to your own interpretation of another person's behavior. Something they say or do goes against your standards of what is acceptable or just, and so you feel angry. You can learn to convey your angry feelings without hurting, judging, or blaming others by using the communication skills discussed in the next section.

5. *Learn to discriminate different ways of expressing anger, depending on the intensity of your feelings.* If your anger is *very* intense, you're probably not ready to speak to someone yet. Instead, you need a direct and physical mode of expression, such as pounding pillows, screaming

into a pillow, or engaging in a vigorous physical workout. After your anger has lessened as a result of direct physical expression—or if it was moderate in the first place—talk it out with someone. If possible, it is best to share it with a neutral friend first before directly confronting the person with whom you're angry. If no such neutral person is available, use the communication guidelines that follow as well as those outlined in chapter 14, Being Assertive. If, finally, your anger is only a mild irritation, you can use the tried-and-true method of deep breathing and counting to ten to dispel it—or communicate it directly if you wish.

## A Caveat

This section on dealing with anger is intended for you if you have difficulty being aware of or expressing angry feelings. If you tend to withhold your anger, even when you are being taken advantage of or abused, then learning to be more in touch with your angry feelings can be empowering. If you have difficulty standing up for yourself in the face of manipulation or when your boundaries are violated, then appropriate, *assertive* communication of your anger is something that you will certainly want to learn.

On the other hand, if you feel angry often and find that your angry feelings interfere with your relationships, then you don't need instructions on how to identify and express your anger. If you're tired of the emotional and physical toll that frequent anger outbursts can take, you're looking for a different solution. *When any emotion is excessive or destructive, the solution lies not in expressing it more but in changing the self-talk and mistaken beliefs that aggravate that emotion.* In brief, while this chapter will be useful if you have difficulty acknowledging or expressing feelings, *a more cognitive approach is needed for any feeling that seems excessive or destructive to you.* Thus it may be useful, if anger comes too easily and interferes with your relationships, to review chapters 8 and 9 and examine self-talk and mistaken beliefs that predispose you to be angry.

## Anger Is a Perception

*Anger, like all other emotions, is determined by your perceptions and interpretations.* Other people and situations don't, *in themselves,* "make" you angry: it is your interpretations of what others do and say, and your internal commentary about them, that stimulate anger. Often these interpretations and self-talk contain an element of distortion. Any of the following cognitive distortions can trigger anger:

- *Global labeling:* When you describe someone to yourself as a "bum" or a "jerk," you write her or him off in a way that ignores the whole person.

- *Black-or-white thinking:* You see things in extreme terms so that people or situations are either all good or all bad; there are no shades of gray. Thus, you may lose sight of the truth of a situation.

- *Magnification:* When you blow something out of proportion, you increase your sense of being wronged and victimized. This is a common way of fueling and maintaining anger.

- *Entitlement:* When you believe that you should always get what you want, everything should come easily, or life should always be fair, your thinking rests on the mistaken belief that you are *naturally entitled* to complete gratification of your needs all the time. This kind of misconception can lead to a lot of self-defeating anger and blame.

The above examples are just four among several types of distorted thinking that can lead to excessive and destructive anger. A more complete discussion of distorted thinking and mistaken beliefs that can trigger anger may be found in the book *When Anger Hurts* by Matthew McKay, Peter Rogers, and Judith McKay. If excess anger is interfering with your well-being and relationships, this book can help.

## Communicating Your Feelings to Someone

Communicating your feelings, for the purposes of this chapter, means letting others know that your feelings have something to do with what they said or did. This level of dealing with your feelings is usually riskier than simply expressing them to a third party or writing them down on paper. Yet when you let someone know how you feel toward him or her, you have the greatest likelihood of being able to work through or resolve the feeling—in short, to be done with it. You can live in fear or anger toward someone for a long time without any change until you finally let the person know how you feel. Once you do, you no longer need to "hold" the feeling in secret or silence. Sometimes the person you have feelings toward is no longer available or alive, in which case you can still communicate your feelings by writing a letter (see exercise 3 at the end of this chapter).

There are two important rules for communicating your feelings:

1. Be sure that the person you disclose your feelings to is *willing* to hear you out and listen.

2. Avoid blaming or belittling the person you're addressing.

The first rule is important because your feelings are an intimate part of you that deserves respect. If someone isn't truly ready or willing to hear you, you're likely to go away feeling discounted and misunderstood. Your sadness, fear, or anger toward the person may even increase. When you're ready to tell someone how you feel, ask her or him to make time to listen to you. You might say, "I have something important to say and I'd appreciate it if you would listen." If the other person interrupts you, you might say, "Would you please wait until I'm finished?" When others truly listen to you, it means that they give you their undivided attention, don't interrupt, and don't offer any advice, opinions, or judgments. They just listen—silently and attentively. If they have any comments, these can wait until after you're finished with your communication. The only appropriate interruption by the other person might be an occasional summary of what you've said, just to confirm that he or she heard you accurately. This occasional summarizing by the listener is called *active listening* and is a skill that you can learn about in any basic book or course on communication. Good listening skills on the part of the person you're addressing will actually *enhance* your ability to disclose and communicate what you're feeling.

The second rule is important because the person you're speaking to can best listen if you respect him or her and refrain from blaming or making him or her responsible for your feelings.

Three skills are needed to accomplish this: 1) using first-person statements, 2) referring how you feel to the other's *behavior* rather than to him or her personally, and 3) avoiding judging the other person.

1.  *Use first-person statements.* When you communicate how you feel to someone, begin what you say with the expression "I feel…" or "I'm feeling…" In this way, you take responsibility for your feelings rather than putting them off onto the other person. The moment you tell someone "You make me feel…" or "You caused me to feel…" you relinquish your responsibility and put the other person on the defensive. Even if part of you wants to cast blame, you'll get your feelings across more easily and get a better hearing if you begin with "I feel…"

2.  *Refer to the other person's behavior rather than making a personal attack.* What do you have feelings about? Although initially it may seem that you're angry at or scared of the other person, this almost invariably turns out to be an overgeneralization. On further reflection, you'll find that you're angered or frightened by something specific that was *said* or *done*. Before communicating your feelings, it's important to determine what that something was. Then, when you actually speak, complete your first-person statement with a reference to that specific behavior or statement.

    "I'm feeling angry because you didn't call when you said you would."

    (*Not* "I had a panic attack because you didn't call—not that you'd care" or "You didn't call, you jerk, and it made me feel awful.")

    "I felt threatened when I saw you dancing with your secretary at the party."

    (*Not* "How could you dance with her when you knew how humiliated I'd feel?" or "You're so completely insensitive to my feelings.")

    "I feel scared when you talk about leaving."

    (*Not* "How can you talk to me like that when you know how vulnerable I am?")

    Although right and wrong ways of stating your feelings can involve little more than a difference in wording, it is an important difference. Referring your feelings to people rather than their behavior results in putting either them or yourself in a one-down position. In the first example, dumping anger on the other person is likely to make him or her feel guilty or angry. Calling someone a jerk—a negative label—will certainly put him or her on the defensive. In the third example, telling someone you're afraid of her or him may make *you* feel more defensive and create more distance in the relationship. In brief, referring your feelings to a specific statement or behavior lets other people know that you're upset with *something they can change*—rather than with *who they are as a person.*

3.  *Avoid judgments.* This point speaks for itself and is an extension of the previous point. When telling people how you feel about what they said or did, avoid judging them. Your problem is with their behavior, not them. Refraining from judging others will greatly increase the likelihood of their hearing you out.

# Exercises

The following three exercises offer direct ways to express your feelings.

## *Exercise 1: Establish a Listening Partner*

Make an arrangement with your spouse, your partner, or a close friend to set aside an hour or more each week for listening to each other. Then do a trade-off. First, your partner gives you his or her undivided attention for a half hour, while you express what you've been feeling during the week. Then you switch roles. As a speaker in this process, you need to focus on how you've actually been *feeling* about what's happening in your life, not just chat about or describe it. If you are the listener, you need to give the speaker your undivided attention without interruptions. For the duration of the period that you're listening, refrain altogether from offering your advice, opinions, or comments. You may ask the speaker for clarification if you're confused about what he or she is saying. It also helps to occasionally summarize what you hear the speaker say, beginning with, "Let's see if I'm following you. You said..." Providing the speaker with occasional brief summaries of what you hear her or him saying is called *active listening*.

## *Exercise 2: The Feeling Journal*

Set aside a notebook whose sole purpose is to provide a place where you can express your feelings. Make entries whenever you feel the need to release frustration, anger, anxiety, fear, sadness, or grief, as well as positive feelings such as joy, love, and excitement. Begin each entry with the words "I feel" or "I felt" and refer to *The Feeling List* earlier in the chapter to help identify the specific feelings you are experiencing.

## *Exercise 3: Write a Letter Communicating Your Feelings*

Write a letter communicating your feelings to someone who is not available in person. Good candidates for this would be an ex-spouse or lover or a deceased parent. Make time to express *all* of your feelings toward this person, both positive and negative. Remember to refrain from judgments and use only first-person statements. Persist with the process until you feel that you've said everything you need to say. It's not uncommon for such a letter to run on for several pages.

When you've completed the letter, read it to a close friend or counselor, which will help make it more real. It's all right, on the other hand, if you prefer to keep the letter private.

*Optional:* You may want to write a letter to someone who is available but to whom, for various reasons, you've avoided communicating your feelings. You might want to consult with a close friend or, even better, a counselor, before deciding to *actually send* such a letter. In some cases, it may be best to stick with writing out your feelings toward the person *without sending* them a letter that could potentially provoke conflict. Again, seek guidance on this from a thoughtful (hopefully neutral) friend or counselor.

## Summary of Things to Do

1.  Reread the section "Recognize the Symptoms of Suppressed Feelings" (under the main section, "Identifying Your Feelings") until you're familiar with both psychological and bodily signs of suppressed feelings: free-floating anxiety, depressed moods, psychosomatic symptoms such as headaches or acid stomach, muscle tension, and so on.

2.  If you have difficulty identifying your feelings, use *The Feeling List* to help you identify specifically what you're feeling.

3.  Practice expressing your feelings on a frequent basis. Find a "listening partner," preferably a good friend, with whom you can trade off talking out your feelings regularly. Or you can keep a feeling journal. (Notice changes in your level of bodily tension and mood after expressing what you feel.)

4.  If anger is an especially difficult feeling to deal with, reread "Some Guidelines for Learning to Deal with Anger." Practice getting comfortable expressing your anger to a neutral person or in a journal before attempting to communicate anger directly.

5.  In communicating anger or any other feeling to people directly, remember to 1) make sure that they're willing to listen to you, 2) use first-person statements, 3) refer your feeling to their behavior (or statements) rather than to them personally, and 4) avoid judging them.

6.  Write a letter communicating your feelings to someone who was or is important in your life. Discuss with a trusted friend, counselor, or therapist whether you wish to send the letter.

## Further Reading

Gendlin, Eugene. *Focusing.* New York: Bantam Books, 2007.

McKay, Matthew, Martha Davis, and Patrick Fanning. *Messages: The Communication Skills Book.* 4th ed. Oakland, CA: New Harbinger Publications, 2018.

———, Peter Rogers, and Judith McKay. *When Anger Hurts.* 2nd ed. Oakland, CA: New Harbinger Publications, 2003.

Peck, M. Scott. *The Road Less Traveled.* 25th anniversary ed. New York: Touchstone/Simon and Schuster, 2003.

Rubin, Theodore I. *The Angry Book.* New York: Touchstone Books, 1998.

Tavris, Carol. *Anger: The Misunderstood Emotion.* Rev. ed. New York: Touchstone/Simon and Schuster, 1989.

# 14

# Being Assertive

Being assertive is an attitude and a way of acting in any problem situation where you need to

- Ask explicitly for what you want, or

- Say no to something you don't want

Becoming assertive involves self-awareness and knowing what you want. Behind this knowledge is the belief that you have the right to ask for what you want. When you are assertive, you are conscious of your basic rights as a human being. You give yourself and your particular needs the same respect and dignity you'd give anyone else's. Acting assertively is a way of developing self-respect and self-worth.

If you are phobic or anxiety-prone, you may act assertively in some situations but have difficulty making requests or saying no to family members or close friends. Having perhaps grown up in a family where you felt the need to be perfect and please your parents, you may have remained a "people pleaser" as an adult. With your spouse or others, you may often end up doing many things you don't really want to do. This creates resentment, which in turn produces tension and sometimes open conflict in your relationships. By learning to be assertive, you can begin to express your true feelings and needs more easily. You may be surprised when you begin to get more of what you want as a result of your assertiveness. You may also be surprised to learn that assertive behavior brings you increased respect from others.

## Alternative Behavior Styles

Assertiveness is a way of acting that strikes a balance between two extremes: submissiveness and aggressiveness.

### Nonassertive or Submissive Style

*Nonassertive or submissive behavior* involves yielding to someone else's preferences while discounting your own rights and needs. You don't express your feelings or let others know what you want. The result is that they remain ignorant of your feelings or wants (and thus can't be blamed for not responding to them). Submissive behavior also includes feeling guilty—or as if you are imposing—when you do attempt to ask for what you want. If you give others the message that you're *not sure* you have the right to express your needs, they will tend to discount them. Phobic and anxiety-prone people are often submissive because, as previously mentioned, they are overly invested in being "nice" or "pleasing" to everybody. Or they may be afraid that the open expression of their needs will alienate a spouse or partner on whom they feel dependent.

## Aggressive Style

*Aggressive behavior,* on the other hand, may involve communicating in a demanding, abrasive, or even hostile way with others. Aggressive people typically are insensitive to others' rights and feelings and will attempt to obtain what they want through coercion or intimidation. In being aggressive, one succeeds by sheer force, creating enemies and conflict along the way. This often puts others on the defensive, leading them to withdraw or fight back rather than cooperate. For example, an aggressive way of telling someone you want a particular assignment at work would be to say, "That assignment has my name written on it. If you so much as look at the boss when she brings it up during the staff meeting, you're going to regret it."

## Passive-Aggressive Style

As an alternative to being openly aggressive, many people act *passive-aggressively.* If this is your style, instead of openly confronting an issue, you express angry, aggressive feelings in a covert fashion through passive resistance. You're angry at your boss, so you're perpetually late to work. You don't want to comply with your spouse's request, so you procrastinate or "forget" about the request altogether. Instead of asking for or doing something about what you really want, you perpetually complain or moan about what is lacking. Passive-aggressive people seldom get what they want because they never get it across. Their behavior tends to leave other people angry, confused, and resentful. A passive-aggressive way of asking for a particular assignment at work might be to point out how inappropriate someone *else* is for the job or saying to a coworker, "If I got more interesting assignments, I might be able to get somewhere in this organization."

## Manipulative Style

A final nonassertive behavior style is being *manipulative.* Manipulative people attempt to get what they want by making others feel sorry for or guilty toward them. Instead of taking responsibility for meeting their own needs, they play the role of victim or martyr in an effort to get others to take care of them. When this doesn't work, they may become openly angry or feign indifference. Manipulation only works as long as those at whom it is targeted fail to recognize what is happening. The person being manipulated may feel confused or "crazy" up to a point; afterward, they become angry and resentful toward the manipulator. A manipulative way of asking for a particular assignment at work would be to tell your boss, "Gee, if I get that assignment, I think my boyfriend will finally have some respect for me," or to tell a coworker, "Don't say a word about this—but if I don't get that assignment, I'm going to finally use that bottle of sleeping pills I've been saving up."

## Assertive Style

*Assertive behavior*—in contrast to the styles described above—involves asking for what you want (or saying no) in a simple, direct fashion that does not negate, attack, or manipulate anyone else. You communicate your feelings and needs honestly and directly while maintaining respect and consideration for others. You stand up for yourself and your rights without apologizing or feeling guilty. In essence, being assertive involves taking responsibility for getting your own needs met in a way that preserves the dignity of other people. Others feel comfortable when you're assertive because they know where you stand. They respect you for your honesty and forthrightness. Instead of demanding or commanding, an assertive statement makes a simple, direct request, such as "I would really like that assignment" or "I hope the boss decides to give that particular assignment to me."

Which of the above five descriptions (nonassertive/submissive, aggressive, passive-aggressive, manipulative, or assertive) fits you most closely? Perhaps, depending on the situation, more than one behavior style applies. The following exercise will assist you in identifying your preferred behavior mode when you want something.

## Your Behavior Style

Think about each of the following situations, one at a time. How would you typically handle it? Would your approach be nonassertive (in other words, you wouldn't do anything about it), aggressive, passive-aggressive, or manipulative—or would you respond assertively? Note the behavior style you believe you would most likely use in your response to each situation. Just write the name of the style of behavior you'd most likely use (submissive, aggressive, passive-aggressive, manipulative, or assertive) next to each situation. When finished, add up the number of times you believe your response to the situation would be assertive.

1. You're being kept on the phone by a salesperson who is trying to sell you something you don't want.

2. You would like to break off a relationship that is no longer working for you.

3. You're sitting in a movie and the people behind you are talking.

4. Your doctor keeps you waiting more than thirty minutes.

5. Your teenager has the stereo on too loud.

6. Your neighbor next door has the stereo on too loud.

7. You would like to return something faulty to the store and get a refund.

8. You're standing in line, and someone moves in front of you.

9. Your friend has owed you money for a long time—money you could use—and is unresponsive to your phone calls.

10. You receive a bill that seems unusually high for the service you received.

11. Your home repair person is demanding payment but has done unsatisfactory work.

12. You receive food at a restaurant that is over- or undercooked.

13. You would like to ask a major favor of your partner or spouse.

14. You would like to ask a major favor of your friend.

15. Your friend asks you for a favor that you don't feel like doing.

16. Your son/daughter/spouse/roommate is not doing his or her fair share of the work around the house.

17. You would like to ask a question but are concerned that someone else might think it's silly.

18. You're in a group and would like to speak up, but you don't know how your opinion will be received.

19. You would like to strike up a conversation at a gathering, but you don't know anyone.

20. You're sitting/standing next to someone who is smoking, and the smoke is beginning to bother you.

21. You find the behavior of your partner/spouse unacceptable.

22. You find your friend's behavior unacceptable.

23. Your friend drops by unexpectedly, just before you were about to leave to run some errands.

24. You're talking to someone about something important, but he or she doesn't seem to be listening.

25. Your friend stands you up for a lunch meeting.

26. You return an item you don't want to the deparment store and request a full refund. The clerk diverts your request and offers to exchange the item for another.

27. You're speaking and someone interrupts you.

28. A solicitor arrives at the door, and you're not interested in what the person has to sell.

29. Your partner or spouse "talks down" to you as if you were a child.

30. You receive an unjust criticism from someone.

If you have fewer than twenty-five out of thirty "assertive" responses (that is, your likely response is inclined to be submissive, aggressive, passive-aggressive, or manipulative), it would be useful for you to work on developing a more assertive behavior style.

# Learn to Be Assertive

Learning to be assertive involves working on learning and practicing the following seven areas:

1. *Learn and develop nonverbal behaviors* of various types that convey an assertive posture.

2. *Recognize and exercise your basic rights* as a human being, as listed in the *Personal Bill of Rights* later in this chapter.

3. *Identify your unique problem situations* that call for being more assertive. For which types of *life situations* and for which types of *people* do you need to become more assertive?

4. *Rehearse assertive responses through writing them out.* Use the *Assertiveness Exercises* later in this chapter to assist with writing out your responses. (You might also practice assertive responses by *role-playing* them with a partner, close friend, or counselor.)

5. *Practice making assertive requests that you could use for real-life situations* where you'd like to be assertive, using the behaviors and skills you'll learn in this chapter.

6. *Develop skills to deal with unexpected situations when you suddenly or spontaneously need to be assertive*—a kind of "assertiveness-on-the-spot."

7. *Learn skills for saying "no"* in situations where you need to turn down a request.

Each of these areas is discussed in more detail below.

# Develop Nonverbal Assertive Behaviors

Acting in an assertive manner depends not only on what you say but also on your body language. Other people can pick up your approach to asking them for something by the way you hold your body as well as what you express in your facial features. Some of the nonverbal aspects of assertiveness include these:

- *Look directly at* people when addressing them. Looking down or away conveys the message that you're not quite sure about asking for what you want. The opposite extreme, staring, is also unhelpful because it may put the other person on the defensive.

- Maintain an *open* rather than closed *posture.* If you're sitting, don't cross your legs or arms. If standing, stand erect and on both feet. Face the person you're addressing directly rather than standing off to the side.

- *Do not back off or move away* from the other person while communicating assertively. The expression "stand your ground" applies quite literally here.

- *Stay calm.* Avoid getting overly emotional or excited. If you're feeling angry, discharge your angry feelings *somewhere else* before you attempt to be assertive. A calm but assertive request carries much more weight with most people than an angry outburst.

Try practicing these nonverbal skills with a friend by role-playing situations that call for an assertive response. Refer back to the list of thirty situations calling for assertiveness in *Your Behavior Style*. If possible, have a friend role-play a situation, such as denying your request, and then you make an assertive response, utilizing appropriate nonverbal behaviors. If no one is available to role-play, an alternative would be to practice nonverbal assertive behaviors in front of a mirror.

## Recognize and Exercise Your Basic Rights

As adult human beings, we all have certain basic rights. Often, though, either we have forgotten them or else as children we were never taught to believe in them. Learning to be assertive involves recognizing that you, just as much as anyone else, have a right to all of the things listed under the *Personal Bill of Rights* that follows. Assertiveness also involves taking responsibility to *exercise* these rights in situations where they are threatened or infringed upon. Read through the *Personal Bill of Rights* and reflect on your willingness to believe in and exercise each one.

### *Personal Bill of Rights*

1.  I have the right to ask for what I want.

2.  I have the right to say no to requests or demands I can't meet.

3.  I have the right to express all of my feelings, positive or negative.

4.  I have the right to change my mind.

5.  I have the right to make mistakes and not have to be perfect.

6.  I have the right to follow my own values and standards.

7.  I have the right to say no to anything when I feel I am not ready, it is unsafe, or it violates my values.

8.  I have the right to determine my own priorities.

9.  I have the right *not* to be responsible for others' behavior, actions, feelings, or problems.

10.  I have the right to expect honesty from others.

11.  I have the right to be angry at someone I love.

12.  I have the right to be uniquely myself.

13.  I have the right to feel scared and say "I feel afraid."

14.  I have the right to say "I don't know."

15. I have the right not to give excuses or reasons for my behavior.

16. I have the right to make decisions based on my feelings.

17. I have the right to my own needs for personal space and time.

18. I have the right to be playful and frivolous.

19. I have the right to be healthier than those around me.

20. I have the right to be in a non-abusive environment.

21. I have the right to make friends and be comfortable around people.

22. I have the right to change and grow.

23. I have the right to have my needs and wants respected by others.

24. I have the right to be treated with dignity and respect.

25. I have the right to be happy.

Photocopy the *Personal Bill of Rights* or download a copy of it from the publisher's website (see the end of this book for details), and post it in a conspicuous place. By taking time to carefully read through the list every day, you will eventually learn to accept that you are entitled to each one of these rights.

## Identify Your Problem Situations

On a blank sheet of paper, write down two or three situations of high priority where you feel you would like to act more assertively. Choose situations that are current and important for you. Describe the situation in detail and specify the person or people to whom you wish to act assertively. Here are some examples, by no means complete, of types of people and types of situations that might be involved in acting more assertively.

People

- Spouse

- Parents

- Significant other

- Children

- Relatives

- Close friends

- Acquaintances

- Fellow workers or classmates

- Salespeople or clerks

- Strangers

Situations

- Asking for help

- Asking for service

- Asking for a favor

- Having to "say no" to a request

- Stating a difference of opinion

- Speaking up about something that annoys you

- Dealing with a person who refuses to cooperate with your wishes

- Having to take charge of a situation

- Making a request of an authority figure

- Negotiating with someone to resolve a difficult situation

- Protesting a purchase that you consider a "rip-off"

- Proposing a new idea

- Asking for a date

# Practice Assertive Responses in Writing—or by Role-Playing—First

Writing out assertive responses before you face a real-life situation can be helpful if you are not used to being assertive. This step is not mandatory but can be quite useful. A trial run in writing can help you develop a greater degree of preparation and confidence for when you actually confront a situation in real life. To practice assertiveness responses in writing, see the exercises below.

# Assertiveness Exercises

The exercises below are designed to give you practice in responding assertively to situations that call on you to be assertive. Here are a few things to keep in mind as you write your responses.

- Evaluate your legitimate rights. (For help, review the *Personal Bill of Rights* above.)

- Keep your request simple and specific.

- Object to the other individual's behaviors that concern you—not their personalities.

- Use I-statements and make a simple request, not a demand or command.

- Don't apologize for your request.

- Explain your request to the other person in terms of its consequences for you, if the person doesn't fully understand your request.

(For further details on these items as well as additional ways to make an assertive request, see the section "Practice Assertive Requests That You Could Use in Real Life," which follows these exercises.)

## Exercise: Write (or Role-Play) Assertive Responses

The situations presented below are common ones that you may have encountered before in your life. The task is to fill in the blank with an assertive response for each situation.

1.  You take your car to the garage for an oil change and receive a bill for that plus wheel alignment and new spark plugs. You say,

_____

_____

2.  You arrange to take turns driving to work with a friend. Each day you drive, she has an errand to run on the way home. When she drives, there are no stops ever made. You say,

_____

_____

3.  When you entertain your coworkers, the conversation always turns to shoptalk. You are planning a party and prefer to avoid the usual topics. You say,

_____

_____

4.  You're in the bank. The teller asks, "Who's next?" It's your turn. A woman who came in after you says, "I am." You say,

_____

_____

5.    You're in a taxi and you suspect that the driver is taking you by a roundabout route. You say,

_____

_____

6.    You're in a restaurant that typically has no-smoking signs posted. A person at the bar nearby lights up a cigarette. You say,

_____

_____

7.    You've frequently had adverse reactions to medications in the past. Your doctor gives you a prescription without telling you what side effects to expect. You say,

_____

_____

8.    You're buying some new clothes. The saleswoman is pressuring you into buying something that makes you look ten pounds heavier. You say,

_____

_____

9.    You're playing miniature golf with your spouse. You're not doing very well but are having a good time. Your spouse is continually telling you how to do it "right." You say,

_____

_____

10.    You've settled in for a quiet Sunday at home, the first in a long time. Your parents call and invite you over for the day. You don't want to go. You say,

_____

_____

11.    You receive a notice informing you that your child has been placed in the classroom of a teacher whom you know to be notoriously incompetent. You call the principal and you say,

_____

_____

12. Someone rings your doorbell, wanting to convert you to his religion. You're not interested. You say,

_____

_____

13. A friend asks you to babysit for her, but you have other plans for the day. You say,

_____

_____

14. You're feeling lonely and "left out." Your spouse is in the living room, reading. You say,

_____

_____

15. You've been rushing about all day. It's very hot and you don't have air conditioning. You prepare a salad for dinner because you don't want to turn the oven on. Your spouse comes home hungry and wants a hot meal. You say,

_____

_____

16. Some friends dropped by without an invitation at five o'clock. It is now seven and you want to serve dinner to your family. You don't have enough to include the guests. You say,

_____

_____

An alternative to writing out assertive responses is to practice them in a more real-life setting by role-playing with a trustworthy partner, friend, or counselor. Your partner plays the role of either 1) disagreeing with your request or 2) making a demand that you don't wish to meet. Your job is to continue making your assertive request without judging or blaming your partner or friend. Again, consult the list for practicing assertive behavior at the beginning of *Assertiveness Exercises* above. Keep in mind that it's helpful to rehearse assertive behaviors in advance to gain skill in becoming more assertive in real life.

# Practice Assertive Requests That You Could Use in Real Life

Based on all the previous sections on learning to be assertive, that is, being aware of nonverbal assertive behaviors, recognizing your basic rights listed in the *Personal Bill of Rights*, identifying situations and/or people with whom you need to be assertive, and rehearsing assertive responses in writing or by doing role-plays, *you are now at last ready to practice being assertive in real life.* Acting in an assertive way includes, at first, the following four major *strategies.* Note that the fourth strategy, the key strategy where you actually *make your assertive request*, is followed by a number of *guidelines* on how to make an assertive request in real life.

1. **Evaluate your legitimate rights** with respect to the situation at hand, which you already have learned to do by utilizing the *Personal Bill of Rights.*

2. **Decide to whom you will make your request.** It is preferable to direct your request toward the person you wish to address, rather than going through a secondary person. Granted, there may be certain situations—such as an upper-level boss at work or an ill relative—where it may be preferable to make your request through a secondary person. In some cases, it may be preferable to ask a friend or relative of the person who is involved. Yet, in a majority of cases, it's best, if possible, to directly address the person whom you most want to impact.

3. **Determine your preferred mode of communication:** email, text, voicemail, live phone conversation, formal letter, or a face-to-face meeting with the person at a mutually agreeable time. You may prefer to utilize a less direct form of communication first and then follow up with a more direct method. For example, you could leave a voicemail requesting a live conversation by phone or in person.

4. **Make your request.** This is the *key* step in being assertive. You simply ask for what you want (or don't want) in a direct, straightforward manner. Observe the following guidelines for making assertive requests:

   - *Utilize assertive nonverbal behaviors,* as you already know how to do. Stand squarely, establish eye contact, maintain an open posture, and work on staying calm and self-possessed if you are speaking to someone in person.

   - *Keep your request simple.* One or two easy-to-understand sentences will usually suffice: "I would like you to take the dog out for a walk tonight," or "I want us to go to a marriage counselor together."

   - *Avoid asking for more than one thing at a time.*

   - *Be specific.* Ask for *exactly* what you want—or the person you're addressing may misunderstand. Perhaps you're working on a phobia of driving freeways. Instead of saying, "I'd like you to help me with my practice sessions," be specific in asking for what you want, such as "I'd like you to go with me when I practice driving on the freeway every Saturday morning." Or instead of "I would like you to come home by a reasonable hour," specify "I would like you to come home by twelve midnight."

- *Object to behaviors—not personalities.* When objecting to what someone is doing, object to the *specific behavior—not to the individual's personality.* Let the person know you're having a problem with something he or she is doing (or not doing), not with who he or she is as a person.

  It's preferable to say, "I have a problem when you don't call to let me know you're going to be late," rather than "You're inconsiderate for not calling me to let me know you'll be late."

- *Use "I-statements":*

  *"I would like..."*

  *"I want to..."*

  *"I would appreciate it if..."*

- *It's important to avoid using "you-statements" when you make a request.* Statements that are potentially threatening ("You'll do this or else") or coercive ("You have to...") will put the person you're addressing on the defensive and decrease the likelihood of your getting what you want.

- *Make requests, not demands or commands.* Assertive behavior always respects the humanity and rights of the other person. Thus, an assertive response is always a request rather than a demand. Demanding and commanding are aggressive modes of behavior based on the false assumption that you are always right or always entitled to get everything your way.

- *If you feel so inclined, let the other person know how you feel.* If you're confused or ambivalent about your feelings, take time to clarify them first by writing them out or talking them out with a supportive friend or counselor. If your feelings are clear, you may choose to disclose them when making an assertive request. Even if the person you're addressing disagrees with your position, he or she may at least appreciate your strong feelings on an issue. In expressing your feelings, it's important to own them and use "I-statements" to convey them. See chapter 13, Dealing with Feelings, for further assistance in identifying and communicating your feelings.

- *Don't apologize for your request.* When you want to ask for something, do so directly. Say, "I would like you to..." instead of "I know this might seem like an imposition, but I would like you to..." When you want to decline a request, do so directly but politely. Don't apologize or make excuses. Simply say, "No, thank you," "No, I'm not interested," or "No, I'm not able to do that." If the other person's response is one of enticement, criticism, an appeal to guilt, or sarcasm, just repeat your statement firmly until you've made your point.

- *Optional: State the positive consequences of cooperation.* If it feels appropriate, you may choose to tell the person you're addressing the consequences of gaining his or her cooperation. You might want to let the person know how positive cooperation will be beneficial for both of you. Be careful, though, about mentioning consequences of *not* obtaining cooperation. This can be difficult to do without making some kind of warning or threat (even if veiled). You want to avoid veiled threats in you communications whenever possible.

## Example: Jean's Assertive Request for Quiet Time

Jean would like a half hour of uninterrupted peace and quiet while she does her relaxation exercise. Her husband, Frank, has had the tendency to disrupt her quiet time with questions and other attention-getting maneuvers. Before confronting him, she wrote out this assertive request.

1. *Evaluate your rights, relying on the Personal Bill of Rights:* "I have a right to have some quiet time to myself." "I have a right to take care of my need for relaxation." "I have a right to have my husband respect my needs."

2. *Decide how you wish to communicate your request* (for example, direct telephone conversation in advance or a real-life encounter). "I will call Frank about my concerns first, before speaking to him directly in person."

3. *Address the person directly, if possible.* "In this situation, as he is my husband, I need to speak to Frank directly."

4. *Make your request, keeping it simple and specific.* Be sure to address the person's behavior that is of concern, not their entire personality: "I would like to be uninterrupted during the time my door is closed, other than in cases of emergency. I'd like you to respect my right to have half an hour of quiet time each day."

    - Refrain from blaming or labeling the other person. In this case, Jean would avoid telling Frank: "It's annoying when you interrupt my quiet time."

    - Use "I-statements" such as "I would like..." or "I would appreciate..." "Frank, I would appreciate it if you would respect my need to have some quiet time on my own in the evening."

    - Don't apologize for making your request. Avoid statements like "I hate to bother you, Frank, but..."

    - You may also want to explain to the person how their behavior led to your need to make your assertive request. For example, "I've let you know several times that I need a half hour each day on my own for relaxation, and I've even shut the door, but you still come in and ask me questions. This disturbs my concentration and interferes with an important part of my program for managing my anxiety."

- You may also state your feelings about the situation as long as you don't blame or judge the other person, for example: "I feel frustrated when my attention is disrupted" or "I feel angry when you don't respect my right to have some quiet time for relaxation."

- State the consequences of gaining cooperation. "If you respect my need to have some quiet time, I'll be much better able to spend some time with you afterward and be a good companion."

Now it's your turn.

## Exercise: Write Out Assertive Requests for Real-Life Situations

Select two or three of the problem people or situations you previously described and write out your assertive request following the guidelines in "Practice Assertive Requests That You Could Use in Real-Life Situations" above.

Once you've written out in detail your assertive request to one or more particular problem situations, you'll find that you feel more prepared and confident when you confront the situation in real life. This process of methodically writing out a preview of your assertive request is especially helpful during the time when you're learning to be assertive. Later on, when you have a fair degree of mastery, you may not need to write out your request in advance every time. It's never a bad idea, though, to prepare your request, especially when a lot is at stake. Attorneys do so as a way of life because they typically assert the rights of their clients in high-stakes situations.

## Assertiveness on the Spot

Many situations arise in the course of everyday life that challenge you to be assertive spontaneously. Someone blasts loud music while you're trying to go to sleep. Or someone insists on smoking in an area that is designated "nonsmoking." Perhaps at the grocery store, someone cuts in front of you in line. You can use the following brief set of guidelines for coming up with a spontaneous assertive request.

1. *Evaluate your rights.* Do you feel there has been a legitimate infringement on your rights?

2. *Make a specific, direct request to the other person using an "I-statement,"* such as "I would like...," "I would appreciate...", "Would you please..." Make a simple request that is non-blaming and nonjudgmental of the other person.

3. *State the problem in terms of its consequences on you.* If you feel the person you're addressing might be puzzled by your request, you may want to explain why his or her behavior has an adverse effect on you. For example, you might say, "Everyone here, including myself, has been waiting in line. Would you mind taking your turn and allowing the other people already waiting to go ahead?"

4. *Optional: Express your feelings.* If you're dealing with a stranger with whom you don't wish to have any further relationship, it's usually okay to omit this step. On the other hand, it may be a good idea to express your feelings when you need to be assertive on the spot with your spouse, child, or close friend ("I'm really disappointed that you didn't call when you said you would" or "I'm feeling too tired to clean up the kitchen right now").

5. *Optional: State the consequences of gaining (or not gaining) cooperation.* With strangers, this step usually won't be necessary. On rare occasions, when someone is resistant to a very reasonable request, you may choose to state negative consequences ("If you continue smoking, I may have an asthma attack" or "Please notice that there is a sign posted here for no smoking"). With family and friends, a statement of positive consequences may be used to strengthen your request ("If you get in bed by eight-thirty, I'll read you a story").

The key to being assertive on the spot is to make your request as simple, specific, and straightforward as possible. Whether you choose to mention the consequences on you of the other person's behavior will largely depend on the situation. Mention consequences when you want the other person to better appreciate your situation. If you know someone well, you might also express your feelings if you want the other person to understand how strongly you feel. For example, "I'm really disappointed that you didn't call when you said you would."

# Learning to Say No

An important aspect of being assertive is your ability to say no to requests that you don't want to meet. Saying no means that you *set limits* on other people's demands for your time and energy when such demands conflict with your own needs and desires. It also means that you can do this without feeling guilty.

In some cases, especially if you're dealing with someone with whom you don't want to promote a relationship, just saying "No, thank you" or "No, I'm not interested" in a firm, polite manner should suffice. If the other person persists, just repeat your statement calmly without apologizing. If you need to make your statement stronger and more emphatic, you may want to 1) look the person directly in the eyes, 2) raise the level of your voice somewhat, and 3) assert your position: "I said no, thank you."

In many other instances—with acquaintances, friends, and family—you may want to give the other person some explanation for turning down the request. Here it's often useful to follow a four-step procedure:

1.  Acknowledge the other person's request by repeating it.

2.  Explain your reason for declining.

3.  Say no.

4.  *Optional:* If appropriate, suggest an alternative proposal where both your and the other person's needs can be met.

Use step 4 only if you can easily see a way for both you and the other person to meet each other halfway.

## Examples

"I understand that you'd really like to get together tonight (*acknowledgment*). It turns out I've had a really long day and feel exhausted (*explanation*), so I need to pass on tonight (*saying no*). Would there be another night later this week when we could get together?" (*alternative option*).

"I hear that you need some help with moving (*acknowledgment*). I'd like to help out, but I promised my boyfriend we would go away for the weekend (*explanation*), so I'm not going to be available (*saying no*). I hope you can find someone else."

Note that in this latter example, the speaker not only acknowledges her friend's need, but indicates that she would have liked to help out if the circumstances had been different. Sometimes you may wish to let someone know that under different conditions you would have willingly accepted their request.

"I realize you would like to go out with me again (*acknowledgment*). I think you're a fine person, but it seems to me that we don't have enough in common to pursue a relationship (*explanation*), so I have to say no (*saying no*)."

"I know that you'd like me to take care of Johnny for the day (*acknowledgment*), but I have some important errands I have to attend to (*explanation*), so I can't babysit today (*saying no*)."

Are there any particular types of situations where you repeatedly have trouble saying no? Make a list of these situations in the space below:

Now take a sheet of paper and write a hypothetical assertive response for each of these situations where you say no, following the four-step procedure outlined above.

The following additional suggestions may also be helpful in learning to say no (adapted from Matthew McKay, Peter Rogers, and Judith McKay's book *When Anger Hurts*):

1. *Take your time.* If you're the type of person who has difficulty saying no, give yourself some time to think and clarify what you want to say before responding to someone's request (for example, "I'll let you know by the end of the week" or "I'll call you back tomorrow morning after sleeping on it").

2. *Don't overapologize.* When you apologize to others for saying no, you give them the message that you're "not sure" that your own needs are just as important as theirs. This opens the door for them to put more pressure on you to comply with what they want. In some cases, they may even try to play upon your guilt to obtain other things or to get you to "make it up to them" for having said no in the first place.

3. *Be specific.* It's important to be very specific in stating what you will and won't do. For example, "I'm willing to help you move, but because of my back I can only carry light-weight items" or "I can take you to work, but only if you can meet me by 8:15."

4. *Use assertive body language.* Be sure to face the person you're talking to squarely and maintain good eye contact. Work on speaking in a calm but firm tone of voice. Avoid becoming emotional.

5. *Watch out for guilt.* You may feel the impulse to do *something else* for someone after turning down a request. Take your time before offering to do so. Make sure that your offer comes out of genuine desire rather than guilt. You've fully mastered the skill of saying no to others when you reach the point that you can do so without feeling guilty.

## Summary of Things to Do

Learning to be assertive can enable you to obtain more of what you want and will help minimize frustration and resentment in your relationships with partners, family, and friends. It can also help you take more risks and ask more of life, adding to your sense of autonomy and self-confidence.

Becoming assertive does, however, take *practice*. When you first attempt to act assertively with family and friends, be prepared to feel awkward. Also be prepared for them not to understand what you're doing and possibly even to take offense. If you explain as best you can and give them time to adjust to your new behavior, you may be pleasantly surprised when they come to respect you for your newfound directness and honesty.

To get the most out of this chapter, consider doing the following:

1. Determine your dominant behavior style (submissive, aggressive, passive-aggressive, manipulative, or assertive) by asking yourself what behavior style you would likely choose for each of the thirty situations listed in the *Your Behavior Style* questionnaire.

2. Make a copy of the *Personal Bill of Rights* and post it in a conspicuous place. Read it over a number of times until you feel thoroughly familiar with all of the rights listed.

3. Write out assertive responses to the *Assertiveness Exercises* or practice assertiveness by role-playing assertive responses with a trusted friend or counselor.

4. Review all four strategies described in "Practice Making Assertive Responses You Could Use in Real Life," particularly #4, "Make Your Request," which offers specific guidelines for making your request. Become thoroughly familiar with the guidelines for making an assertive request: keeping your request simple, being specific, using first-person statements, objecting to behaviors (not personalities), not apologizing for being assertive, making requests instead of demands, stating your feelings about your assertive request (especially to people with whom you are close), and mentioning, if appropriate, the positive consequences of obtaining cooperation with your assertive request.

5. Look at the example for making an assertive request ("Jean's Assertive Request for Quiet Time"), as well as your responses to the exercise *Write Out Assertive Requests for Real-Life Situations,* and then think about all you've learned in this chapter and how you can use these assertiveness skills in your own life.

6. Review the section "Assertiveness on the Spot" to assist you with any situations that arise in the course of daily life and that require a spontaneous assertive response.

7. Review the section "Learning to Say No" and, with a friend or counselor, role-play saying no to unreasonable requests.

8. Consult the books listed below under "Assertiveness Skills" for a more thorough coverage of the topic. If you feel the need to seek extra help beyond these books, look for podcasts or YouTube videos demonstrating assertiveness skills.

9. Consult the books listed below under "Communication Skills" or take a class in communication to back up your assertiveness training with other important interpersonal skills, such as listening, self-disclosure, and negotiating.

# Further Reading

## Assertiveness Skills

Alberti, Robert E., and Michael Emmons. *Your Perfect Right*. 10th ed. Oakland, CA: Impact Publishers, 2017.

Davis, Martha, Elizabeth Robbins Eshelman, and Matthew McKay. *The Relaxation & Stress Reduction Workbook*. 7th ed. Oakland, CA: New Harbinger Publications, 2019.

McKay, Matthew, Peter Rogers, and Judith McKay. *When Anger Hurts*. 2nd ed. Oakland, CA: New Harbinger Publications, 2003.

Smith, Manuel J. *When I Say No, I Feel Guilty*. New York: Bantam, 1975.

## Communication Skills

Fisher, Roger, and William Ury. *Getting to Yes: Negotiating Agreement Without Giving In*. Rev. ed. New York: Penguin, 2011.

McKay, Matthew, Martha Davis, and Patrick Fanning. *Messages: The Communication Skills Book*. 4th ed. Oakland, CA: New Harbinger Publications, 2018.

# 15

# Self-Esteem

Self-esteem is a way of thinking, feeling, and acting that implies that you accept, respect, trust, and believe in yourself. When you *accept* yourself, you can live comfortably with both your personal strengths and your weaknesses without undue self-criticism. When you *respect* yourself, you acknowledge your own dignity and value as a unique human being. You treat yourself well in much the same way you would treat someone else you respect. *Self-trust* means that your behaviors and feelings are consistent enough to give you an inner sense of continuity and coherence despite changes and challenges in your external circumstances. To *believe* in yourself means that you feel you deserve to have the good things in life. It also means that you have confidence that you can fulfill your deepest personal needs, aspirations, and goals. To get a sense about your own level of self-esteem, think of someone (or imagine what it would be like to know someone) whom you *fully* accept, respect, trust, and believe in. Now ask yourself to what extent you hold these attitudes toward yourself. Where would you place yourself on this scale?

| Very Low | | | | | | | | | | | | Very High |
|---|---|---|---|---|---|---|---|---|---|---|---|---|
| Self-Esteem | 0 | 1 | 2 | 3 | 4 | 5 | 6 | 7 | 8 | 9 | 10 | Self-Esteem |

A fundamental truth about self-esteem is that it needs to come from *within*. When self-esteem is low, the deficiency creates a feeling of emptiness that you may try to fill by latching on—often compulsively—to something external that provides a temporary sense of satisfaction and fulfillment. When the quest to fill your inner emptiness by appropriating something from outside becomes desperate, repetitive, or automatic, you have what is called an *addiction*. Broadly defined, addiction is an attachment to something or someone outside yourself that you feel you need to provide a sense of inner satisfaction or relief. Frequently, this attachment substitutes preoccupation with a substance or an activity for healthy human relationships. It may also substitute a temporary feeling of control or power for a more lasting sense of inner confidence and strength.

A healthy alternative to addiction is to work on building your self-esteem. Growing in self-esteem means developing confidence and strength from within. While still enjoying life fully, you no longer need to appropriate or identify with something or someone outside yourself to feel okay. The basis for your self-worth is internal. As such, it is much more lasting and stable.

# Ways to Build Self-Esteem

There are many pathways to self-esteem. It is not something that develops overnight or as a result of any single insight, decision, or modification in your behavior. Self-esteem is *built gradually* through a willingness to work on a number of areas in your life. This chapter considers—in three parts—a variety of ways to build self-esteem:

- Taking care of yourself

- Developing support and intimacy

- Other pathways to self-esteem

Most fundamental to your self-esteem are your willingness and ability to take care of yourself. This means first that you can *recognize* your basic needs as a human being and then *do* something about meeting them.

Part I of this chapter focuses on this theme of taking care of yourself. It begins by enumerating a variety of dysfunctional family situations that can cause low self-esteem. Following this is a discussion of basic human needs, to help you identify those needs that are most important to address in your life right now.

Part II of this chapter is an extension of part I. Finding support and intimacy in your life is obviously a major part of taking care of yourself. Other people can't give you self-esteem, but their support, acceptance, validation, and love can go a long way toward reinforcing and strengthening your own self-affirmation. This part is divided into four sections. The first addresses the importance of developing a support system. The second presents ten conditions that are critical to genuine intimacy. The third section offers a discussion of interpersonal boundaries. Having boundaries in your relationships is essential both to intimacy and to self-esteem. A final section underscores the relevance of assertiveness to self-esteem.

Part III presents four additional aspects of self-esteem:

- Personal wellness and body image

- Emotional self-expression

- Self-talk and affirmations for self-esteem

- Personal goals and a sense of accomplishment

Although these pathways to self-esteem are diverse among themselves, they can all be viewed as an extension of the basic idea of taking care of yourself.

# Part I: Taking Care of Yourself

Taking care of yourself is the foundation on which all other pathways to self-esteem rest. Without a basic *willingness* and *ability* to care for, love, and nurture yourself, it is difficult to achieve a deep or lasting experience of self-worth.

Perhaps you had the good fortune to receive the love, acceptance, and nurturing from your parents that could provide you with a solid foundation for self-esteem as an adult. Presently, you are free of any deep-seated feelings of insecurity, and your path to self-esteem is likely to be simple and short, involving certain changes in attitude, habits, and beliefs. For those who have carried a lifelong sense of insecurity, though, the way to self-worth involves developing the ability to give yourself what your parents could not. *It's possible to overcome deficits from your past by developing a constructive relationship with yourself in the present.* Two ways to do so are 1) acknowledging and making time for your basic needs, and 2) making time for small acts of self-nurturing on a daily basis.

## Some Causes of Low Self-Esteem

What are some of the childhood circumstances that can lead you to grow up with feelings of insecurity or inadequacy?

1. **Overly critical parents.** Parents who were constantly critical or set impossibly high standards of behavior may have left you feeling guilty, or that somehow you could "never be good enough." As an adult, you will continue to strive for perfection to overcome a long-standing sense of inferiority. You may also have a strong tendency toward self-criticism.

2. **Significant childhood loss.** If you were separated from a parent as a result of death or divorce, you may have been left feeling abandoned. You may have grown up with a sense of emptiness and insecurity that can be restimulated very intensely by losses of significant people in your adult life. As an adult, you may seek to overcome old feelings of abandonment by overdependency on a particular person or an addiction to food, drugs, work, or whatever works to cover the pain.

3. **Parental abuse.** Physical, emotional, and/or sexual abuse are extreme forms of deprivation. They may leave you with a complex mix of feelings, including inadequacy, insecurity, lack of trust, guilt, and/or rage. Adults who were physically abused as children may become perpetual victims or may themselves develop a hostile posture toward life, victimizing others. Adults—especially men—who were sexually abused as children sometimes express their rage by turning to rape and abuse as adults. Or they may turn that rage inward in deep feelings of self-loathing and inadequacy. Survivors of abusive childhoods often, and understandably, have difficulty with intimate relationships in their adult lives. While less flagrant, constant verbal abuse can have equally damaging effects.

4. **Parental alcoholism or drug abuse.** Much has been written in recent years on the effects of parental alcoholism on children. Chronic drinking or substance abuse creates a chaotic, unreliable family atmosphere in which it is difficult for a child to develop a basic sense of trust or security. The attendant denial of the problem, often by both parents, teaches the child to deny his or her own feelings and pain connected to the family situation. Many such children grow up with poor self-esteem or a poor sense of personal identity. Fortunately, support groups are presently available to help adult children of alcoholics

heal the adverse effects of their past. If one or both of your parents were alcoholic, you may wish to read the following books: *Adult Children of Alcoholics* by Janet Woititz, and *Recovery: A Guide for Adult Children of Alcoholics* by Herbert Gravitz and Julie Bowden. You may also want to join a support group or therapy group for adult children of alcoholics in your area.

5. **Parental neglect.** Some parents, because they are preoccupied with themselves, their work, or other concerns, simply fail to give their children adequate attention and nurturing. Children left to their own devices often grow up feeling insecure, worthless, and lonely. As adults, they may have a tendency to discount or neglect their own needs.

6. **Parental rejection.** Even without physical, emotional, sexual, and/or verbal abuse, some parents impart a feeling to their children that they are unwanted. This profoundly damaging attitude teaches a child to grow up doubting his or her very right to exist. Such a person has a tendency toward self-rejection or self-sabotage. Adults with such pasts must learn to love and care for themselves if they are to overcome what their parents didn't give them.

7. **Parental overprotectiveness.** The child who is overprotected may never learn to risk independence and trust the world outside of the immediate family. As an adult, such a person may feel very insecure and afraid to venture far from a safe person or place. Through learning to acknowledge and care for their own needs, overprotected individuals can gain the confidence to make a life of their own and discover that the world is not such a dangerous place.

8. **Parental overindulgence.** The "spoiled" child of overindulgent parents is given insufficient exposure to deferred gratification or appropriate limits. As adults, such people tend to be bored, lack persistence, or have difficulty initiating and sustaining individual effort. They tend to expect the world to come to them rather than taking responsibility for creating their own lives. Until they are willing to take personal responsibility, such people feel cheated and very insecure because life does not continue to provide what they learned to expect during childhood.

Do any of the above categories seem to fit you? Does more than one? You may initially find it difficult to acknowledge problems in your past. Our memory of childhood is often hazy and indistinct—especially when we do not *want* to recall what actually happened. The point of remembering and acknowledging what happened to you as a child is not so that you can blame your parents. Most likely, your parents did the best they could with their available personal resources, which may have been severely limited as a result of deprivations they experienced with *their* parents. The purpose of remembering your past is to *release* it and *rebuild your present*. Old patterns based on fear, guilt, or anger will tend to interfere with your present life and relationships until you can identify and release them. Once you acknowledge and ultimately forgive your parents for what they were unable to give you, you can truly begin the journey of learning to care for yourself. In essence, this means becoming a good parent to yourself. The balance of this section will consider two important ways in which you can learn to take better care of yourself:

1. Acknowledging and meeting your basic needs

2. Making time for small acts of self-nurturing on a daily basis

## *Your Basic Needs*

*Basic human needs* conjures an association with shelter, clothing, food, water, sleep, oxygen, and so on—in other words, what human beings require for their physical survival. It was not until the twentieth century that higher-order *psychological needs* were identified. While not necessary for survival, meeting these needs is essential to your emotional well-being and a satisfying adjustment to life. The psychologist Abraham Maslow proposed five levels of human needs, with three levels beyond primary concerns for survival and security. He arranged these levels into a hierarchy:

Self-Actualization Needs (fulfillment of your potential in life, wholeness)

↑

Esteem Needs (self-respect, mastery, a sense of accomplishment)

↑

Belongingness and Love Needs
(support and affection from others, intimacy, a sense of belonging)

↑

Safety Needs (shelter, stable environment)

↑

Physiological Needs (food, water, sleep, oxygen)

In Maslow's scheme, taking care of higher-level needs is dependent on having satisfied lower-level needs. It's difficult to satisfy belongingness and esteem needs if you're starving. On a subtler level, it's difficult to fulfill your full potential if you're feeling isolated and alienated for lack of having met needs for love and belongingness. Writing in the 1960s, Maslow estimated that the average American satisfied perhaps 90 percent of physiological needs, 70 percent of safety needs, 50 percent of love needs, 40 percent of esteem needs, and 10 percent of the need for self-actualization.

Although Maslow defined esteem narrowly in terms of a sense of accomplishment and mastery, full self-esteem is dependent on *recognizing and taking care of all of your needs*.

How do you recognize what your needs are? How many of the following important human needs are you aware of?

1. Physical safety and security

2. Financial security

3. Friendship

4. The attention of others

5. Being listened to

6. Guidance

7. Respect

8. Validation

9. Expressing and sharing your feelings

10. Sense of belonging

11. Nurturing

12. Physically touching and being touched

13. Intimacy

14. Sexual expression

15. Loyalty and trust

16. A sense of accomplishment

17. A sense of progress toward goals

18. Feeling competent or masterful in some area

19. Making a contribution

20. Fun and play

21. Sense of freedom, independence

22. Creativity

23. Spiritual awareness—connection with a Higher Power

24. Unconditional love

Now go back over the list carefully and ask yourself how many of these needs you are actually getting fulfilled at this time. In what areas do you come up short? What concrete steps can you take in the next few weeks and months to better satisfy those needs that are going unmet? You may, for example, want to work to overcome your phobias, which will help you meet needs #17 and #18. Going dancing or to a movie will help in a small way with your need for fun and play.

The point is that learning to take care of yourself involves being able to 1) *recognize* and 2) *meet* your basic needs as a human being. The above list may give you ideas on areas of your life that need more attention. Use the following chart to plan what you will actually do in the next month about five (or more) of your needs that could be better met.

| *Need* | *What I'm willing to do in the next month to better meet this need* |
| --- | --- |
| | |

## Self-Nurturing Activities

Identifying your most important psychological needs (from Maslow's list) and paying attention to those that may have gone unattended is an important first step. More specifically, you can practice specific self-nurturing activities that help enhance your relationship with yourself. Not all of the activities on the list may be relevant or useful, but you might attempt to find at least three or more self-nurturing activities to help increase your feelings of self-worth and self-respect.

The following list has been very helpful to many of my clients who suffer from anxiety disorders or depression. By performing at least one or two items from the list every day, or anything else you find pleasurable, you can cultivate a more constructive relationship with yourself. You have nothing to lose but your sense of insecurity and inadequacy—and nothing to gain except increased self-esteem.

1. Take a warm bath or shower.

2. Have breakfast in bed.

3. Take a sauna.

4. Get a massage.

5. Buy yourself a rose.

6. Take a bubble bath.

7. Go to a pet store and play with the animals.

8. Walk on a scenic path in a park.

9. Visit a zoo.

10. Have a manicure or pedicure.

11. Stop and smell some flowers.

12. Wake up early and watch the sunrise.

13. Watch the sunset.

14. Relax with a good book and/or soothing music.

15. Go rent a funny video.

16. Play your favorite music and dance to it by yourself.

17. Go to bed early.

18. Sleep outside under the stars.

19. Take a "mental health day" off from work.

20. Fix a special dinner just for yourself and eat by candlelight.

21. Go for a walk.

22. Call a good friend—or several good friends.

23. Go out to a fine restaurant just with yourself.

24. Go to the beach.

25. Take a scenic drive.

26. Meditate.

27. Buy new clothes.

28. Browse in a book or record store for as long as you want.

29. Buy yourself a cuddly stuffed animal and play with it.

30. Write yourself a love letter and mail it.

31. Ask a special person to nurture you (feed, cuddle, and/or read to you).

32. Buy yourself something special that you can afford.

33. Go see a good film or show.

34. Go to the park and feed the ducks, swing on the swings, and so on.

35. Visit a museum or another interesting place.

36. Give yourself more time than you need to accomplish whatever you're doing (let yourself dawdle).

37. Work on your favorite puzzle or puzzle book.

38. Go into a hot tub or Jacuzzi.

39. Make a recording of affirmations.

40. Write out an ideal scenario concerning a goal, then visualize it.

41. Read an inspirational book.

42. Write a letter to an old friend.

43. Bake or cook something special.

44. Go window shopping.

45. Buy a meditation CD or download one.

46. Listen to a positive, motivational recording.

47. Write in a special diary about your accomplishments.

48. Exercise, specifically engaging in a type of exercise you enjoy.

# Part II: Developing Support and Intimacy

While self-esteem is something we build within ourselves, much of our feeling of self-worth is determined by our significant personal relationships. Others cannot give you a feeling of adequacy and confidence, but their acceptance, respect, and validation of you can reaffirm and strengthen your own positive attitude and feelings about yourself. Self-love becomes narcissistic in isolation from others. Let's consider four pathways to self-esteem that involve relationships with others:

- Close friends and support

- Intimacy

- Boundaries

- Assertiveness

## Close Friends and Support

When surveys of human values have been done, many people rank close friends near the top, along with career, a happy family life, and health. Each of us needs a support system of at least two or three close friends in addition to our immediate family. A close friend is someone you can deeply trust and confide in. It is someone who comfortably accepts you as you are in all your moods, behaviors, and roles. It is also someone who will stand by you no matter what is happening in your life. A close friend allows you the opportunity to share your feelings and perceptions about your life outside your immediate family. Such a person can help bring out aspects of your personality that might not be expressed with your spouse, children, or parents. At least two or three close friends of this sort, whom you can confide in on a regular basis, are an essential part of an adequate support system. Such friends can help provide continuity in your life through times of great transition, such as moving away from home, divorce, or the death of a family member.

How many close friends of the type just described do you have? If you don't have at least two, what could you do to cultivate such friendships?

## Intimacy

While some people seem content to go through life with a few close friends, most of us seek a special relationship with one particular person. It is in intimate relationships that we open ourselves most deeply and have the chance to discover the most about ourselves. Such relationships help overcome a certain loneliness that most of us would eventually feel—no matter how self-sufficient and strong we may be—without intimacy. The sense of belonging that we gain from intimate relationships contributes substantially to our feelings of self-worth. However, self-worth cannot be derived entirely from someone else. A healthy intimate relationship simply reinforces your own self-acceptance and belief in yourself.

Much has been written on the topic of intimacy and on what ingredients contribute to lasting intimate relationships. Some of the most important of these are listed below (not ranked in any order):

1. Common interests, especially leisure time and recreational interests. (A few differences in interests, though, can add some novelty and excitement.)

2. A sense of romance or "magic" between you and your partner. This is an intangible quality of attraction that goes well beyond the physical level. It's usually very strong and steady in the first three to six months of a relationship. The relationship then requires the ability to renew, refresh, or rediscover this magic as it matures.

3. You and your partner need to be well matched in your relative needs for togetherness versus independence. Conflict may arise if one of you has a much greater need for freedom and "space" than the other, or if one of you has a need for protection and coziness that the other doesn't want to provide. Some partners may hold a double standard—in other words, they're unwilling to allow you what they require for themselves (such as trust and freedom).

4. Mutual acceptance and support of each other's personal growth and change. It is well known that when only one person is growing in a relationship, or when one person feels invalidated in his or her growth by the other, the relationship often ends.

5. Mutual acceptance of each other's faults and weaknesses. After the initial romantic months of a relationship are over, each partner must find enough good in the other to tolerate and accept the other's faults and weaknesses.

6. Regular expressions of affection and touching. An intimate relationship cannot be healthy without both partners being willing to overtly express affection. Nonsexual expressions such as hugging and cuddling are just as important as a sound sexual relationship.

7. Sharing of feelings. Genuine closeness between two people requires emotional vulnerability and a willingness to open up and share your deepest feelings.

8. Good communication. Entire books and courses are devoted to this subject. While there are many different aspects to good communication, the two most important criteria are that

   • *The partners are genuinely willing to listen to each other,* and

   • *Both are able to express their feelings and ask for what they want directly* (as opposed to complaining, threatening, demanding, and otherwise attempting to manipulate the other to meet their needs).

9. A strong sense of mutual trust. Each person needs to feel that he or she can rely on the other. Each also trusts the other with his or her deepest feelings. A sense of trust does not come automatically; it needs to be built over time and maintained.

10. Common values and a larger sense of purpose. An intimate relationship has the best opportunity to be lasting when two people have common values in important areas of life, such as friendships, education, religion, finances, sex, health, and family life. The strongest relationships are usually bound by a common purpose that transcends the personal needs of each individual—for example, raising children, running a business, or a commitment to a spiritual ideal.

How many of the above ten characteristics are present in your intimate relationship? Are there any, in particular, that you would like to work on?

## Boundaries

Just as important as intimacy is the need for each of us to maintain appropriate boundaries within both intimate and other relationships. Boundaries simply mean that you know where you end and the other person begins. You don't define your identity in terms of the other person. And above all, you don't derive your sense of self-worth and self-authority by attempting to take care of, rescue, change, or control the other person. The term "codependent" (or expressions like "women who love too much") has often been used to define those people who, because they lack a solid, internal basis of self-worth, attempt to validate themselves through taking care of, rescuing, or simply pleasing another person. The classic case of this is the person who attempts to organize his or her life around "rescuing" an alcoholic or otherwise addicted spouse or close relative. But loss of boundaries can occur in any relationship in which you attempt to gain self-worth and security by overextending yourself to take care of, control, rescue, or change someone else. Your own needs and feelings are set aside and discounted in the process. A good indication of loss of boundaries is when you spend more time talking or thinking about another's needs or problems than your own.

Two excellent books—*Women Who Love Too Much* and *Codependent No More*—are recommended if you want to further explore boundary issues in your own relationships. In her best-selling book *Women Who Love Too Much*, Robin Norwood advocates the following guidelines in overcoming codependency in a close relationship:

- Learning to stop managing, controlling, or "running the life" of another or others you love

- Making recovery from codependency your highest priority

- Going for outside help, such as from a counselor—giving up the idea that you can handle it alone

- Learning to let go of playing the game of "rescuer" and/or "victim" with the other person

- Finding a support group of peers who understand the problem, for example, an Al-Anon or Codependents Anonymous group

- Facing and exploring your own personal problems and pain in depth

- Cultivating yourself: developing a life of your own and pursuing your own interests

- Developing a personal spiritual life that allows you to let go of self-will and rely on a Higher Power

- Becoming "selfish"—not in the unhealthy sense of egotism but in the sense that you put *your* well-being, desires, work, play, plans, and activities first instead of last

- Sharing what you have learned with others

In *Codependent No More,* Melody Beattie carefully defines codependency and provides a series of steps for overcoming the problem of codependency. Some of her recommendations include these:

- Practicing "detachment"—letting go of obsessively worrying about someone else

- Letting go of the need to control someone else—respecting that person enough to know that he or she can take responsibility for his or her own life

- Taking care of yourself, which includes finishing up "unfinished business" from your own past and learning to nurture and cherish the needy, vulnerable child within

- Improving communication—learning to state what you want and to say no

- Dealing with anger—giving yourself permission to feel and express anger at loved ones when you need to

- Discovering spirituality—finding and connecting with a Higher Power

Is codependency an issue for you? Have you considered joining a support group that focuses on codependency issues, such as Al-Anon or Codependents Anonymous?

## Assertiveness

Cultivating assertiveness is critical to self-esteem. If you're unable to clearly get across to others what you want or do not want, you will end up feeling frustrated, helpless, and powerless. If you do nothing else, the practice of assertive behavior in and of itself can increase your feeling of *self-respect*. Honoring your own needs with other people in an assertive manner also increases *their* respect for you, and quickly overcomes any tendency on their part to take advantage of you.

The concept of assertiveness, along with exercises for developing an assertive style of communication, is presented in chapter 14 of this workbook.

# Part III: Other Pathways to Self-Esteem

The first two parts of this chapter focused on taking care of your needs and developing support and intimacy in your relationships. In this final part, four other pathways to self-esteem that involve different levels of your whole being are described.

- Body: physical well-being and body image

- Feelings: emotional self-expression

- Mind: positive self-talk and affirmations for self-esteem

- Whole self: personal goals and a sense of accomplishment

Although these areas have been considered elsewhere in this workbook, they are discussed briefly here for their relevance to self-esteem.

## Physical Well-Being and Body Image

Physical health and a sense of personal wellness, vitality, and robustness comprise one of the most important foundations of self-esteem. It's often difficult to feel good about yourself when you're feeling physically weak, tired, or ill. Current evidence points to the role of physiological imbalances—often caused by stress—in the genesis of panic attacks, agoraphobia, generalized anxiety, and obsessive-compulsive disorder (see chapter 2). Improving your physical well-being will have a direct impact on your particular problem with anxiety, as well as contribute substantially to your self-esteem. The chapters on relaxation, exercise, and nutrition relate directly to physical well-being. Reading them and putting into practice the suggestions and guidelines offered will go a long way toward upgrading your personal wellness. The questionnaire below is intended to give you an overview of how you are doing in this area.

## Personal Wellness Questionnaire

1. Are you exercising for at least one half hour three to five times per week?

2. Do you enjoy the exercise you do?

3. Do you give yourself the opportunity to deeply relax each day through progressive muscle relaxation, visualization, meditation, or some other relaxation method?

4. Do you give yourself at least one hour of downtime or leisure time each day?

5. Do you manage your time so that you are not perpetually rushed?

6. Do you handle stress, or do you feel that it has control of you?

7. Do you give yourself solitary time for personal reflection?

8. Do you get at least seven to eight hours of sleep every night?

9. Are you satisfied with the quality and quantity of your sleep?

10. Are you eating three solid meals each day, including a good-size breakfast?

11. Are you minimizing your consumption of stress-producing foods (those containing caffeine, sugar, or salt, or processed "junk" foods)?

12. Do you take vitamin supplements on a regular basis to augment your diet—such as a multivitamin tablet, and extra vitamin B-complex and vitamin C when you're under physical or emotional stress?

13. Do you like your living environment? Is the place where you live comfortable and relaxing?

14. Does smoking tobacco interfere with your physical well-being?

15. Does excessive use of alcohol or so-called recreational drugs compromise your well-being?

16. Are you comfortable with your present weight? If not, what can you do about it?

17. Do you value your personal appearance through good hygiene, grooming, and dressing in a way that feels comfortable and attractive?

18. Do you like your body and the way you appear?

## Emotional Self-Expression

When you're out of touch with your feelings, it's hard to know who you are. You tend to feel internally detached from yourself and often fearful. By identifying and expressing the full range of your feelings, you can become better acquainted with your unique needs, desires, and yearnings. Literally you begin to *feel* yourself—your whole self—rather than walking around in a cloud of worried thoughts, fantasies, and anticipations. Learning to own and express your feelings takes time, courage, and a willingness to be vulnerable in the presence of others whom you trust. (See chapter 13 of this book for further information on identifying and expressing feelings.)

## Constructive Self-Talk and Affirmations for Self-Esteem

What you tell yourself and your beliefs about yourself contribute in an obvious and literal way to your self-esteem. If you are feeling inadequate and powerless, it's likely because you *believe* that you are. By the same token, you can raise your self-esteem *simply* by working on changing your self-talk and basic beliefs about yourself.

Exercises for identifying and altering your negative self-talk and mistaken beliefs have been presented in chapters 8 and 9. The sections that follow highlight certain parts of those chapters that are relevant to self-esteem. First, consider four different types of unconstructive self-talk, which chapter 8 describes in terms of four "subpersonalities": the Worrier, Critic, Victim, and Perfectionist. Second, consider using affirmations, like the ones provided under "Affirmations for Self-Esteem" (in the following section) to overcome negative beliefs and assumptions about yourself.

Of the four types of self-talk described in chapter 8—the Worrier, the Critic, the Victim, and the Perfectionist—the Critic and the Victim are the most potentially destructive to your self-esteem. Indeed, people with low self-esteem invariably have a strong Critic or a strong Victim consciousness, or both. It's the Critic's specific function to talk you down into feeling inadequate, inferior, and incompetent. Then the Victim's self-talk may add insult to injury by telling you that you're hopeless and powerless.

First, go back to chapter 8 and review the section "Types of Negative Self-Talk" and the exercise *What Are Your Subpersonalities Telling You?* with particular attention to the Critic and the Victim. Complete the worksheets for countering the destructive self-talk of each of these subpersonalities, if you haven't already. Then, when you catch yourself engaging in self-critical or self-victimizing inner dialogues, follow these three steps:

1. **Disrupt the chain of negative thoughts** with some method that diverts your attention away from your mind and helps you be more in touch with your feelings and body. Any of the following may work:

   • *Physical activity*—for example, household chores or exercise

   • *Taking a brisk walk outside*

   • *Abdominal breathing*

   • *Five to ten minutes of progressive muscle relaxation*

   • *Shouting "Stop!" aloud or silently, several times in succession, if necessary*

   The point of these disruption strategies is to help you move away from overthinking in your mind and move into your physical body in a way that helps you slow down, giving you a bit of distance from your negative thoughts.

2. **Challenge your negative self-talk** with appropriate questioning, if necessary. Good questions to raise with your Critic or Victim might be "What's the evidence for this?" "Is this *always* true?" and "Am I looking at all sides of this issue?" Review the list of Socratic questions in chapter 8 for other examples of questions.

3. **Counter your negative inner dialogue** with positive, self-supportive statements. You may want to design your own positive statements specifically tailored to refute your Critic's or Victim's statements, one by one. Alternatively, you can draw positive counterstatements from the following list of affirmations meant to promote self-esteem.

# *Affirmations for Self-Esteem*

## What I Am

I am lovable and capable.

I fully accept and believe in myself just the way I am.

I am a unique and special person. There is no one else quite like me in the entire world.

I accept all the different parts of myself.

I'm already worthy as a person. I don't have to prove myself.

My feelings and needs are important.

It's okay to think about what I need.

It's good for me to take time for myself.

I have many good qualities.

I believe in my capabilities and value the unique talents I can offer the world.

I am a person of high integrity and sincere purpose.

I trust in my ability to succeed at my goals.

I am a valuable and important person, worthy of the respect of others.

Others perceive me as a good and likable person.

When other people really get to know me, they like me.

Other people like to be around me. They like to hear what I have to say and know what I think.

Others recognize that I have a lot to offer.

I deserve to be supported by the people who care for me.

I deserve the respect of others.

I trust and respect myself and am worthy of the respect of others.

I now receive assistance and cooperation from others.

I'm optimistic about life. I look forward to and enjoy new challenges.

I know what my values are and am confident of the decisions I make.

I easily accept compliments and praise from others.

I take pride in what I've accomplished and look forward to what I intend to achieve.

I believe in my ability to succeed.

I love myself just the way I am.

I don't have to be perfect to be loved.

The more I love myself, the more I am able to love others.

## What I Am Learning

Every day I am learning to love myself more.

I am learning to believe in my unique worth and capabilities.

I am learning to trust myself (and others).

I am learning to recognize and take care of my needs.

I am learning that my feelings and needs are just as important as anyone else's.

I am learning to ask others for what I need.

It's okay to say no to others when I need to.

I am learning to take life one day at a time.

I am learning to approach my goals one day at a time.

I am learning to take better care of myself.

I am learning how to take more time for myself each day.

I am learning to let go of doubts and fear.

I am learning to let go of worry.

I am learning to let go of guilt (or shame).

I am learning that others respect and like me.

I am learning how to be more comfortable around others.

I am learning to feel more confident in _____ (name situation).

I am learning that I have a right to _____ (specify).

I am learning that it's okay to make mistakes.

I am learning that I don't have to be perfect to be loved.

Today I'm learning to accept myself just the way I am.

There are several ways you might want to work with the above list. Chapter 9 on mistaken beliefs contains a number of suggestions for working with affirmations. The following two methods are easy to implement:

- Select your favorite affirmations from the list and write them down individually on 3 by 5 index cards. Then read through the stack slowly and with feeling once or twice a day. Doing this while alternately looking at yourself in a mirror can be a helpful practice. You may also want to reword each affirmation in the second person—"You are lovable and capable" rather than "I am lovable and capable"—when repeating the phrases to your mirror image.

- Alternatively, you can record the affirmations. Repeat each affirmation slowly and leave about five to ten seconds between different statements. Listen to the recording once a day when you feel relaxed and receptive. You are most likely to internalize affirmations when you focus your attention on them fully while in a relaxed state. (Note that you may wish to construct your own list of self-esteem affirmations, drawing on those that are most meaningful to you from the above list or making up new ones of your own.)

## Personal Goals and a Sense of Accomplishment

Accomplishment of personal goals always adds to your self-esteem. If you look back over your life to the times when you felt most confident, you'll find that they often followed the accomplishment of important personal goals. Although external achievements can never be the *sole* basis of a sense of self-worth, they certainly contribute to how you feel about yourself.

If you are dealing with phobias or panic attacks, a most significant accomplishment is the ability to enter into and handle situations that you previously avoided. An even more unassailable sense of achievement is reached when, in addition to confronting phobic situations, you become confident that you can handle any panic reaction that might arise. The mastery of phobias and panic reactions is a main theme of this book and is dealt with in detail in chapters 6 and 7. If you have fully recovered from agoraphobia, social phobias, or panic disorder through conscientiously facing the very things you feared most, you know how much self-confidence and inner strength there is to be gained. Facing your phobias (including the phobia of panic itself) through a process of gradual exposure will, *in and of itself,* add considerably to your self-esteem.

Beyond the important goal of overcoming phobias and panic, however, are all the other goals you might have in your life. Your sense of self-esteem depends on the feeling that you're making progress toward *all* of your goals. If you feel "stuck" and unable to move toward something important that you want, you may begin to doubt yourself and feel somewhat diminished.

Beyond the issue of recovery from phobias and panic, then, you might ask yourself two questions:

1.   What are the most important things I want out of life—now and in the future?

These are your most important personal values.

2.   What specific goals do I need to set to fulfill my most important values?

To answer these questions and work on setting and achieving your most important personal goals, see the section "Finding and Fulfilling Your Unique Purpose" in chapter 21 (Personal Meaning).

## Remembering Previous Accomplishments

In identifying your most important values and goals for the future, it's important not to lose sight of what you've already accomplished in your life. It's common to forget about past attainments at those times when you're feeling dissatisfied with yourself. You can raise your self-esteem in a few minutes by thinking about your life and giving yourself credit for those goals you've already achieved.

The following exercise is designed to help you do this. Think about your entire life as you review each area and make a list of your accomplishments. Keep in mind that while it's gratifying to have external, "socially recognized" achievements, the most important attainments are more intangible and internal. What you've given to others (for example, love, assistance, or guidance) and the life lessons you've gained on the road to maturity and wisdom are ultimately your most important accomplishments.

# *List of Personal Accomplishments*

For each of the following areas, list any accomplishments you've had up to the present. Use a separate sheet of paper if you need to.

*School*

*Work and career*

*Home and family* (for example, raising a child or taking care of a sick in-law)

*Athletics*

*Arts and hobbies*

*Leadership*

*Prizes or awards*

*Personal growth and self-improvement*

*Charitable activities*

*Intangibles given to others*

*Important life lessons learned*

*Other*

# Summary of Things to Do

So many different strategies for raising your self-esteem have been presented in this chapter that it would be impractical to summarize each one of them here. The following worksheet is intended to help you organize what you've learned from this chapter and decide which particular strategies for building self-esteem you want to try out in the immediate future.

## *Strategies for Building Self-Esteem*

Go back through the chapter and decide which of the following strategies you want to implement in raising your self-esteem over the next month. Stick with no more than three or four strategies listed below and devote at least one week to each. In the spaces provided below, or on a separate sheet of paper, write out specifically what actions you'll take with respect to each strategy. When you're finished, design your own four-week self-esteem program by writing down which strategy you'll work with over each of the next four weeks.

1. Identify no more than three or four needs from the list of needs mentioned earlier in this chapter (see "Your Basic Needs") to which you'd like to give special attention. Then take action to do something about meeting those needs you've singled out. What specifically will you do?

2. Do one or more things from the list of self-nurturing activities, if possible on a daily basis. What will you do for yourself each day of a given week?

3. Work on building your support system. How, specifically, will you do this?

4. Work on cultivating or enhancing an intimate relationship (for example, spending quality time with your partner, taking a course in communication skills, attending a marriage enrichment weekend). How will you do this?

5. Work on improving your understanding and ability to maintain appropriate boundaries (for example, read the suggested books by Robin Norwood and Melody Beattie; attend Al-Anon

or Codependents Anonymous meetings; attend a workshop on codependency). How, specifically, will you do this?

6. Learn and practice assertiveness skills (see chapter 14). What specifically will you do?

7. Work on upgrading your personal wellness and body image (for example, implement relaxation, exercise, and nutritional improvements in your life—see chapters 4, 5, and 16). What are you willing to do in the next month?

8. Work on identifying and expressing your feelings (see chapter 13). What specifically will you do?

9. Counter the negative self-talk of your Critic or Victim subpersonalities (use the *Critic and Victim Worksheets* in chapter 8).

10. Work with self-esteem affirmations by

    • Writing one or two of them out several times each day

    • Reading them daily from a list

    • Putting them on a recording that you listen to daily

    Which one will you do?

11. List personal accomplishments you've achieved to date, using the worksheet in this chapter.

## *Four-Week Self-Esteem Program*

Which of the above interventions will you implement over the next four weeks?

Week 1:

Week 2:

Week 3:

Week 4:

# Further Reading

Beattie, Melody. *Codependent No More*. 25th anniversary ed. Center City, MN: Hazelden, 1992.

Branden, Nathaniel. *The Psychology of Self-Esteem*. 32nd anniversary ed. San Francisco: Jossey-Bass, 2001.

Gravitz, Herbert, and Julie Bowden. *Recovery: A Guide for Adult Children of Alcoholics*. New York: Touchstone, 1987.

Jeffers, Susan. *Feel the Fear and Do It Anyway*. 20th anniversary ed. New York: Ballantine Books, 2006.

McKay, Matthew, and Patrick Fanning. *Self-Esteem*. 4th ed. Oakland, CA: New Harbinger Publications, 2016.

Norwood, Robin. *Women Who Love Too Much*. New York: Pocket Books, 2008.

Schiraldi, Glenn R. *The Self-Esteem Workbook*. 2nd ed. Oakland, CA: New Harbinger Publications, 2016.

Woititz, Janet G. *Adult Children of Alcoholics*. 2nd expanded ed. Deerfield Beach, FL: Health Communications, 1990.

# 16

# Nutrition

Relatively little has been written on the subject of nutrition and anxiety disorders. Yet if it is assumed that there is at least some biological basis for panic attacks and anxiety, the subject of nutrition becomes important. What you eat has a very direct and significant impact on your physiology and biochemistry.

In the last thirty years, the relationship between diet, stress, and mood has been well documented. It's known that certain foods and substances tend to create additional stress and anxiety, while others promote a calmer and steadier mood. Certain natural substances have a directly calming effect and others are known to have an antidepressant effect. You may not yet recognize connections between how you feel and what you eat. You simply may not notice that the amount of coffee or cola beverages you drink aggravates your anxiety level. Or you may be unaware of any connection between your consumption of sugar and your anxiety, depression, or PMS symptoms. This chapter may clarify some of these connections and help you make positive changes in the way you feel.

The discussion of nutrition in this chapter covers three main topics:

- Foods, substances, and conditions that aggravate anxiety

- Dietary guidelines for reducing anxiety

- Supplements for reducing anxiety

The information in these sections is based on my personal experience and reading in the field of nutrition. It is intended to be suggestive only—not prescriptive. If you wish to make an in-depth assessment and reevaluation of your diet, consult with a nutritionist or a holistic physician who is knowledgeable about nutrition.

## Substances That Can Increase Anxiety

### Stimulants: Caffeine

Of all the dietary factors that can aggravate anxiety and trigger panic attacks, caffeine is the most notorious. Several of my clients can trace their first panic attack to an excessive intake of caffeine. Many people find that they feel calmer and sleep better after they've reduced their caffeine consumption. Caffeine has a directly stimulating effect on several different systems in your body. It increases the level of the neurotransmitter norepinephrine in your brain, causing you to feel alert and awake. It also produces the very same physiological arousal response that is triggered when you are subjected to stress—increased sympathetic nervous system activity and a release of adrenaline.

In short, too much caffeine can keep you in a chronically tense, aroused condition, leaving you more vulnerable to generalized anxiety, as well as panic attacks. Caffeine further contributes to stress by causing a depletion of vitamin $B_1$ (thiamine), which is one of the so-called antistress vitamins.

Caffeine is contained not only in coffee but also in many types of tea, soda beverages, chocolate candy, cocoa, and over-the-counter drugs. Pseudoephedrine in many over-the-counter drugs may have a stimulant effect equivalent to caffeine.

Use the *Caffeine Chart* provided in this chapter to track your caffeine intake. If you are prone either to generalized anxiety or to panic attacks, consider reducing your total caffeine consumption to *less than 100 mg per day*. For example, one cup of percolated coffee or one diet cola beverage a day would be a maximum. For coffee lovers, this may seem like a major sacrifice, but you may be surprised to find how much better you feel if you can wean yourself down to a single cup in the morning. The sacrifice may well be worth it if you have fewer panic attacks. If you are very sensitive to caffeine, eliminating it altogether would be advisable.

Please note that there are tremendous individual differences in sensitivity to caffeine. As with any addictive drug, chronic caffeine consumption leads to increased tolerance and a potential for withdrawal symptoms. If you have been drinking five cups of coffee a day and abruptly cut down to one a day, you may have withdrawal reactions, including fatigue, depression, and headaches. It's better to taper off gradually over a period of a few months—for example, from five cups to four cups per day for a month, then two or three cups per day for the next month, and so on. Some people like to substitute decaffeinated coffee, which has about 3 mg of caffeine per cup, while others drink herbal teas such as green tea. At the opposite extreme of the sensitivity continuum are people who are made jittery by a single cola or cup of tea. Some of my clients have found that even small amounts of caffeine predispose them to panic or a sleepless night. So it's important that you experiment to find out what your own optimal daily caffeine intake might be. For most people prone to anxiety or panic, this turns out to be less than 100 mg per day, and sometimes none at all.

## Nicotine

Nicotine is as strong a stimulant as caffeine. It causes increased physiological arousal and vasoconstriction, and makes your heart work harder. Smokers often object to this notion and claim that having a cigarette tends to calm their nerves. Research has proven, however, that smokers tend to be more anxious than nonsmokers, even when there are no differences in their intake of other stimulants, such as coffee and over-the-counter drugs. They also tend to sleep less well than nonsmokers. After quitting, smokers not only feel healthier and more vital but are also less prone to anxiety states and panic. In short, if you presently smoke, here is one more reason for stopping.

# Caffeine Chart

| Coffee | _____ cups | @ _____ mg = _____ mg |
| Tea | _____ cups | @ _____ mg = _____ mg |
| Cola drinks | _____ cups | @ _____ mg = _____ mg |
| Over-the-counter drugs | _____ tablets | @ _____ mg = _____ mg |

Other sources (chocolate, 25 mg per bar; cocoa, 13 mg per cup)   _____ mg

Daily Total   _____ mg

Caffeine content of coffee, tea, and cocoa (milligrams per cup)

| Coffee, instant | 66 mg |
| Coffee, percolated | 110 mg |
| Coffee, drip | 146 mg |
| Tea bag—five-minute brew | 46 mg |
| Tea bag—one-minute brew | 28 mg |
| Loose tea—five-minute brew | 40 mg |
| Cocoa | 13 mg |
| Decaffeinated coffee | 4 mg |

Caffeine content of cola beverages (milligrams per 12-ounce can)

| Coca-Cola | 65 mg |
| Dr Pepper | 61 mg |
| Mountain Dew | 55 mg |
| Diet Dr Pepper | 54 mg |
| Diet Coke | 49 mg |
| Pepsi | 43 mg |

## Stimulant Drugs

Some over-the-counter medicines have a stimulant effect, especially cold and cough medicines containing pseudoephedrine and phenylpropanolamine. In addition to these medicines, you should be aware of prescription drugs that contain amphetamines, including Adderall, Adderall XR, and Dexedrine. Ritalin and Ritalin LA, Concerta, and Vyvanse are also stimulant drugs. Being strong stimulants, they can be risky to use if you have a history of anxiety or panic attacks.

The same is especially true for cocaine and methamphetamine, recreational drugs whose use has become widespread. Use of either recreational drug can become the initial cause of recurring panic attacks for numerous people. If you are at all concerned about panic, these are definitely drugs to avoid.

## Substances That Stress the Body

### Salt

Excessive salt (sodium chloride) stresses the body in two ways: 1) it can deplete your body of potassium, a mineral that's important to the proper functioning of the nervous system, and 2) it raises blood pressure, putting extra strain on your heart and arteries and hastening arteriosclerosis. You can reduce the amount of salt you consume by avoiding the use of table salt, using a natural salt substitute (such as tamari) both in cooking and on the table, and limiting, as much as possible, salty meats, salty snack foods, and other processed foods containing salt. As a rule of thumb, it's good to limit your salt intake to one teaspoon per day (or 5.7 grams). If you must buy processed foods, choose those that are labeled low sodium or salt-free.

### Preservatives

There are presently about five thousand chemical additives used in commercial food processing. Common artificial preservatives include nitrites such as sodium nitrite, nitrates, sulfites such as sodium sulfite, sodium benzoate, monosodium glutamate (MSG), BHT, BHA, high fructose corn syrup, aspartame, potassium bromate, propyl paraben, and artificial colorings and flavorings. Our bodies are simply not equipped to handle these artificial substances, and, in most cases, very little is known about their long-term biological effects. To date, some that have been thoroughly tested have been found to be carcinogenic and thus have been removed from the market. Others currently in use, especially monosodium glutamate, nitrites, and nitrates, produce allergic reactions in many people. Worse yet, associations have been found between these additives and diabetes and neurodegenerative diseases. For example, high use of aspartame over time, in most diet soda beverages, has been associated with increased risk of brain damage. It is known that traditional societies that eat strictly whole foods without additives have a lower incidence of cancer and other illnesses. You should try to eat whole, unprocessed foods as much as possible—the foods your body was designed to handle. Try to purchase vegetables and fruits that haven't been treated with pesticides (organically grown) if these are available in your area.

### Hormones in Meat

Red meat, pork, and most commercially available forms of chicken are derived from animals that have often been fed steroid hormones to promote fast weight gain and growth. There is evidence that such hormones stress these animals (steers and hogs sometimes die of heart attacks on the loading platform). While there is at present no conclusive evidence, many people believe that these hormones might also have harmful effects for the human consumers of meat and meat products.

Try to reduce your consumption of red meat, pork, and commercially available poultry, replacing it with organically raised beef, poultry, and nonfarmed fish such as cod, halibut, salmon, snapper, sole, trout, or turbot. Tilapia, a common menu item, is almost always farmed.

# Stressful Eating Habits

Stress and anxiety can be aggravated not only by what you eat but also by the way you eat. In our modern, fast-paced society, many of us simply do not give ourselves enough time for eating. Any of the following habits can aggravate your daily level of stress:

- Eating too fast or on the run

- Not chewing food at least fifteen to twenty times per mouthful (food must be partially predigested in your mouth to be adequately digested later)

- Eating too much, to the point of feeling stuffed or bloated

- Drinking too much fluid with a meal, which can dilute stomach acid and digestive enzymes; one cup of fluid with a meal is sufficient

All of the above put a strain on your stomach and intestines in their attempt to properly digest and assimilate food. This adds to your stress level in two ways:

1. Directly, through indigestion, bloating, and cramping

2. Indirectly, through *malabsorption* of essential nutrients

If food is not properly digested in your mouth and stomach, much of it will pass undigested through your intestines and will subsequently putrefy and ferment—causing bloating, cramps, and gas. The result is that you will get only a limited portion of the nutrition potentially available in your food, leading to a subtle form of undernourishment that you're not likely to be aware of.

So, in addition to reconsidering what you eat, you can decrease stress and a probable malabsorption problem by giving yourself adequate time to eat, chewing your food thoroughly, and not overtaxing your body by eating excessive amounts.

# Sugar, Hypoglycemia, and Anxiety

Among nutritionally conscious people these days, sugar has become somewhat of a dirty word. The fact is, however, that your body and brain need glucose—a naturally occurring product of the breakdown of sugar—in order to operate. Glucose is the fuel your body burns; it provides the energy that sustains life. Much of this glucose is derived from carbohydrate foods in your diet such as bread, cereal, potatoes, vegetables, fruits, and pasta. The starches in these foods are broken down into glucose.

Simple sugars, on the other hand, such as refined white sugar, brown sugar, and honey, break down *very quickly* into glucose. These simple sugars can cause problems because they tend to overload your system with too much sugar too quickly. Our bodies are simply not equipped to process large amounts of sugar rapidly; in fact, it was not until the twentieth century that most of us (other than the very wealthy) consumed large amounts of refined sugar. Today, the standard American diet includes sugar in most beverages (coffee, tea, cola), sugar in cereal, sugar in salad dressings, and sugar in processed meat, along with one or two desserts per day and perhaps a donut or a cookie on coffee breaks. In fact, the average American consumes about *120 pounds* of sugar per year! The result of continually bombarding the body with this much sugar is the creation of a chronic dysregulation in sugar metabolism. For some people, this dysregulation can lead to excessively high levels of blood sugar, or diabetes (the prevalence of which has increased dramatically in the present century, to nearly one in five people). For other individuals, the problem is just the opposite—periodic drops in blood sugar level *below* normal, a condition that is popularly termed *hypoglycemia*.

The symptoms of hypoglycemia tend to appear when your blood sugar drops below 50 to 60 milligrams per deciliter—or when it drops very rapidly from a higher to a lower level. Typically, this occurs about two to three hours after eating a meal. It can also occur *simply in response to stress*, since your body burns up sugar very rapidly under stress. The most common subjective symptoms of hypoglycemia are:

- Light-headedness

- Anxiety

- Trembling

- Feelings of unsteadiness or weakness

- Irritability

- Palpitations

Do the symptoms look familiar? All of them are symptoms that can accompany a panic attack. In fact, for *some* people, panic reactions may actually be caused by hypoglycemia. Generally, such people recover from panic simply by having something to eat. Their blood sugar rises and they feel better. (In fact, an informal, nonclinical way to diagnose hypoglycemia is to determine whether you have any of the above symptoms three or four hours after a meal, and whether they then go away as soon as you have something to eat.)

The majority of people with panic disorder or agoraphobia find that their panic reactions do *not* necessarily correlate with bouts of low blood sugar. Yet hypoglycemia can aggravate both generalized anxiety and panic attacks that have been caused for other reasons.

What causes blood sugar to fall below normal is an excessive release of insulin by the pancreas. Insulin is a hormone that causes sugar in the bloodstream to be taken up by the cells. (Insulin is used in the treatment of diabetes to lower excessive blood sugar levels.) In hypoglycemia, the pancreas tends to overshoot in its production of insulin. This can happen if you ingest too much sugar, with the result that you feel a temporary sugar high followed a half hour later by a crash. This can also happen in response to sudden or chronic stress. Stress can cause a rapid depletion of blood sugar. You then experience confusion, anxiety, spaciness, and tremulousness because 1) your brain is not getting enough sugar and 2) a secondary stress response occurs. When blood sugar falls too low, your adrenal glands kick in and release adrenaline and cortisol, which causes you to feel more anxious and hyper. It also has the specific purpose of causing your liver to release stored sugar in order to bring your blood sugar level back to normal. So the subjective symptoms of hypoglycemia arise from both a deficit of blood sugar and a secondary stress response mediated by the adrenal glands.

Hypoglycemia can be formally diagnosed through a clinical test called the six-hour glucose tolerance test. After a twelve-hour fast, you drink a highly concentrated sugar solution. Your blood sugar is then measured at half-hour intervals over a six-hour period. You will likely get a positive result on this test if you have a moderate to severe problem with hypoglycemia. Unfortunately, many *milder* cases of hypoglycemia are missed by the test. It's quite possible to have subjective symptoms of low blood sugar and to test negative on a glucose tolerance test. Any of the following subjective symptoms are suggestive of hypoglycemia:

- You feel anxious, light-headed, weak, or irritable several hours after a meal (or in the middle of the night); these symptoms disappear within a few minutes of eating.

- You get a high feeling from consuming sugar, and this changes to a depressed, irritable, or spacey feeling twenty to thirty minutes later.

- You experience anxiety, restlessness, or even palpitations and panic in the early morning hours, between four and seven. (Your blood sugar is lowest in the early morning because you have fasted all night.)

How do you deal with hypoglycemia? Fortunately, it's quite possible to overcome problems with low blood sugar by 1) making several significant dietary changes and 2) taking certain supplements. If you suspect that you have hypoglycemia or have had it formally diagnosed, you may want to implement the following guidelines. Doing so may result in a calmer disposition— less generalized anxiety, less emotional volatility, and less vulnerability to panic. You may also notice that you are less prone to depression and mood swings.

## Dietary Modifications for Hypoglycemia

- Eliminate as much as possible all types of simple sugar from your diet. This includes foods that obviously contain white sugar, such as candy, ice cream, desserts, Coke, or Pepsi. It also includes subtler forms of sugar, such as honey, corn syrup, corn sweeteners, molasses, and high fructose corn syrup. Be sure to read labels on any and all processed foods to detect these various forms of sugar.

- Substitute fruits (other than dried fruits, which are too concentrated in sugar) for sweets. Avoid fruit juices or dilute them 1:1 with water. It's particularly important to eliminate beverages and other foods containing pure fructose or high fructose corn syrup. (Naturally occurring fructose in organic fruits is okay.)

- Reduce or consume only small amounts of simple starches such as pasta, refined cereals, potato chips, and white bread. Substitute instead complex carbohydrates such as whole-grain breads and cereals, vegetables, and brown rice or other whole grains. Eat these complex carbohydrates in moderate amounts.

- Have a protein snack (nuts or organic cheese, for example) halfway between meals— around ten-thirty to eleven in the morning and especially around four to five in the afternoon. If you awaken early in the morning at four or five, you may also find that a small snack will help you get back to sleep for a couple of hours. As an alternative to snacks between meals, you can try having four or five small meals per day no more than two to three hours apart. The point of either of these alternatives is to maintain a steadier blood sugar level.

## Supplements

1. Vitamin B-complex: 50 mg of each of all eleven B vitamins once per day with meals. (For some people, lower doses, such as 25 mg or 10 mg of each of the B vitamins in a B-complex supplement, is sufficient.)

2. Vitamin C: 1000 mg once or twice per day with meals.

3. Chromium picolinate (often called *glucose tolerance factor*): 200 micrograms per day. This is available at your local health food store.

4. Optional: A combination of glycogenic amino acids (including L-glycine, L-glutamic acid, L-tyrosine, L-leucine, L-alanine, L-methionine, and L-lysine). These combinations are available at many health food stores under the name of *hypoglycemia balancer* or *glycemic factors*. Take it as recommended either on the bottle or by a qualified nutritionist. In your regular diet, be sure to combine starches such as bread or white rice with a protein, such as cheese or organic meat (including nonfarmed fish).

Vitamin B-complex and vitamin C help increase your resiliency to stress, which can aggravate blood sugar swings. The B vitamins also help regulate the metabolic processes that convert carbohydrates to sugar in your body.

The mineral chromium and the glycogenic amino acids have a direct, stabilizing effect on your blood sugar level. (If you have an alcohol problem, it helps reduce cravings for alcohol as well.) Alcohol consumption by itself can aggravate hypoglycemia.

If you're interested in exploring the subject of hypoglycemia in greater depth, you might want to read the book *Sugar Blues* by William Dufty.

## Food Allergies and Anxiety

An allergic reaction occurs when the body attempts to resist the intrusion of a foreign substance. For some people, certain foods affect the body like a foreign substance, causing not only classic allergic symptoms such as runny nose, mucus, and sneezing but also a host of psychological or psychosomatic symptoms, including any of the following:

- Anxiety or panic

- Depression or mood swings

- Dizziness

- Irritability

- Insomnia

- Headaches

- Confusion and disorientation

- Fatigue

Such reactions occur in many individuals only when they eat an excessive amount of a particular food, eat a combination of offending foods, or have excessively low resistance due to a cold or an infection. Other people are so highly sensitive that only a small amount of the wrong food can cause debilitating symptoms. Often the subtler, psychological symptoms have a delayed onset, making it difficult to connect them with the offending foods.

In our culture, the two most common foods causing allergic reactions are milk or dairy products and wheat. It is casein in milk and gluten in wheat that tend to cause problems. Other foods that can be a source of allergic response include alcohol, chocolate, citrus fruits, corn, eggs, garlic, peanuts, yeast, shellfish, soy products, and tomatoes. One of the most telling signs of food allergy is addiction. You tend to crave and are addicted to the very foods you are allergic to. While chocolate is the most flagrant example of this, you might also take pause if you find yourself tending to crave bread (wheat), dairy products, or another specific type of food. Many people go for years without recognizing that the very foods they crave the most have a subtle but toxic effect on their mood and well-being.

How can you find out whether food allergies are aggravating your problems with anxiety? As in the case of hypoglycemia, there are both formal tests you can obtain from a nutritionally oriented doctor as well as informal tests you can conduct on your own.

Doctors often use a combination of skin testing and blood testing to evaluate food allergies. One common test is the "scratch test." Allergists usually perform skin tests on your forearm or back. The allergist then waits fifteen to twenty minutes to see if reddish, raised spots occur, indicating an allergy.

A less formal and expensive way to assess food allergies is to conduct your own elimination tests. If you want to determine whether you are allergic to wheat, simply eliminate all products containing wheat from your diet for two weeks and notice whether you feel better. Then, at the end of the two weeks, suddenly eat a large amount of wheat and carefully monitor any symptoms that appear in the next few hours. After trying out wheat, you might want to try out milk and milk products. It's important to experiment with only one potentially allergic type of food at a time so that you don't confound your results.

It's also a good idea to keep a diary of symptoms comparing how you feel before, during, and following the elimination of a particular food type. Many people feel worse immediately after they eliminate a food for a few days, as though their body is going through withdrawal symptoms. This is a telltale sign of food allergy. In severe cases, such withdrawal symptoms may persist for several weeks, and the period for eliminating the food may need to be lengthened. If this happens, consult a qualified nutritionist or allergist to assist you in conducting elimination tests.

An alternative way to test for food allergies is to take your pulse after eating a meal. If it is elevated more than ten beats per minute above your normal rate, it's possible that you ate something you're allergic to.

The good news is that you do not have to permanently abstain from a food to which you are allergic. After a period of several months away from a food, it is possible to eat it again *occasionally* without adverse effects. For example, instead of having whole-grain bread at almost every meal, you'll find that you feel better having it only two or three times per week.

For some people, food allergies can definitely be a contributing factor to excessive anxiety and mood swings. If you suspect this to be a problem, try experimenting with the elimination method and/or consult a qualified nutritionist.

**Note:** Although the emphasis of this section has been on food allergies, many people have allergic symptoms to other environmental substances, both organic and inorganic, which can precipitate a host of psychological symptoms, *including anxiety and panic.* Offending substances can include food preservatives, natural gas, synthetic fabrics, household cleaners and detergents, hydrocarbons in smog, gasoline fumes, insect sprays, molds, newspaper print, kerosene, turpentine, tar or asphalt, asbestos, cosmetics, shampoos, perfumes, colognes, hair sprays, and, quite commonly, hay fever in response to grasses and trees (especially in the spring), to name a few. If you suspect that you might be sensitive to any of these substances, you might want to consult an allergy specialist.

# Move Your Diet in the Direction of Vegetarianism

It has been frequently observed that vegetarians tend to be somewhat calmer and more easygoing than their meat-eating counterparts. It might be argued that low-stress, laid-back types are more attracted to vegetarianism in the first place. However, impressions from clients and personal experience suggest otherwise. A dietary change toward vegetarianism can definitely promote a calmer, less anxiety-prone disposition.

If you're used to eating meat, dairy, cheese, and egg products, it is not necessary—or even advisable—to give up *all* sources of animal protein from your diet. Giving up red meat alone, for example—or restricting your consumption of cow's milk (and using rice or almond milk instead)—can have a noticeable and beneficial effect.

How can vegetarianism lead to a calmer disposition? Earlier in this chapter, it was mentioned that steroid hormone residues in red meat can exert an effect not unlike the body's own steroid hormones, activating natural defenses against stress and suppressing immunity. Another reason, however, is that meat, poultry, dairy and cheese products, and eggs—along with sugar and refined flour products—are all *acid-forming* foods. These foods are not necessarily acid in composition, but they leave an acid residue in the body after they are metabolized, making the body itself more acid. This can create two kinds of problems:

*When the body is more acid, the transit time of food through the digestive tract can increase to the point where vitamins and minerals are not as fully assimilated.* This selective malabsorption of vitamins—especially B vitamins, vitamin C, and minerals—can subtly add to the body's stress load and eventually lead to low-grade malnutrition. Taking supplements will not necessarily correct this condition unless you are able to adequately digest and absorb them.

*Acid-forming foods, especially meats, can create metabolic breakdown products that are congestive to the body.* This is especially true if you are already under stress and unable to properly digest protein foods. The result is that you tend to end up feeling more sluggish or tired and may have excess mucus or sinus problems. Although it's true that this congestion is not exactly the same thing as anxiety, it can certainly add stress to the body, which in turn aggravates tension and anxiety. The freer your body is from congestion due to acid-forming foods, the lighter and more clear-headed you'll be likely to feel. Be aware, also, that many medications have an acid reaction in the body and may lead to the same types of problems as acid-forming foods.

To maintain a proper acid-alkaline balance in the body, it helps to decrease consumption of acid-forming foods—most animal-based foods, sugar, and refined flour products—and increase the amount of *alkaline-forming* foods in your diet. Prominent among alkaline foods are all vegetables; most fruits, except plums and prunes; whole grains such as brown rice, millet, couscous, and buckwheat; and bean sprouts. Ideally, about 50 to 60 percent of the calories you consume should come from these foods, although in the winter it is okay to eat a slightly higher percentage of animal proteins. Try including more of the alkaline foods in your diet and see if it makes a difference in the way you feel.

## Increase Protein Relative to Carbohydrates

Years ago, many nutritionists advocated eating a high amount of complex carbohydrates (whole grains, pastas, bread)—as much as 70 percent of total calories. The prevailing idea was that too much fat promoted cardiovascular disease and too much protein led to excessive acidity and toxicity in the body. The ideal diet was thought to consist of 15 to 20 percent fat, 15 to 20 percent protein, and the rest carbohydrates.

More recently, however, evidence has mounted against the idea of eating high quantities of carbohydrates, especially by themselves. Carbohydrates are used by the body to produce *glucose,* the form of sugar the body and brain use for fuel. In order to transport glucose to the cells, your pancreas secretes insulin. Eating high levels of carbohydrates means your body produces higher levels of insulin, and too much insulin has an adverse effect on some of the body's most basic hormonal and neuroendocrine systems, especially prostaglandins and serotonin.

In brief, eating high amounts of cereals, breads, pastas, or even starches such as white rice, corn, and potatoes can raise your insulin levels to the point that other basic systems are thrown out of balance. The answer is not to eliminate complex carbohydrates but to reduce them *proportionately* to the amount of protein and fat you consume, *without increasing the total number of calories in your diet.* By doing this, you won't end up eating a diet that is too high in fat or protein. Instead, you'll continue to eat fat and protein in moderation *while decreasing the amount of carbohydrates you have at each meal relative to the amount of fat and protein.* An optimal ratio may be 40 percent carbohydrates, 30 percent protein, and 30 percent fat.

Dr. Barry Sears, in his book *Enter the Zone,* presents considerable research supporting the value of reducing the proportion of carbohydrates relative to protein and fat. Many people report that they feel better and have more energy when they increase the ratio of protein to carbohydrates in their diets. Several clients of mine have noticed that increasing protein relative to carbohydrates at each meal had a favorable effect on both anxiety and depression. This isn't surprising because anxiety and mood disorders often involve deficiencies in neurotransmitters, especially serotonin. The body has no way to make neurotransmitters (and serotonin in particular) without a steady supply of amino acids, which are derived from protein. Whether or not you agree with Dr. Sears's approach or choose to adopt a 40:30:30 diet, it's a good idea that you have some protein (preferably in the form of wild fish, organic poultry, eggs, tofu, tempeh, or beans and grains) at every meal. On the other hand, aim not to exceed 30 percent of your calories as protein—especially in the form of meat, chicken, or fish—as this may tend to make your body overly acidic.

## What to Do When You Eat Out

The pressures and constraints of modern life require that many of us eat lunch or dinner out. Unfortunately, most restaurant food, even at its best, provides too many calories, too much saturated fat, and too much salt, and often includes food that has been cooked in stale or rancid oils. Much restaurant food is less fresh than what you can obtain on your own. For the most part, eating in restaurants is not optimal for taking care of your health.

If you need to eat in restaurants often, observe the following guidelines:

- Avoid all fast food or "junk food" concessions.

- Whenever possible, eat out at natural food or health food restaurants that use whole, preferably organic foods.

- If natural food restaurants are unavailable, go to high-quality seafood restaurants and order fresh wild fish, preferably broiled without butter or oil. Accompany the fish with fresh vegetables, potatoes or rice, and a green salad. On the salad, avoid creamy or dairy-based dressings.

- As a third choice, try a high-quality Chinese or Japanese restaurant and have a meal consisting of rice, vegetables, and fresh fish or tofu (bean curd). In Chinese restaurants, be sure to ask your server to leave off MSG (monosodium glutamate), a flavor enhancer to which many people are allergic.

- As a general rule, when eating out, have no more than one roll with one pat of butter, and minimize ordering cream-based soups, such as clam chowder. Get your salad dressings on the side, using oil and vinegar or a low-fat Italian dressing. Stick with simple entrées such as chicken (preferably organic) or whitefish without elaborate sauces or toppings. Organic poultry or wild fish are preferable. If possible, try to avoid high-fat desserts. Don't hesitate to ask your server for assistance in having food prepared according to your needs. Learn to enjoy the subtle tastes of simple foods. You'll find this becomes easier and desirable after a while when you omit rich, high-fat, and sugary foods.

As you think back over all of the guidelines for improving your nutrition, keep in mind that it's unnecessary to try to adopt them all at once. Begin by decreasing your caffeine and sugar consumption, which will have the most direct impact on reducing your vulnerability to stress and anxiety. Beyond these suggestions, go at your own pace in upgrading your diet. You're more likely to *maintain* a dietary change that you've decided you truly *want* to make, instead of one you've pressured yourself into.

## Summary: Low Stress/Anxiety Dietary Guidelines

As with the rest of the information in this chapter, the following guidelines are intended to be suggestive rather than prescriptive. These guidelines are not intended to take the place of a detailed dietary assessment, recommendations, and the creation of a meal plan by a competent nutritionist or nutritionally oriented physician. Although all of the guidelines below are important, they are listed in order of their direct relevance to anxiety reduction.

1. Eliminate as far as possible the stimulants and stress-inducing substances described in the first section of this chapter—caffeine, regular tea, nicotine, other stimulants, salt (down

to one teaspoon per day, or 5.7 grams), and preservatives. (Elimination of caffeine and nicotine is the most critical for reducing anxiety.) Instead of black tea, try green tea (lower amount of caffeine) or herbal teas.

2.  Eliminate or reduce to a minimum your consumption of refined sugar, brown sugar, honey, sucrose, dextrose, and other sweeteners such as corn syrup, corn sweeteners, and high fructose corn syrup. Replace desserts, sugary beverages, and sweet snacks with fresh fruit and sugar-free beverages. Moderate alcohol consumption, since your body converts alcohol to sugar. Also eliminate artificial sweeteners such as aspartame (NutraSweet) and saccharin. Aspartame, in particular, can aggravate panic attacks and may, over time, cause damage to the nervous system. For a natural sweetener with no proven adverse effects, try stevia.

3.  Reduce or eliminate refined and processed foods from your diet as much as possible. Replace them with whole and fresh foods (preferably organic). Even many apparent "health food" items, such as protein powder, are highly processed. Instead of sodas, try fresh (unprocessed) fruit juices, or better yet, whole fruits themselves.

4.  Eliminate or reduce to a minimum any food that you establish as an allergen. Notice particularly how you feel if you eliminate wheat and/or dairy products from your diet. Be mindful of any food that causes you to feel tired or produce mucus after eating it.

5.  Reduce consumption of red meat as well as poultry containing steroid hormones and other chemicals. Replace these with organic poultry and/or wild seafood (fish such as wild halibut, salmon, snapper, sole, trout, and turbot are recommended). Avoid large sea fish, such as swordfish, marlin, and tuna, which contain excessive levels of mercury. Try to avoid tilapia, which is almost always farmed.

6.  Increase your intake of dietary fiber by eating whole grains, bran, raw vegetables, and high-fiber fruits such as apples. (Note, though, that too much fiber can cause gas and bloating and interfere with the body's ability to absorb protein.)

7.  Drink the equivalent of at least six 8-ounce glasses of bottled spring water or purified water per day. Reverse osmosis and activated carbon are good methods of filtration. When possible, avoid drinking water sold in plastic bottles. If you do, drink all of the water after opening the bottle—don't leave water in a plastic bottle for days (even in the refrigerator) to have later.

8.  Increase your intake of raw, fresh vegetables. A mixed-vegetable salad every day is an excellent idea. Include one fresh (not frozen or canned) cooked vegetable in your diet each day.

9.  Whenever possible, buy produce that is organic.

10. Keep all fat in your diet (oils, nuts, salad dressings, and so on) to 30 percent of your total calories. Animal fat and cholesterol-containing foods such as red meat, organ meats, gravy, cheeses, butter, eggs, whole milk, and shellfish should make up no more than 10 percent of your total calories. Avoid foods containing trans-fatty acids altogether (contained in deep-fried foods, chips, mayonnaise, margarine, most doughnuts, cookies, crackers, cakes, and all processed foods that contain partially hydrogenated oils).

11. To avoid excessive weight gain, consume only as much energy (calories) as you expend. Decrease caloric intake and increase aerobic exercise if you're already overweight.

12. Select foods from the four major food groups: 1) fruits and vegetables (four to five servings daily), 2) whole grains, including whole-grain rice and whole-grain breads (two to three servings daily), 3) animal proteins, emphasizing organic poultry, seafood, and eggs, or legume equivalents if you are vegetarian (two to three servings daily), and 4) dairy products, emphasizing low-fat or nonfat dairy products (one serving daily). If you are lactose intolerant or otherwise sensitive to cow's milk, try substituting rice or almond milk instead. Your diet should emphasize the first two categories and moderate amounts of the latter two. In general, it's a good idea to move your diet in the direction of vegetarianism and away from excess consumption of animal-based foods. At the same time, you should increase the ratio of protein to carbohydrates in your diet. Protein should make up approximately 30 percent of what you eat; healthy fat, 20 to 30 percent (or less if your cholesterol is above 250); and complex carbohydrates, about 40 to 50 percent.

Use the *Food Diary* on the next page to monitor what you eat for at least three days. In what ways might you improve your dietary habits? What would you actually be willing to change in the next month?

# Food Diary

*Instructions:* Use the following chart to evaluate your eating habits for three days. The areas in which your average daily consumption varies the most from the ideal are the areas in which you can make the greatest improvement in what you eat. Make copies of this form (or download the blank version available online—see the back of the book for information) so that you can track your diet for two or three weeks.

For three days, keep track of how many servings you have of each of these food categories. For each category, divide the total servings, days 1 to 3, by 3 to get your daily average for the period. Compare your eating pattern to the ideal, specified in the left column.

| Week of: _____ (dates) | Day one servings | Day two servings | Day three servings | Average servings per day | Ideal servings per day |
|---|---|---|---|---|---|
| **Caffeine** serving = 1 cup coffee or black tea, or regular tea (1 serving) | | | | | |
| **Sweets** serving = 1 candy bar, 1 piece of pie, 1 cup ice cream (1 serving) | | | | | |
| **Alcohol** serving = 1 beer, 1 glass of wine, or 1 cocktail (1 serving) | | | | | |
| **Vegetables and fruits** serving = 1 cup string beans, 1 apple, medium potato (5 to 10 servings per day) | | | | | |
| **Whole-grain breads and cereal** serving = 1 slice bread; ¾ cup cereal; ¾ cup rice, oats, or quinoa (4 to 6 servings per day) | | | | | |
| **Milk, cheese, yogurt** serving = 1 cup milk, 1 medium slice cheese, 1 carton of yogurt (2 to 3 servings per day) | | | | | |
| **Meat, poultry, fish, eggs, beans, and nuts** serving = 3 oz lean meat or fish, 2 eggs, 1¼ cups cooked beans, ¾ cup nuts (2 to 3 servings per day) | | | | | |

# Supplements for Anxiety

## *B Vitamins[1] and Vitamin C*

It is widely known that *during times of stress* your body tends to rapidly deplete stores of B vitamins and vitamin C. In general, it's recommended that you take a high-potency B-complex vitamin and a two-gram dose of vitamin C every day. Doing so may make a noticeable difference in your energy level and resilience to stress. The B vitamins are necessary to help maintain the proper functioning of your nervous system. Deficiencies, especially of vitamins $B_1$, $B_2$, $B_6$, and $B_{12}$, can lead to anxiety, irritability, restlessness, fatigue, and even emotional instability. It's best to take all eleven of the B vitamins together in a B-complex supplement, since they tend to work together synergistically. Vitamin C is well known for enhancing the immune system and promoting healing from infection, disease, and injury. Less well known is the fact that vitamin C helps support the adrenal glands, whose proper functioning is necessary to your ability to cope with stress. Vitamin $B_5$ (pantothenic acid) also supports the adrenal glands, and many people find that it is helpful in dealing with excess stress.

The following doses of B-complex and vitamin C are recommended on a regular basis:

- B-complex: 25 to 50 mg each of all eleven B vitamins once a day (twice a day under high stress)

- Vitamin C: 1000 mg in a time-release form, twice a day (double this dose under high stress). Vitamin C-complex, in combination with the bioflavonoids, rutin and hesperidin, is preferred.

Please note that it's not easily possible to overdose on B vitamins, since they are water soluble. The one exception to this is vitamin $B_6$. It is important not to exceed 100 mg per day if you're taking $B_6$ on a long-term basis. (Higher doses of $B_6$ may be taken on a short-term basis to relieve premenstrual symptoms, however.) High daily doses of vitamin C are generally harmless and a good hedge against infections and colds. However, repeated daily doses in *excess of 5000 mg per day* have been associated with stomach complaints, diarrhea, and even kidney stones in some people.

It's important that you take B vitamins, vitamin C, and other vitamins *with meals*. Stomach acids and enzymes produced while digesting food are necessary to help break down and assimilate vitamins. Do not take vitamins on an empty stomach (with the exception of amino acids, as discussed in the section on amino acids). Capsule forms of vitamins are generally easier on the stomach than tablets.

---

1   B vitamins include thiamine ($B_1$), riboflavin ($B_2$), niacin or niacinamide ($B_3$), pantothenic acid ($B_5$), pyridoxine ($B_6$), biotin, folic acid, choline, inositol, cyanocobalamin ($B_{12}$), and PABA (para-aminobenzoic acid).

## Calcium

It is widely known that calcium can act as a tranquilizer, having a calming effect on the nervous system. Calcium, along with neurotransmitter substances, is involved in the process of transmitting nerve signals across the synapses between nerve cells. Depletion of calcium can result in nerve cell overactivity, which may be one of the underlying physiological bases of anxiety. It's important that you get at least 1000 mg of calcium per day, either in calcium-rich foods, such as dairy products, eggs, and leafy vegetables, or by taking calcium supplements (chelates are preferred to calcium carbonate). If you take a calcium supplement, be sure to take it in combination with magnesium, as these two minerals balance each other and work in tandem. For some people, magnesium can have a relaxing effect equal to that of calcium. In your supplement, the ratio of calcium to magnesium should be either two to one or one to one.

**Note:** You may want to have your nutritionist or holistic doctor perform a hair analysis test if you are concerned about having a deficiency of calcium or other minerals. Utilizing a hair sample, the test detects deficiencies of a large number of different minerals. The presence of certain mineral deficiencies can be used to detect other conditions. For example, too little chromium suggests a problem in carbohydrate metabolism and possible hypoglycemia. Too little cobalt suggests a possible vitamin $B_{12}$ deficiency. The test can also detect excesses of toxic metals such as aluminum, lead, or mercury in your body. High levels of mercury, in particular, have been associated with anxiety.

## Antioxidants

Your body needs antioxidants in order to combat inflammatory processes that can lead to a variety of diseases, especially cardiovascular disease. Good antioxidant foods include beans (kidney, pinto, and black beans), berries (organic blueberries, raspberries, and strawberries), apples, walnuts, pecans, and artichoke hearts. Good antioxidant supplements include vitamin C (up to two grams per day), vitamin E (400 IU per day), selenium (100 mg per day), $CoQ_{10}$ (100 mg per day), resveratrol (also found in red wine), and natural astaxanthin (starting at 4 mg, and going up to 12 mg, per day).

## Relaxing Herbs

Herbs have been used for hundreds of years to promote calmness and relaxation. While usually not as potent as prescription tranquilizers, such as Xanax or Klonopin (with the exception of kava), they have few side effects and are nonaddictive. Many people benefit from using herbs for mild to moderate states of anxiety. The following herbs have been most helpful to my clients.

### Kava: Relaxing Herb from the Pacific Islands

Kava (or kava kava) is a natural tranquilizer that has been popular in the United States for several years. Some clients of mine have testified that it's as potent a relaxer as Xanax. A member of the pepper tree family, kava is native to the South Pacific. Polynesians have used it for centuries both in ceremonial rituals and as a social relaxer. Small doses produce a sense of well-being, while large doses can produce lethargy and drowsiness and reduce muscle tension.

In European countries, such as Germany, kava has been approved for treatment of insomnia and anxiety. It appears from the limited research available that kava may tone down the activity of the limbic system, particularly the amygdala, which is a brain center associated with anxiety (see chapter 2). Detailed neurophysiological effects of kava are not known at this time.

Kava's principal advantage over such tranquilizers as Xanax or Klonopin is that it's not addictive. It's also less likely to impair memory or aggravate depression, as tranquilizers sometimes can. Research indicates that it is an effective treatment for mild to moderate anxiety (not panic attacks), insomnia, headaches, muscle tension, and gastrointestinal spasms and can even help relieve urinary tract infections.

When buying kava, it's preferable to obtain a standardized extract with a specified percentage of kavalactones, the active ingredient. The percentage of kavalactones can vary from 30 to 70 percent. If you multiply the total number of milligrams of kava in each capsule or tablet by the percentage of kavalactones, you get the actual strength of the dose. For example, a 200 mg capsule with 70 percent kavalactones would actually be a 140 mg dose.

Most kava supplements at your health food store contain on the order of 50 to 70 percent kavalactones per capsule. Research in Europe has found that taking three or four doses of this strength daily may be as effective as a tranquilizer.

At present, there is little hard data on the long-term effects of taking kava on a daily basis. In the Polynesian islands, where residents use kava in high doses daily for long periods of time, skin discoloration can occasionally occur. Sometimes this progresses to scaling dermatitis, which is relieved when the use of kava is discontinued. If you notice any ill effects, please stop using kava immediately, and do not resume without consulting a naturopath or an informed physician. It's preferable that you not use kava on a *daily* basis for more than six months. On an intermittent basis, however, you can use it indefinitely.

In general, it's not a good idea to use kava in combination with tranquilizers. While not dangerous, such a combination can produce grogginess and even disorientation. Especially if you're taking a moderate to high dose of Xanax or Klonopin (more than 1.5 mg a day), refrain from using kava.

Kava should also not be taken if you have Parkinson's disease, are pregnant, or are breastfeeding. It should be used with caution before driving or operating machinery.

Several years ago there were widespread concerns that kava might cause liver problems. In Europe, some manufacturers used the stems and leaves of the kava plant, which contain a liver toxin, and a few people subsequently developed liver disease. American-based companies then used and now continue to use only the root of the plant (as the Polynesians have done for centuries), which is considered to be safe. Kava has never been banned in the United States, though it is currently restricted in some countries. The FDA cautions that people with a history of liver problems should not use kava without first consulting with their physician.

## Valerian

Valerian is an herbal tranquilizer and sedative that is widely used in Europe. In recent years, it has gained popularity in the United States. Clinical studies, mostly in Europe, have found it to be as effective as tranquilizers in alleviating mild to moderate anxiety and insomnia, as Jonathan Davidson and Kathryn Connor discuss in *Herbs for the Mind*. Yet it has fewer side effects and is nonaddictive.

Valerian is also not as likely as prescription tranquilizers to impair memory and concentration or cause lethargy and drowsiness. It will generally not cause a hangover the next day if used for sleep, though a few people have reported being affected that way. In general, valerian can work well for mild to moderate anxiety but may be less effective for more severe cases.

Derived from the plant *Valeriana officinalis*, valerian has numerous chemical constituents, including essential oil, iridoids, and alkaloids. No one of these constituents is responsible for its sedative properties; the overall impression is that all of the components work synergistically. It's therefore unlikely that a single component will be isolated and manufactured synthetically.

Valerian has a good reputation for promoting sleep. Numerous studies have shown that it can reduce the time it takes to get to sleep, as well as improve the quality of sleep. If you try valerian for sleep and it doesn't seem to work, don't give up. Some studies indicate that it may take from two to three weeks of regular use for the herb to achieve its full benefit, whether you're taking it for insomnia or anxiety.

Valerian can be obtained at most health food stores in three forms: capsules, liquid extract, or tea. In treating anxiety or insomnia, try each of these forms to see which you like best, following the instructions given on the bottle or package. Capsules are the most convenient, but some people swear by the efficacy of the tinctures and teas. Frequently, you'll find valerian combined with other relaxing herbs such as passionflower, skullcap, hops, or chamomile. You may find these combinations to be more palatable or effective.

The effective dose for valerian ranges from 200 to 400 mg for anxiety relief during the day and 400 to 800 mg for help with sleeping at night. For sleep, it's best to take it about an hour before retiring. For mild to moderate anxiety during the day, you might take two or three doses in the 200 to 400 mg range.

Be sure to buy a valerian product with sufficient potency. Generally, a statement on the bottle indicating that the product has been standardized to at least 0.5 percent of *valerenic acid* is an indication that it has reasonable potency. Also note the expiration date, as older products tend to lose potency. If the product contains other herbs or ingredients besides valerian, it should offer a complete listing of these along with the amount in each recommended dose. Avoid products that don't provide a full listing of ingredients.

As a general rule, you should avoid using valerian daily for over six months. Long-term use at high doses has been associated with side effects such as headache, excitability, restlessness, agitation, and heart palpitations. You can use it three to four times per week, however, indefinitely. Also, valerian should not be taken together with benzodiazepine tranquilizers such as Xanax (alprazolam), Ativan (lorazepam), and Klonopin (clonazepam), or with sedatives such as Restoril (temazepam), Ambien (zolpidem), and Sonata (zaleplon). It can be combined with other herbs, such as kava, Saint-John's-wort, and especially hops or passionflower.

A long history of use in Europe indicates, valerian is an especially safe herb. Still, there are occasional reports of paradoxical reactions of increased anxiety, restlessness, or heart palpitations, possibly due to allergy. Stop using valerian or any other herb if it causes such reactions.

## Saint-John's-Wort

Saint-John's-wort (*Hypericum perforatum*) also has a long history of use. It was recommended by Hippocrates for anxiety more than two thousand years ago. Currently, it is being used widely in Europe and the United States to treat symptoms of mild to moderate depression, as well as anxiety.

Saint-John's-wort has a direct effect on relieving depression and appears to reduce anxiety as a secondary effect. European studies have found it to have antianxiety properties nearly comparable to tranquilizers. There is evidence that Saint-John's-wort enhances levels of all three neurotransmitters implicated in anxiety disorders: serotonin, norepinephrine, and dopamine. On this basis, it might be seen as preferable to SSRI antidepressants, which raise only serotonin levels.

Saint-John's-wort is available in health food stores and many drugstores. Be sure to obtain brands that are standardized to contain 0.3 percent hypericin, the active ingredient. The standard dose is three 300 mg capsules per day.

When starting out, you may want to try two capsules per day to get used to the herb, then raise the dose to three capsules, or 900 mg, per day. If you find it upsets your stomach, take each dose with a meal.

It's important to keep in mind that Saint-John's-wort takes four to six weeks to reach therapeutic effectiveness. If you're not seeing any benefit in the first two to three weeks, don't get discouraged and stop; you need to stick with it for at least one month.

Saint-John's-wort has had a very good safety record over the hundreds of years it has been used. For some people, though, it can cause photosensitivity, an increased sensitivity to sunlight. If you are using it and are in direct sunlight frequently, you may want to limit your exposure or use a sunscreen with 30 SPF or higher.

If you're already taking an SSRI or tricyclic antidepressant and want to switch to Saint-John's-wort, it's best to wean yourself off the prescription drug before starting to take the herb. In general, *do not take an SSRI and Saint-John's-wort together* without your doctor's approval.

It's okay to take Saint-John's-wort in conjunction with relaxing herbs such as kava or valerian. There is no strong evidence against combining it with tranquilizers, such as Xanax and Klonopin, though some doctors are wary of doing so. However, if you are taking an MAO-inhibitor antidepressant, such as Nardil or Parnate, do *not* take Saint-John's-wort. In general, because it interacts with a number of different drugs, it's a good idea to check with your doctor before taking it.

In conclusion, Saint-John's-wort is likely to be helpful if you're dealing with mild to moderate depression. It may also alleviate mild to moderate levels of anxiety after four to six weeks' use, although it is probably not effective in relieving panic attacks, obsessive-compulsive disorder, or symptoms of post-traumatic stress disorder. If you are suffering from more severe anxiety symptoms and have not obtained sufficient help from cognitive behavioral therapy and other natural strategies, consult a qualified psychiatrist and consider a trial of an SSRI medication (see chapter 18).

For further information on Saint-John's-wort, see the book *Hypericum and Depression* by Harold Bloomfield, Mikael Nordfors, and Peter McWilliams.

## Other Helpful Herbs

### Passionflower

Passionflower is a good natural tranquilizer considered by many to be as effective as valerian. In higher doses, it is often used to treat insomnia, as it both relieves nervous tension and relaxes muscles. It's available either in capsules or in liquid extract at your health food store. Sometimes you'll find products that combine it with valerian or other relaxing herbs. Use as directed on the bottle or package.

### Gotu Kola

Gotu kola has been popular for thousands of years in India. It has a mildly relaxing effect and helps revitalize a weakened nervous system. It has been found to help improve circulation and memory function, and it has also been found to promote healing following childbirth. You can find it in most health food stores in capsules or extracts.

### Ginkgo Biloba

Derived from the ginkgo tree, ginkgo biloba can indirectly help reduce anxiety by improving concentration and mental clarity. It does this by increasing the flow of blood, oxygen, and nutrients to the brain. Studies have found that it can improve mental function in elderly people and can also help tinnitus, or "ringing in the ears." It's typically available in 60 mg tablets; consider taking one or two 60 mg doses per day. If you're taking aspirin regularly, limit your use of ginkgo, since the combination can inhibit blood clotting.

In using any of the herbs described above, be sure not to exceed the recommended dose. For further information on herbs, consult the books by Harold Bloomfield, Michael Tierra, or Earl Mindell listed at the end of this chapter or see a doctor (usually a holistic physician or naturopath) who is well versed in the use of herbs.

### SAMe: Fast-Acting Natural Antidepressant

Unlike the herbs just described, S-adenosyl-L-methionine (abbreviated SAMe, pronounced "Sammy") is a substance that occurs naturally in the body. Widely popular in Europe for over three decades, it first became available in the United States in 1999. Extensive research done in Europe has found it is sometimes as effective in treating depression as prescription SSRI antidepressants.

SAMe appears to work by increasing serotonin and dopamine activity in the brain. While healthy people manufacture enough of their own SAMe, research has found that clinically depressed people are often deficient.

A major advantage of SAMe is that it has almost no side effects. Since it occurs naturally in the body, adverse reactions are rare. Some people occasionally report nausea or queasiness when starting it, but this tends to go away after a few days. SAMe also works very quickly. Unlike prescription antidepressants and Saint-John's-wort, the benefits are usually felt within a few days of starting to take it.

Combining SAMe with prescription SSRIs is somewhat controversial. Be sure to talk with your doctor if you're thinking of combining SAMe with an SSRI medication.

In addition to helping with depression, SAMe has been found useful in the treatment of osteo-arthritis and fibromyalgia. It appears to restore and maintain healthy joint function by contributing to regeneration of cartilage. SAMe also has potent antioxidant properties. It's used by the body to help synthesize glutathione, an important antioxidant involved in protecting cells from free-radical damage. Finally, SAMe is beneficial to the liver and can assist in detoxifying the body from alcohol, drugs, and environmental toxins.

At present, information on the use of SAMe to treat anxiety is limited. Most available research has evaluated its effectiveness as an antidepressant. If it functions at all like the SSRIs, it would be expected to have antianxiety as well as antidepressant effects.

SAMe is available in most health food stores and drugstores in 200 mg tablets. The recommended dose for depression is 400 to 1200 mg a day. Because it can cause nausea and gastro-intestinal (GI) disturbances for some people, start with 200 mg per day at first (for this reason, enteric-coated tablets are preferable). After two days, raise the dose to 200 mg twice per day. If you do not experience benefits after a week at this dose, you can raise the dose again to 800 to 1200 mg per day. If you're taking it primarily for arthritis or fibromyalgia, 800 mg per day is probably sufficient.

People with bipolar disorder (manic depressives) should take SAMe only under the supervision of a knowledgeable physician, as it can aggravate manic states.

For detailed information on SAMe, see the book *Stop Depression Now* by Dr. Richard Brown.

## Amino Acids

In the past few decades, amino acids, which are the natural constituents of protein, have come into use in the treatment of both anxiety disorders and depression. Many people prefer them to prescription drugs because they have fewer side effects and are nonaddictive. You may wish to talk to a holistic doctor, a naturopath, or the staff at your local health food store to expand on the information presented below.

### Tryptophan

The amino acid tryptophan (or L-tryptophan) is a natural precursor to the neurotransmitter serotonin. Serotonin is involved in regulating many body functions, including mood, sleep, appetite, and pain threshold. It produces a feeling of calmness and well-being, and deficiencies have been linked to anxiety.

Some studies have found tryptophan to be as effective as prescription antidepressants and sedatives in relieving insomnia, generalized anxiety, and depression.

Tryptophan is available in two forms: 5-hydroxytryptophan (5-HT) and L-tryptophan. You can find 5-HT in most health food stores. The recommended dose is 50 to 100 mg two or three times per day (or in a single combined dose at bedtime for insomnia), with or without food. L-tryptophan was widely used in the 1980s and then taken off the market in 1989 by the FDA: an impurity in the manufacturing process at a single company caused a rare blood disease that resulted in severe illness for several thousand people. In the mid-90s, L-tryptophan was reintroduced in the United States under strict manufacturing standards and only by prescription.

In recent times, it has become available again to the public and can be obtained at some health food stores and over the Internet. Many people find L-tryptophan to be more sedating than 5-HT and so prefer it for insomnia. The recommended dose is 1000 to 2000 mg at bedtime, taken with a carbohydrate snack or fruit juice. If you take either 5-HT or L-tryptophan, effectiveness can be improved by taking it along with vitamin $B_3$ (niacinamide) (100 to 500 mg) and vitamin $B_6$ (100 mg). If you are taking an SSRI, SNRI, tricyclic, or MAO-inhibitor antidepressant, *do not take either form of tryptophan except under the supervision of a physician.*

## Theanine

The amino acid theanine was discovered as a constituent of green tea in 1949. Subsequently, it was used in a variety of foods.

Able to cross the blood-brain barrier, theanine's primary effect is to increase the overall level of the brain inhibitory neurotransmitter GABA, leading to reduced anxiety and stress. Theanine has also been found to promote alpha wave production in the brain. It is thought that supplemental theanine, being a precursor to GABA, reaches the brain more easily than supplemental GABA, described below. A few studies have found that theanine may have a beneficial effect on immune function.

A study in 2007 by the NIH (National Institutes of Health) found that oral intake of theanine could have antistress effects via the inhibition of cortical neuron excitation.

Currently, theanine is widely used as a mild natural tranquilizer. It is available in 100 mg capsules both at health food stores (under amino acids) and through online vitamin distributors. The recommended dose for mild to moderate anxiety is one or two 100 mg capsules. For some people, higher doses may be helpful in getting to sleep. Few side effects have been reported for doses in the range of 100 to 200 mg.

## Gamma-Aminobutyric Acid

As an alternative to tryptophan, you may want to consider trying gamma-aminobutyric acid (GABA, for short), an amino acid that is available at many health food stores. GABA has a mildly tranquilizing effect, and some people have used it as an alternative to prescription tranquilizers such as Xanax and Ativan. Although it is not as potent as prescription drugs, GABA does have the advantage of having few side effects and being nonaddictive.

The usual dose of GABA recommended for its calming effect is 200 to 500 mg. It is fine to take it in this dose once or twice per day (do not exceed 1000 mg in a twenty-four-hour period).

It's a good idea to take GABA with a carbohydrate snack (such as a piece of toast, crackers, cereal, or rice cakes). Carbohydrate foods actually enhance the calming or sedative effect. Avoid taking GABA with protein. There is nothing harmful in doing so, but the protein (which is made up of many different amino acids) will tend to compete with absorption of GABA.

## Tyrosine

Since depression frequently accompanies anxiety, you may want to consider an amino acid that has been used in some cases to treat depression. Tyrosine increases the amount of neurotransmitter substances in the brain known as *norepinephrine and dopamine*, substances whose deficiency has been implicated as a contributing cause of depression. Since earlier editions of this book, research on tyrosine for treatment of depression has been mixed. Yet many people report benefits in taking tyrosine for depression. Tyrosine has also been known to increase alertness, attention, and focus. Tyrosine is found in many foods, especially cheese, as well as turkey, chicken, and fish.

Tyrosine is available in 250 mg or 500 mg capsules or tablets in many health food stores as well as online. If you are interested in experimenting with it, please observe the following guidelines:

- Do not take tyrosine if you are pregnant, have PKU (a disease requiring a phenylalanine-free diet), or are taking an MAO-inhibitor medication (such as Nardil or Parnate). If you have high blood pressure, take it only under a doctor's supervision.

- Take 500 mg to 1000 mg of tyrosine once in the morning, preferably before exercise. It's better that you avoid taking tyrosine right after a protein-heavy meal, as it cannot cross the blood-brain barrier if there are competing amino acids (as found in protein). It's best to take tyrosine on an empty stomach. If you do, start with just a 500 mg dose before trying 1000 mg. If taking tyrosine causes any side effects, such as headache, nausea, or increased anxiety, discontinue it.

- You may experience some benefit from tyrosine after a few weeks, if taken at the right dosage. Do not exceed 1000 mg per day except under the supervision of a doctor who is familiar with the use of amino acid therapy. If you are severely depressed and/or have suicidal thoughts, do not rely on amino acids alone to deal with your problem. Please consult a psychiatrist.

An in-depth discussion of the use of amino acids in the treatment of depression can be found in the books by Joan Mathews Larson and Julia Ross listed at the end of this chapter.

## *Omega-3 Fatty Acids*

Omega-3 fatty acids, especially DHA and EPA, are important for brain and neurological health. Without sufficient levels of omega-3 fatty acids, nerve cell membranes are less fluid and may cause nerve cells to react slowly and misfire. Recent studies have found omega-3 supplementation to be helpful in diminishing symptoms of depression. The best source of omega-3 fatty acids is wild fish (especially salmon and sardines). Taking fish oil in liquid (two tablespoons per day) or in one-gram capsules (two or three per day, or a combined dose of 1000 to 2000 mg per day) may help alleviate depression and mood instability. Oils should be stored in the freezer or refrigerator to protect them from damaging oxidations. Taking 400 international units (IU) daily of vitamin E (mixed tocopherol form) can also provide protection from oxidation.

## Hormone Supplements

Certain hormones are available to supplement presumed deficiencies. You've probably seen them at your local drugstore or health food store. Some may promote relaxation and aid sleep. One of the most common, melatonin, is discussed below.

### Melatonin

Melatonin is a hormone secreted at night by the pineal gland to signal the brain that it is time to go to sleep. Supplemental melatonin can help regulate sleep cycles. It is taken in doses from 0.5 to 5 mg. While some people find it useful, others say that they get no benefit from it and that it leaves them feeling groggy in the morning.

# Summary of Things to Do

1.  Evaluate the amount of caffeine in your diet using the *Caffeine Chart* in this chapter, and attempt to gradually reduce your intake to less than 100 mg per day. If you are especially sensitive, you may want to eliminate caffeine altogether, substituting decaf coffee, green tea, or even herbal tea without caffeine.

2.  Stop smoking. In addition to significantly reducing your risk for cardiovascular disease and cancer, you will lower your susceptibility to panic attacks and anxiety.

3.  Reduce your consumption of substances that stress your body. Decrease your intake of salt to one teaspoon (5.7 grams) per day. Replace processed foods containing preservatives with (preferably organic) vegetables and fruits and whole grains. If possible, substitute organic beef, poultry, and fish for commercially available meats. Avoid processed meats.

4.  Allow eating to be a relaxing activity. Avoid eating on the run or eating excessively. Chew your food thoroughly and limit your fluid intake during a meal to eight ounces.

5.  Evaluate whether you experience the subjective symptoms of hypoglycemia—such as light-headedness, anxiety, depression, weakness, or shakiness—three or four hours after a meal (or in the early morning hours) and whether they are quickly relieved by eating. You may want to follow this up with a formal six-hour glucose tolerance test. If you suspect that hypoglycemia is contributing to your problem with anxiety, strive to eliminate from your diet all forms of white sugar as well as brown sugar, honey, corn syrup, corn sweeteners, molasses, and high fructose corn syrup. Avoid NutraSweet (aspartame). A recent study found a link between this substance and panic disorder for certain people. Most fresh, whole fruits (not dried) are fine if you're hypoglycemic, although fruit juices should be diluted with water. Observe the "Dietary Modifications for Hypoglycemia" recommended in this chapter and consider taking the suggested supplements. You may want to consult a qualified nutritionist to assist you in setting up an appropriate dietary and supplement regime.

6. Evaluate your susceptibility to food allergies. Take note of any types of food that you crave (paying attention particularly to wheat and dairy products) and try eliminating that food from your diet for two weeks. Then reintroduce the food and notice if you have any symptoms.

7. Work toward complying with the "Low Stress/Anxiety Dietary Guidelines" described in this chapter. Use the *Food Diary* to monitor your intake of caffeine, fats, sweets, and alcohol, and try for a balanced number of servings of each major food group for several weeks. *Avoid pushing yourself to radically change your diet all at once*, or you may end up rebelling against the idea of making any changes. Introduce one small change each week—or perhaps even each month—so that you gradually modify your dietary habits.

8. Consider taking the supplements recommended for anxiety and stress, especially the B vitamins, vitamin C, calcium-magnesium, and antioxidants. You may want to consult with a nutritionist or physician who is supportive of the idea of high-potency vitamins (not everyone is) to assist you in this.

9. You may want to try the herbs kava or valerian as a mild tranquilizer to relieve anxiety. Or you may want to try SAMe or Saint-John's-wort as a treatment for mild to moderate depression. Fish oil capsules (high in omega-3 fatty acids) can also be helpful for depression. All of these substances can usually be found at your local drugstore, health food store, or online. Avoid exceeding recommended levels unless you consult with a knowledgeable professional.

10. You may want to explore whether amino acids can be helpful—specifically, theanine, GABA, or tryptophan for anxiety, and tyrosine for depression. Consult the books by Joan Mathews Larson and Julia Ross listed below for in-depth information on the use of amino acids to treat anxiety and depression.

11. Of the many things your brain needs in order to function properly, the following three criteria are of particular importance to people who have panic attacks, phobias, and/or anxiety:

    - *An adequate level of serotonin.* Adequate levels can be accomplished, if necessary, via the selective serotonin reuptake inhibitor medications, such as Prozac, Zoloft, Paxil, Lexapro, or Celexa (see chapter 18). Natural alternatives for increasing serotonin include the use of the herb Saint-John's-wort, S-adenosyl-L-methionine (SAMe), or the amino acid tryptophan. You can also increase your serotonin levels by eating tryptophan-rich foods such as turkey, tuna, eggs, or milk, getting plenty of exercise, getting at least one hour per day of exposure to sunshine, and, last but not least, having that magic ingredient in your life known as love and affection.

    - *An adequate, stable level of blood sugar.* Review the sections on hypoglycemia and dietary guidelines for hypoglycemia. Eliminate sweets other than organic fruits from your diet. Always have a nonsugar snack such as unsalted nuts or crackers and cheese with you (in your car, at work, and so on) should you start to experience hypoglycemic symptoms. Be sure to take supplemental B-complex and chromium.

- *Sufficient light.* Review the section in chapter 17 on seasonal affective disorder to determine whether light deficiency is an issue for you. If so, read the book by Norman Rosenthal listed below. In the meantime, increase your exposure to sunlight or bright light during fall and winter, if possible.

# Further Reading

Balch, Phyllis. *Prescription for Nutritional Healing.* 5th ed. Garden City Park, NY: Avery Trade, 2010. (A comprehensive reference book.)

Bloomfield, Harold. *Healing Anxiety Naturally.* New York: HarperPerennial, 1999.

———, Mikael Nordfors, and Peter McWilliams. *Hypericum and Depression.* Los Angeles: Prelude Press, 1997.

Bourne, Edmund J., Arlen Brownstein, and Lorna Garano. *Natural Relief for Anxiety.* Oakland, CA: New Harbinger Publications, 2004.

Brown, Richard, Theodore Bottiglieri, and Carol Colman. *Stop Depression Now.* New York: Berkley, 2000.

Davidson, Jonathan, and Kathryn Connor. *Herbs for the Mind.* New York: The Guilford Press, 2000.

Dufty, William. *Sugar Blues.* Reissue. New York: Grand Central Life & Style, 1986. (Classic popular book on hypoglycemia.)

Haas, Elson M., and Buck Levin. *Staying Healthy with Nutrition.* 1st ed. Berkeley, CA: Celestial Arts, 2006.

Larson, Joan Mathews. *Depression-Free, Naturally.* New York: Ballantine, 2001.

Mindell, Earl. *Earl Mindell's New Vitamin Bible.* New York: Grand Central Life & Style, 2011.

Robbins, John. *The Food Revolution.* 10th anniversary ed. San Francisco: Conari Press, 2011.

Rosenthal, Norman. *Winter Blues: Everything You Need to Know to Beat Seasonal Affective Disorder.* 4th ed. New York: Guilford Press, 2012.

Ross, Julia. *The Mood Cure.* New York: Penguin Books, 2003.

Sears, Barry. *Enter the Zone.* New York: HarperCollins, 1995.

Tierra, Michael. *The Way of Herbs.* Rev. ed. New York: Pocket Books, 1998.

Weil, Andrew. *Natural Health, Natural Medicine.* Rev ed. New York: Houghton Mifflin Harcourt, 2004.

# 17

# Health Conditions That
# May Contribute to Anxiety

It's likely that rather than having one identifiable cause, your anxiety springs from a variety of lifestyle, physical, and psychological factors. This chapter examines a number of common physical conditions that can aggravate anxiety or tax your system and make you more vulnerable to its effects. These conditions include adrenal fatigue, thyroid imbalance, body toxicity, premenstrual syndrome, menopause, seasonal affective disorder, and insomnia. Hypoglycemia and food allergies, discussed in chapter 16, can have similar effects. In order to adequately address your problem with panic, phobias, generalized anxiety, or depression, it's important to deal with these conditions as well, since any one or more of them can aggravate your anxiety problems. While this list is by no means exhaustive of all of the conditions that can complicate anxiety, it includes some of the more common ones. Some of these conditions are obvious, while others are not. You know it if you can't sleep or if you suffer from PMS, but you (and your therapist) may not be aware of conditions such as adrenal fatigue, body toxicity, thyroid imbalances, or seasonal affective disorder. Anyone who suffers from anxiety should be aware of the symptoms, causes, and treatments of all of the disorders discussed in this chapter.

## Adrenal Fatigue and "Burnout"

Prolonged and unremitting stress may affect your adrenal glands. In *The Stress of Life*, stress expert Hans Selye describes how protracted stress on the adrenal glands results in a state of chronic underfunctioning or ultimate "exhaustion."

Insufficient adrenal resources, in turn, tend to affect how you handle stressful situations, making it more likely that you will *become anxious in the face of stress*. Inadequate sleep; prolonged exposure to heat or cold; exposure to toxins, pollutants, or substances you're allergic to; and taking cortisone over a period of time can also contribute to adrenal stress. Sudden severe trauma or severe physical illness can initiate or worsen adrenal fatigue. Evidence for an actual persistent reduction in adrenal output due to stress is mixed, so the alternative terms "adrenal fatigue" or "burnout" are used in this chapter. Notice that many of these factors, particularly sudden trauma such as losses or life transitions, also play a role in the onset of anxiety disorders. Anxiety disorders and adrenal fatigue frequently occur together, and are sometimes difficult to disentangle.

Adrenal fatigue appears to develop in stages. When you're combating stress, the adrenal glands tend to hyperfunction, producing large amounts of adrenaline and noradrenaline, as well as steroid hormones such as *cortisol*. According to Hans Selye, as stress becomes prolonged, the glands begin to be overtaxed and go into a state of temporary underfunctioning. If you are relatively healthy, the glands will try to compensate and can actually rebuild themselves to the point of *hypertrophy* (growing larger). However, if high levels of stress continue, the glands will eventually exhaust themselves again and then remain in a chronic state of underfunctioning. At this stage, they can oscillate between overproducing adrenaline, which can cause panic or mood swings, and underproducing adrenaline. The ultimate outcome of prolonged adrenal fatigue can be chronic fatigue syndrome, fibromyalgia, chronic bronchitis or sinusitis, or autoimmune disorders ranging from lupus to rheumatoid arthritis.

Symptoms of adrenal fatigue include:

- Low stress tolerance (little things that didn't use to bother you get to you)

- Lethargy and fatigue (often manifested in difficulty getting up in the morning)

- Light-headedness when standing up quickly (called *postural hypotension*)

- Light sensitivity (difficulty adjusting to bright light outdoors)

- Difficulties with concentration and memory

- Insomnia

- Hypoglycemia

- Allergies (to foods, environmental substances, pollens, molds, and so on)

- Increased symptoms of premenstrual syndrome

- More frequent colds and respiratory conditions

*Hypoglycemia and adrenal fatigue.* Hypoglycemia and adrenal fatigue often go hand in hand. The adrenals function along with the pancreas in helping to maintain stable blood sugar levels. When the adrenals underfunction, blood sugar levels tend to become erratic. As adrenal fatigue worsens, the immune system is compromised, leading to increased susceptibility to allergies, asthma, respiratory infections, and colds.

*Addictions and adrenal fatigue.* Addiction to caffeine, tobacco, alcohol, or recreational drugs (particularly stimulants) is frequently associated with adrenal fatigue, as is the physiological craving for sugar. Continued use of any of these substances tends to worsen the condition. If you have any of these addictions, your risk of adrenal fatigue may be higher than average.

*Your day-to-day life and adrenal fatigue.* A day-to-day life that is chronically stressful and demanding due to perfectionism and self-imposed pressure to achieve may lead to adrenal fatigue.

## Recovery from Adrenal Fatigue

To recover from adrenal fatigue, you have to address it on several different fronts. Certain lifestyle changes, supplementation, and dietary modifications can be helpful. These are outlined below:

**Simplify your life.** Ask yourself which of your habits, practices, and obligations clutter your life rather than enrich it.

**Regularly practice your preferred form of relaxation.** Whether this is progressive muscle relaxation, guided visualization, yoga, or meditation, try to commit to practicing it daily. See chapter 4, Relaxation, for further information on relaxation.

**Give yourself downtime daily.** Remember that downtime is not a luxury; it is necessary for maintaining a vibrant, fulfilling life (see chapter 4). Break up your day with at least two twenty- to thirty-minute periods of relaxation. A full hour of downtime in the evening is even better.

**Strive to get eight hours of sleep at night.** Sufficient sleep is not a luxury, either. Turn in by ten or eleven at night if possible. Whenever you can sleep late in the morning, allow yourself to do so.

**Exercise regularly.** Get twenty to thirty minutes of moderate exercise every day, preferably outdoors (see chapter 5).

**Reduce caffeine and alcohol, and eliminate nicotine and recreational drugs.** Keep coffee to one cup per day, if possible. Keep alcohol consumption to one or two beers, or one six-ounce glass of wine per day. Reduce soda consumption to no more than one bottle or can per day. If you are sensitive to caffeine, substitute herbal teas for caffeinated beverages. Licorice tea is especially good if you're hypoglycemic.

**For two months, eliminate all forms of sugar except xylitol or stevia.** This includes white and brown sugar, honey, chocolate, molasses, pure fructose, refined fructose corn syrup, maple syrup, and dried fruit. Substitute fresh fruits in moderation. Xylitol is a sugar that is made from the fiber of the birch tree. It produces only a small increase in blood sugar and no rise in insulin levels. Stevia is derived from a South American herb and is many times sweeter than sugar. It has no calories and is much safer than artificial sweeteners like aspartame and saccharin. Both xylitol and stevia are available at most health food stores. After two months, you can reintroduce natural sugars such as honey in very small amounts.

**Eat a healthy, balanced diet.** As much as possible, eliminate processed foods and foods to which you're allergic. Emphasize whole grains, fresh vegetables, and fresh fruits in your diet. Eat protein in the form of beans and grains; eggs; organic poultry; free-range, hormone- and antibiotic-free meat; or wild fish. Do not overeat carbohydrates. Reduce your consumption of simple starches: pasta, bread, chips, potatoes, cereal, crackers, rolls, and so on. Combine a healthy fat (such as an olive oil–based salad dressing), protein, and complex carbohydrate source at every meal. Avoid eating just fruit first thing in the morning and avoid processed fruit juices (see chapter 16).

**If you have hypoglycemia, eat the appropriate diet.** Be sure to eat a protein-carbohydrate snack two to three hours after each main meal (see chapter 16).

## Supplements for Adrenal Fatigue

Certain supplements can help relieve adrenal fatigue. Talk to your health professional about taking the supplements and quantities listed below:

- Vitamin C with bioflavonoids: 500 to 1000 mg three times per day with meals

- Zinc picolinate: 30 mg daily

- Vitamin $B_6$: 50 mg twice daily

- Calcium with magnesium (preferably in chelated forms such as citrate or aspartate): 1000 mg calcium to 1000 mg magnesium at bedtime

Some people find licorice, in the form of whole licorice root capsules, to be helpful in treating adrenal fatigue. Do not take licorice, though, if you have high blood pressure or high estrogen levels. Licorice has also been found to be helpful for hypoglycemia.

# Thyroid Imbalances

Your thyroid gland sits above your breastbone and directs metabolic reactions throughout your body. It secretes two hormones, thyroxine and triiodothyronine, which play a role in regulating your body temperature and metabolic rate, among many other things.

The thyroid gland can be out of balance in two ways: either it can become sluggish and not secrete enough hormones, a condition called *hypothyroidism,* or it can become overly active, which, as you might have guessed, is referred to as *hyperthyroidism* (or *thyrotoxicosis*). According to Dr. Ridha Arem, author of *The Thyroid Solution,* approximately 10 to 20 percent of the adult population suffers from some kind of thyroid imbalance.

*Low thyroid function is associated with depression, low energy, weight gain, fatigue, and lethargy.* You may be inclined to feel cold, especially in your hands and feet, and tend to gain weight easily. Other symptoms can include menstrual problems in women, water retention, and poor concentration and memory. *An overly active thyroid, on the other hand, is associated with anxiety, hyperactivity, restlessness, difficulty sleeping, weight loss, increased heart rate, and a tendency toward profuse sweating and elevated body temperatures.*

Hyperthyroidism is a condition that is occasionally mistaken for generalized anxiety. If you're not only anxious but feel "hyper," have recently lost weight despite good or increased appetite, or tend to sweat a lot, it would be a good idea to have your thyroid function evaluated.

If you suspect you might have a thyroid problem, it's best to consult with a physician. Your doctor should do a *complete* thyroid blood panel, preferably one that measures the following four factors:

- *TSH (thyroid stimulating hormone).* A hormone released by your pituitary gland that tells your thyroid gland to make more or less of its hormones. A TSH value of four milli-international units per liter or higher is considered to be indicative of hypothy-roidism. A value below 0.5 milli-international units suggests a hyperthyroid condi-tion. Also high levels of thyroid hormone itself (T3) suggest hyperthyroidism.

- *T4 (free thyroxine).* This is a less active form of thyroid hormone, which you have on hand to convert to the more active thyroid hormone, T3.

- *T3 (free triiodothyronine).* This is the active form of thyroid hormone produced from T4. Low levels of T3 are commonly associated with depression and other symptoms of hypothyroidism. Many doctors may suspect you have a problem even if your T3 level is at the low end of the normal range. High levels are associated with hyperthyroidism.

- *Antithyroglobulin* and *antithyroperoxidase.* These are two factors that measure the number of antibodies you may be making that can attack your thyroid gland and sup-press its function. High levels of these antibodies are indicative of a condition called Hashimoto's thyroiditis, which can lead to either hypo- or hyperthyroid conditions, and needs to be treated medically.

## Treating Thyroid Imbalance

If your thyroid panel indicates abnormal thyroid function, your doctor may choose from among several alternative treatments. If blood test results indicate a *hypothyroid* condition, you will usually be put on a ninety-day trial of thyroid medication, such as Levothroid, Synthroid (levothyroxine), or Cytomel (liothyronine). The correct dose of such medications needs to be adjusted over a period of time. "Natural" thyroid hormone replacement using Armour Thyroid (derived from animal thyroid gland tissue) is sometimes used but is less popular these days due to difficulties with product standardization and numerous adverse drug interactions with birth control pills, blood thinners, insulin, aspirin, steroids, or medications that contain iodine. Some people, however, do fine and prefer natural, bioidentical thyroid hormones.

Beginning thyroid hormone replacement, whether natural or synthetic, is usually accompa-nied by a period of a month or two adjusting the dose upward or downward to determine the precise dose that you need. If you find you're too jittery on the medicine, your doctor will lower the dose to the minimum level you need to relieve symptoms of sluggishness, depression, and weight gain. Or you may try two or three different types of thyroid hormone. Generally, you need to stay on thyroid hormone for a year. At that point, you can try going off and see how you do. About two-thirds of people with hypothyroidism need to keep taking hormone replacement long term.

If thyroid test results indicate *hyperthyroidism,* your doctor will want to perform further tests to rule out problems such as Graves' disease (another type of autoimmune problem). Mild cases of hyperthyroidism may resolve on their own over time. Sometimes beta blockers such as Inderal (propranolol) are given to reduce symptoms of anxiety, rapid heart rate, and sweating. In more severe cases, treatment can involve antithyroid medications, radioactive iodine (which partially destroys the thyroid and thus stops the excessive production of hormones), or surgery to remove part or all of the thyroid. If your thyroid gland has to be removed, you would need to take syn-thetic or natural thyroid hormone indefinitely to avoid developing hypothyroidism.

# Body Toxicity

Excessive body toxicity may not directly increase anxiety, but it adds to the physical stress level of your body and thus makes the impact of anxiety symptoms greater. Body toxicity often aggravates allergies and chemical sensitivities, which in turn can aggravate anxiety. Factors that can cause toxins to build up in your body include consumption of chemicals, additives, and pesticides in food; exposure to environmental pollutants in the air and water; exposure to substances used indoors, such as household cleaners, deodorants, hair sprays, cosmetics, and even carpeting (which may off-gas toxic chemicals); use of either prescription or recreational drugs; and buildup of your own metabolic waste products, which are produced in abundance when you're under stress.

Those who have reached a high level of cumulative toxicity may experience any of the following symptoms frequently:

- Fatigue and low energy

- Joint or muscle pain

- Headaches

- "Brain fog" or mental confusion

- Irritability and moodiness

- Insomnia

- Sensitivity to chemicals in the environment

- Depression

- Heavily coated tongue or abnormal body odor

- Excess mucus (coughing and wheezing)

- Allergies

- Sinus or respiratory problems

The liver and colon are believed to be the organs most affected by toxic buildup. Next to the brain and heart, the liver is probably the most important organ in your body. It is the metabolic "factory" in which hundreds of functions necessary for life take place. Some of the more important ones include:

- Filtration of the blood

- Secretion of bile, which is necessary to digest fats

- Extraction and storage of vitamins (such as vitamins A, D, and E) from nutrients in your bloodstream

- Synthesis of fatty acids from amino acids and sugar

- Oxidation of fat to produce energy

- Storage of sugar in the form of *glycogen,* which can be used when the body is depleted of blood sugar or glucose

- Detoxification of the by-products of digestion (such as ammonia from protein digestion)

- Detoxification of metabolic waste products as well as all chemicals and foreign substances to which you are exposed

Exposure to toxins, some drugs, poor diet, and overeating can cause accumulations of fatty deposits on the liver and interfere with its functioning. Regular consumption of large quantities of alcohol can damage the liver and eventually lead to cirrhosis. Chronic overeating forces the liver to work harder and may weaken it over time, especially if you are eating foods laden with preservatives and additives. Eating a lot of fried or processed foods containing trans fats can also be hard on the liver.

## Detoxifying Your Lifestyle

Some of the most important measures you can take to decrease the level of toxicity in your body and improve everyday diet and lifestyle include these:

**Avoid foods containing preservatives and additives.** Try to eat unprocessed, whole foods as much as possible. Be sure to include plenty of fresh fruits and vegetables, preferably four or five servings a day.

**Reduce or eliminate caffeine, nicotine, sugar, and alcohol.** Aside from other health problems these substances can contribute to, they leave toxic waste products in your body.

**Minimize your use of drugs.** Take only necessary medications prescribed by your physician and avoid recreational drug use.

**Reduce animal proteins (especially red meat) and increase vegetable sources of protein (tofu, tempeh, and beans).** When metabolized, animal proteins can produce toxic by-products, especially if not properly digested.

**Drink purified or filtered water.** Eight 8-ounce glasses a day will assist your kidneys in their natural process of elimination. Your kidneys are critically involved in ridding your body of various toxic waste products.

**Include ample fiber in your diet.** Make sure your diet contains high-fiber foods such as whole-grain cereals, all kinds of bran, most fresh fruits, fresh raw vegetables, nuts and seeds, and legumes such as beans, lentils, or peas. You may also want to take a fiber supplement recommended by your health practitioner.

**Move away from acid-forming, congestive foods toward more alkaline-forming, detoxifying foods.** This means reducing your consumption of red meat, sweets, fried foods, fatty foods, milk, cheese, eggs, refined flour, and salty foods, as well as any foods you know you're allergic to, such as wheat or dairy. See chapter 16, Nutrition, for more information on acid-forming and alkaline-forming foods.

**Increase your consumption of fresh vegetables, fruits, whole grains, beans, nuts, and seeds, and increase the proportion of raw to cooked foods that you eat.** It's good to have some raw, fresh vegetables or fruit at each meal. Be aware that the degree to which you move from acid- to alkaline-forming foods should be tailored to your individual constitution and needs. If you've been highly toxic in your eating habits, make the change *gradually*. You can have one or two days per week in which you take a break from your normal diet of striving to eat more healthy foods.

**Get regular, aerobic exercise.** This helps clear your body of toxins through sweating, and it aids the digestive, renal, and lymphatic systems.

**Discuss the use of antioxidant supplements with your doctor.** These supplements include vitamin C, vitamin E, selenium, zinc, lipoic acid, coenzyme $Q_{10}$, and the amino acids cysteine and methionine.

**Investigate various herbs that can help detoxify your body.** Consult a naturally oriented physician or a qualified nutritionist or herbologist before using any herbs or supplements. Some herbs believed to aid detoxification are milk thistle, dandelion root, burdock, cayenne, ginger, licorice, echinacea, and goldenseal. A high-potency multivitamin and mineral supplement can help combat heavy metal poisoning and help the liver detoxify.

**Support liver detoxification.** Eat foods that protect the liver and improve its function. These include cruciferous vegetables such as cabbage, broccoli, cabbage, kale, bok choy, and brussels sprouts, as well as high-sulfur foods like garlic, onions, eggs, and legumes. Herbs such as dandelion root, burdock, and milk thistle are often used to help detoxify the liver.

# Premenstrual Syndrome

*Premenstrual syndrome* (PMS) involves a constellation of disruptive physical and psychological symptoms that many women experience in the days or week prior to menstruation. PMS can often aggravate a preexisting anxiety or mood disorder. Common physical symptoms of PMS include water retention, breast soreness, bloating, acne, headaches, increased hunger, and a craving for sweets. Psychological symptoms can include depression, irritability, anxiety and tension, mood swings, distractibility and forgetfulness, fatigue, and even a feeling of "going crazy." Up to half of all women experience a premenstrual increase in depression, anxiety, or irritability in addition to some of the above physical symptoms. Panic reactions can also sometimes be a symptom of PMS. The question to ask is whether your panic attacks typically occur—or increase in frequency and intensity—during the days before menstruation. If so, treating your PMS may help reduce or eliminate panic attacks.

Most medical theories relate PMS to an imbalance in the amount of estrogen and progesterone in a woman's body, particularly during the second half of the menstrual cycle. During this fourteen-day period, women with PMS tend to experience elevated estrogen levels, while progesterone is reduced. Insufficient levels of progesterone relative to the amount of estrogen tend to promote water retention, reduced levels of serotonin in the brain, lower endorphin levels, impaired vitamin $B_6$ activity, and alterations in other hormone levels.

Other theories about PMS suggest that menstruation allows the body to throw off excess toxins accumulated through improper diet, as well as from exposure to environmental contaminants and pollutants. Thus the symptoms experienced just prior to menstruation reflect the body's reaction to excess toxicity. The implication is that eating a healthy diet and reducing exposure to other toxins should help lessen PMS symptoms.

Both theories are probably valid. PMS symptoms can definitely be helped by eliminating foods that tend to aggravate them. Symptoms can also be alleviated in many cases with the aid of supplemental vitamins, minerals, and herbs, particularly those that raise the body's level of progesterone. Recommendations for treating PMS follow. Before undertaking any of them, consult a physician, nutritionist, or qualified practitioner of Chinese medicine who is well versed in treating this problem.

## Dietary Help for PMS

Avoid or minimize the following foods:

- Foods high in sugar as well as large amounts of simple carbohydrates (bread, chips, or pasta). It's especially important to avoid the impulse to binge on sweets and carbohydrate foods, including chocolate, for one week before the expected onset of symptoms.

- Salty foods and table salt. This will help reduce bloating and water retention.

- High-fat foods. Reducing calories consumed as fat will help reduce estrogen levels.

- Caffeinated drinks, including coffee, tea, and colas. Caffeine is linked to breast tenderness as well as psychological symptoms such as anxiety, depression, and irritability.

- Alcohol.

Eat plenty of fresh fruits and vegetables, whole-grain breads and cereals, and legumes, nuts, free-range poultry, and wild fish. Consume soy foods, such as tofu or soy milk, in moderation.

## Vitamin and Mineral Supplements for PMS

The following is a list of vitamin and mineral supplements that may help relieve PMS symptoms.

- **Vitamin $B_6$.** The recommended dose is 200 mg daily during the week before menstruation, but you should avoid taking this much vitamin $B_6$ for more than one week out of every month.

- **A high-potency B-complex in conjunction with calcium and magnesium (1000 mg calcium to 1000 mg magnesium).** Supplementing with calcium and magnesium may help reduce menstrual cramps.

- **Zinc.** During the entire month, take 15 to 20 mg per day.

- **Essential fatty acids.** A good source of essential fatty acids can be found in fish oils, which contain both EPA and DHA omega-3 fatty acids. You can take 1000 to 2000 mg per day of combined EPA/DHA in the form of fish oil capsules. An alternative is flax-seed oil, which provides a plant-based form of omega-3 fatty acids; however, the conversion to EPA and DHA is nowhere near as efficient as occurs with fish oils. Borage oil, black currant seed oil, or evening primrose oil are sources of GLA, a special form of omega-6 fatty acid that is essential for humans. You can take 300 to 900 mg of any one of these daily.

## Herbs for PMS

The following herbs are recommended by alternative medicine practitioners to help reduce the physical and psychological symptoms of PMS:

- **Black cohosh.** This is a popular herb used for both PMS and menopause. The recommended dose is usually a 20 or 40 mg tablet or capsule twice per day. It can relieve PMS symptoms such as headaches, mood swings, and insomnia, among others.

- **Dong quai.** This herb can boost energy and stabilize your mood during PMS. It will also help relieve menstrual cramps. It can be taken in capsule form (follow dosage recommendations given on the label), in a tincture, in a liquid extract, or as a tea.

- **Licorice root**, taken three times per day in a powdered root form, as a tea, or as a liquid extract. It will help stabilize hormone levels and blood sugar levels, and can also relieve cramps.

- **Rosemary, cramp bark, and kava** have been known to reduce cramps.

- **Kombucha tea.** This provides energy and stimulates the immune system. It has been reported to be helpful for some women.

## Regular Exercise

A program of regular physical exercise will liven up your metabolism, help your mood, and reduce stress levels. If you can't do vigorous exercise, try walking at least one mile each day. (See chapter 5.)

## Prescription Treatments for PMS

Below is a list of treatments prescribed by doctors to relieve PMS.

**Oral contraceptives.** These may help maintain proper estrogen-to-progesterone balance. Be aware that the effectiveness of oral contraceptives in preventing pregnancy can be reduced by some antibiotics and perhaps by Saint-John's-wort. Oral contraceptives have a number of short- and long-term side effects that you may wish to avoid.

**Diuretics.** These reduce water retention and breast swelling.

**Natural progesterone.** Natural progesterone creams are used effectively by many women to increase levels of progesterone prior to menstruation. These creams are available over the counter, but it's best if you consult with a health professional experienced in the use of these creams before you try one on your own. It's also important to monitor your progesterone levels after using progesterone cream for a month to be sure your progesterone levels aren't elevated and to determine the proper dose and frequency of use of the cream. For further information on PMS and on the use of natural progesterone to treat it, go to womenshealth.gov or webmd.com/women/pms.

**Antidepressants.** Antidepressant medications are sometimes used in treating the mood disturbances associated with PMS.

For additional information on PMS, see the books *Period Repair Manual* or *PMS: Premenstrual Syndrome Self-Help Book* in the "Further Reading" section at the end of the chapter.

# Menopause

Menopause is medically defined as the cessation of menstrual periods for at least six months. On the average, it begins when a woman reaches the age of fifty to fifty-one, though it can start as early as forty or as late as fifty-five. Common symptoms that accompany menopause include:

- Hot flashes

- Headaches

- Mood swings

- Vaginal dryness

- Insomnia

- Bladder or urinary tract infections

- Cold hands and feet

- Forgetfulness and the inability to concentrate

- Reduced libido

- Anxiety and/or depression

The main underlying cause of menopause is reduced production of the two main female hormones, estrogen and progesterone. Interestingly, the undesirable symptoms of menopause appear only in countries where the aging of women is devalued, particularly in the United States and Western Europe. In many traditional cultures, where youthfulness and sex appeal are not worshiped and women receive increasing respect with aging, menopausal symptoms are mostly nonexistent. This is a clear example of the effect of culture on symptomatology, even though the underlying physiological basis of menopause is universal. In the United States, 60 to 85 percent of menopausal women experience hot flashes. Among Mayan Indian women, no one does.

Estrogen replacement therapy, as a treatment for menopause, began back in the 1950s with the administration of synthetic estrogen (such as Premarin) to women. After about twenty years, doctors finally realized that estrogen replacement is associated with up to thirteen times increased risk of developing endometrial cancer. Thus, in the 1970s, it became fashionable to add synthetic progesterone (progestin) to the estrogen, and so the treatment came to be called "hormone replacement therapy." HRT is an effective treatment insofar as it reduces hot flashes and other symptoms of menopause and has the added advantage of reducing women's risk of developing endometrial cancer as well as osteoporosis (loss of bone density that comes with age). After another twenty years, however, it became apparent that HRT significantly increases the risk of breast cancer, especially in women who are already at risk for developing it. Worse yet, a later study (Women's Health Initiative 2002) found that the risk of heart disease and stroke increased with HRT, enough so that investigators halted the study and told all subjects to stop taking Premarin and Provera (brand names of synthetic estrogen and progesterone) immediately. Additional side effects of synthetic estrogen and progesterone can include nausea, breast tenderness, depression, liver disorder, fluid retention, and blood sugar disturbances. Because of all of these problems, some doctors currently do not recommend HRT except for short-term use. As with PMS, menopause symptoms can be helped effectively through a combination of diet, exercise, supplements, and herbs.

You may find any or all of the following to be helpful:

## Bioidentical Hormones

Bioidentical hormones are hormone preparations that have the same chemical formula as those made in the body. Rather than synthesized from animal sources, bioidentical hormones are synthesized from plant chemicals derived from soy and yams. There is a prevalent belief that, because bioidentical hormones are synthesized from plants, they are more natural than synthetic hormones.

These hormones do appear to be helpful to many women for a variety of menopausal symptoms. However, the Mayo Clinic *Health Letter* maintains that there is no consistent evidence that bioidentical hormones are more effective or even safer than traditional hormone therapy for menopause, so consult with your gynecologist before you decide to use them.

Other medications used to help with menopause include low-dose antidepressants, Neurontin, and medications to reduce the risk of osteoporosis.

## Herbs

Many women find *black cohosh* to be an effective herb in reducing symptoms of menopause. Used by American Indians for centuries, black cohosh is effective in reducing hot flashes and other menopausal symptoms such as depression, headaches, and vaginal dryness. If you use black cohosh, it's recommended that you purchase a product standardized to contain at least 1 mg of *triterpenes*, the active ingredient. *Dong quai* (angelica) also can be very helpful in relieving hot flashes and other symptoms of menopause. Licorice and chasteberry are additionally helpful in stabilizing hormone levels, although it's not clear that any herb can actually raise deficient levels of estrogen and progesterone up to normal.

## Supplements

You may find the following supplements to be helpful in alleviating menopause symptoms:

- Vitamin D—400 to 1000 IU per day

- Flaxseed oil

- Calcium and magnesium (1000 mg and 500 mg per day, respectively)

- Red clover

## Diet

Along with the healthy diet recommended in chapter 16, it's good to eat foods that are high in phytoestrogens, which bind to estrogen receptors just like estrogen does in your body. Such foods include soy products, flaxseed oil, apples, whole grains, celery, parsley, and alfalfa. In general, vegetables and plant-based foods tend to be high in phytoestrogens relative to animal-based foods, which may explain why cultures whose diets are predominantly plant-based (including soy) tend to have low incidence of menopausal symptoms.

## Exercise

Regular physical exercise, so helpful in reducing symptoms of anxiety and depression, is also helpful in reducing the severity and frequency of hot flashes.

See the book by Christiane Northrup in "Further Reading" at the end of the chapter for further information on menopause.

# Seasonal Affective Disorder

When the seasons change from spring and summer to fall and winter, do you develop the following symptoms? Check off the symptoms that are familiar.

- Lower energy than usual

- Awakening feeling tired, although you sleep more

- Mood changes such as feeling more anxious, irritable, sad, or depressed

- Diminished productivity or creativity

- Feeling that you have little control over your appetite or weight

- More memory and concentration problems

- Lowered interest in socializing

- Lessened ability to cope with stress

- Less enthusiasm about the future or reduced enjoyment in your life

If you checked off two or more of these, you may be one of the many people affected by *seasonal affective disorder* (SAD) or a milder form of this disorder known as *subsyndromal SAD*. Seasonal affective disorder is a cyclical depression that occurs during the winter months, typically between November and March. It's brought on by insufficient exposure to natural light. As the days get shorter and the angle of the sun changes during the fall, the symptoms of SAD begin to appear. An estimated 20 percent of the American adult population, or 36 million people, are affected by SAD and subsyndromal SAD. The farther from the equator you happen to live, the more susceptible you are.

## Anxiety and SAD

Many individuals dealing with anxiety disorders experience an aggravation of their condition during the late fall and winter. Panic attacks may occur more often, and generalized anxiety may increase along with depression. It's not surprising that this is so, because the same systems of the brain that contribute to the neurobiological basis of depression, the *noradrenergic system* and the *serotonergic system*, are also implicated in anxiety disorders, particularly panic disorder, generalized anxiety disorder, and obsessive-compulsive disorder. Biochemical imbalances in these systems tipped one way may cause depression; tipped the other way, they may aggravate anxiety disorders. For many individuals, unfortunately, problems with anxiety and depression coexist, both becoming aggravated during the winter months.

Whether they manifest as depression or anxiety, the symptoms of SAD are caused by decreased availability of natural light. SAD can be aggravated not only by reduced light outside during the winter months but also by spending too much time in indoor environments that have low levels of light, whether at home or work. SAD symptoms have been reported even in the summer among people who work in environments without windows. They can also occur in sensitive individuals at any time of year after a succession of cloudy days.

It used to be thought that SAD was caused by insufficient suppression of a hormone in the brain called *melatonin*. Melatonin is secreted by the pineal gland in the brain at night after several hours of darkness. It is one of the mechanisms by which your brain lets you know it is time to go to sleep. With light in the morning, melatonin secretion is suppressed, and you know that it's time to wake up. Although popular for many years, the hypothesis that SAD is caused by insufficient melatonin suppression has not been borne out by systematic research. Results of studies have been mixed, and researchers have looked in other directions to find clues to the cause of SAD. The hypothesis that has recently received the most attention is that light insufficiency can cause a reduction in levels of serotonin in the brain. Norman Rosenthal, one of the leading researchers in this field, writes in *Winter Blues* that when susceptible individuals are exposed to too little environmental light—such as during winter—they produce too little serotonin. Rosenthal and others believe that these low levels of serotonin are responsible for the symptoms of SAD.

Issues with serotonin metabolism are frequently associated with symptoms of depression, anxiety, or both; that is why drugs that block the reuptake of serotonin in the brain—drugs such as Prozac (fluoxetine), Zoloft (sertraline), or Paxil (paroxetine)—often alleviate depression and many of the anxiety disorders. But why should reduced light affect serotonin? Why only in certain individuals? The answer to the first question is still being researched. In answer to the second question, there is some evidence that people who are susceptible to SAD may have difficulty receiving or processing light at a neurological level.

During the winter, people with SAD tend to crave sweets and carbohydrates. Eating large amounts of carbohydrates usually increases the amount of *tryptophan* (an essential amino acid derived naturally from protein foods) that gets into the brain. Once in the brain, tryptophan becomes serotonin, the neurotransmitter that is so critical to psychological well-being. Eating sweets and carbohydrates gives tryptophan a competitive edge over the body's other amino acids in getting into the brain. So, if you tend to be drawn to sweets and starches in the wintertime, it may be your body's attempt to raise your levels of serotonin.

## Light Therapy for SAD

The treatment that most effectively reduces the symptoms of SAD is *light therapy*. In principle, it would be possible to reduce SAD in the winter by spending prolonged periods of time outdoors every day. Unless you're a ski instructor or a snowplow operator, however, this is pretty impractical in cold climates. Light therapy involves the use of one or more specific devices indoors to increase your exposure to bright light. Sometimes light-sensitive individuals can experience an improvement simply by increasing normal room light or installing brighter light bulbs. However, most SAD sufferers seem to require exposure to higher light levels—at least four times brighter than normal household and office light.

*Light boxes* are commonly used to alleviate symptoms of SAD. A light box is a set of fluorescent bulbs in a box, with a diffusing plastic screen. Most of these devices deliver between 2,500 and 10,000 lux of light energy—considerably above the usual range of indoor lighting (approximately 200 to 1,000 lux). A typical light therapy session involves sitting within two or three feet of a light box for a period of half an hour to two hours in the morning. It's neither necessary nor advisable to look directly at the light; rather, you can use the time to read, write, eat, sew, or do whatever you need to do. The amount of daily light exposure needed to achieve a reduction in symptoms varies from one person to another. Experiment with varying the duration of exposure according to your own needs.

Light therapy is very effective when administered properly, as Norman Rosenthal documents in his book *Winter Blues*. In experimental trials, it has been shown to help 75 to 80 percent of SAD sufferers within a week if used regularly. Before undertaking light therapy on your own, you should consult with a physician or another health professional who is knowledgeable about this therapy and its application. Although light therapy devices are available without a prescription, you can save yourself time—as well as such possible side effects as headache, eyestrain, irritability, or insomnia—by getting assistance in using them properly.

## Coping with SAD

The National Organization for Seasonal Affective Disorder (NOSAD) offers the following suggestions:

- Discuss your symptoms with your physician. You may be referred to a psychiatrist who may diagnose seasonal affective disorder or subsyndromal SAD and prescribe special light treatments to help relieve your symptoms. Certain SSRI antidepressants also can be helpful in treating some people with seasonal depression.

- If you have a medical diagnosis of SAD or subsyndromal SAD and your doctor prescribes light treatment, do not skip or shorten treatment because you're feeling better; you may relapse. Work with your doctor in adjusting the length of time, time of day, distance, and intensity of light for your own individualized treatment.

- Get as much light as possible and avoid dark environments during daylight hours in winter.

- Reduce mild winter depressive symptoms by exercising daily, preferably outdoors, to take advantage of natural light.

- If you are unable to exercise outdoors in the winter due to extreme cold, exercise inside. If possible, try sitting in sunlight from a south-facing window for short but frequent periods during the day. As an alternative, do indoor exercise in front of a light box.

- Rearrange work spaces at home, and work near a window, or set up bright lights in your work area.

- Stay on a regular sleep/wake schedule. People with SAD report being more alert and less fatigued when they get up and go to sleep at preset hours than when they vary their schedules.

- Be aware of cold outside temperatures and dress to conserve energy and warmth. Many people affected by seasonal changes report sensitivity to extreme temperatures.

- Arrange family outings and social occasions for daytime and early evening in winter. Avoid staying up late, which disrupts your sleep schedule and biological clock.

- Conserve energy by managing time wisely and avoiding or minimizing unnecessary stress.

- Share experiences regarding SAD as a way to get information, understanding, validation, and support.

- If you are able, arrange a vacation during the winter to a warm, sunny climate.

During the winter months you may find it helpful to boost your serotonin levels either naturally or with prescription medication. For the natural approach, try taking 5-hydroxytryptophan (5-HTP). You can start with 50 mg per day and go as high as 300 mg per day (see chapter 16 for more information on tryptophan). If you feel you're not getting help from 5-HTP, you might consult with your doctor about trying a selective serotonin reuptake inhibitor (SSRI) medication such as Zoloft, Celexa, Luvox, Lexapro, or Paxil (see chapter 18 for more information on SSRIs).

# Insomnia

Insomnia affects about 30 percent of adults and is the most common condition that can aggravate anxiety disorders. Anxiety problems of all kinds are generally worse after a poor night's sleep.

Most of us need seven to eight hours of sleep per night, at least six of which are uninterrupted. It is during the early hours of the night that we get the deep sleep needed to replenish our body systems for another day, while during the latter part of the night we get proportionately more REM (rapid eye movement) or dream sleep, which is necessary for the brain to integrate and work through "unfinished business" from the previous day. Sleep actually goes through a series of stages: four stages of progressively deeper sleep, followed by one stage of REM sleep. This five-stage cycle repeats itself three or four times during the night.

If you can't sleep, the problem may be either with *getting* to sleep, in which case it takes you more than twenty minutes to fall asleep, or in *staying* asleep, where you may fall asleep easily but awaken hours before dawn and not be able to get back to sleep. Typically, anxiety is more associated with the first type of problem, while depression is associated with "early morning awakening." However, it's not uncommon to have both types of problems if you're anxious or depressed.

## Ten Common Problems

Why is it that you are unable to sleep? Insomnia is complex and can have a very large variety of causes. In most cases there are, in fact, several causes operating at once. What follows are ten of the more common origins of sleeplessness.

1. *Too much caffeine during the day.* Excessive consumption of coffee, tea, cola beverages, and other foods or medicines containing caffeine is a very common culprit behind insomnia. Everyone, of course, is different. You may be so highly sensitive to caffeine that even one cup of coffee in the morning can keep you awake the following night. At the opposite extreme, you may be able to have coffee at bedtime. As a general rule, it's best to avoid caffeine after noon if you're having problems with sleep, and you may even want to consider cutting down your consumption in the morning. (See the *Caffeine Chart* in chapter 16 to determine how much caffeine you consume in a day.)

2. *Insufficient exercise.* One of the best remedies for insomnia is to do an aerobic workout during the day. Vigorous exercise helps release muscle tension and burn off excess stress hormones (such as adrenaline and thyroxine), both of which can interfere with sleep. It can also release pent-up frustration that can keep your mind racing at night. If you're not working out during the day, you may be surprised to find how much such a workout can help your sleep and help you with your anxiety, as well (see chapter 5). The one precaution is to avoid vigorous exercise within three hours of bedtime, as it can be overstimulating and interfere with getting to sleep.

3. *Excess stimulation in the evening.* Anything that overstimulates you after nine in the evening can keep you from getting to sleep (or staying asleep) later that night. This could include watching a dramatic or violent TV show, surfing the web, doing difficult tasks (including difficult reading), having a stimulating phone conversation, or experiencing a domestic quarrel. You can also keep yourself awake by exposing yourself to bright light (such as a computer screen) late at night. It's best to turn yourself down during the last two or three hours of the day with soothing TV programs, reading, or conversation. Better yet, try a warm bath or shower before bedtime to unwind. Listening to soothing music can help too.

4. *Excess worry about sleep.* Sleep is an automatic process that requires letting go. The more you try to pursue it, the more it tends to get away from you. In general, worrying about sleep will prevent you from falling asleep, whether at bedtime or at four in the morning. Telling yourself to stop worrying probably won't be very helpful, so the best solution is some kind of diversionary tactic. The various relaxation techniques described in chapter 4 can all be helpful toward that end. Progressive muscle relaxation is helpful if your muscles feel tight, while meditation or a guided visualization can be useful for a racing, anxious mind. For some people, just listening to soothing music or the drone of the TV can put them to sleep, while for others a boring novel does the trick. If you find yourself worrying, experiment with different diversionary tactics to redirect your mind away from it.

   A famous, time-honored sleep principle is that if you're lying awake in bed for very long (more than thirty minutes to an hour), don't stay there. Get up and do a relaxation technique, meditation, or light reading in an easy chair or on the couch until you feel genuinely drowsy. Then get back in bed. That way your bed will become associated only with sleep—instead of with wakefulness.

5. *Serotonin and/or melatonin deficiency.* Over time, stress can deplete your brain's stores of the neurotransmitter serotonin and the hormone melatonin. Both are needed for sleep. Serotonin is needed to activate the parts of the brain that are responsible for sleep onset, and it's also needed to make melatonin. Melatonin is made from serotonin by your pineal gland, usually late in the day with the onset of darkness. It's the chemical your brain uses to signal to itself that it's time to sleep. In short, without melatonin, it's hard to get to sleep, and without serotonin, it's hard to make melatonin.

   It's easy to increase your supplies of serotonin or melatonin with natural supplements available at your health food store or drugstore. Tryptophan, in the form of 5-hydroxy-tryptophan (5-HTP; 50 to 150 mg) or L-tryptophan (500 to 1500 mg), is an amino acid that naturally converts to serotonin in your brain. Try 5-HTP first at the suggested dose at bedtime, and if you aren't satisfied with the results, try L-tryptophan, which is available at some health food stores and over the Internet. The effect of tryptophan can be enhanced by taking it with a carbohydrate snack (such as orange juice or crackers) along with 100 mg of vitamin $B_6$. The hormone melatonin is available in health food stores in tablets ranging from 0.5 to 5 mg. Experiment with the dose to determine what is best for you, since people vary a lot in what constitutes an optimal dose. If doses of 2 to 5 mg give you side effects, then lower the dose down to 0.5 or 1 mg. Keep in mind that it's okay to take both tryptophan and melatonin at bedtime to enhance your sleep.

If you find that natural supplements are ineffective in helping you sleep, you may want to consult your doctor about prescription medications that boost serotonin. Any of the selective serotonin reuptake inhibitors (SSRIs, for example Celexa or Zoloft)—medications commonly used to treat anxiety disorders—can also be helpful for insomnia. (See chapter 18 for a more detailed description of SSRIs.) Particularly if you're dealing with protracted depression along with insomnia, you may benefit from trying an SSRI. Generally when you take SSRIs, you need to take them on a daily basis for a period of six months to one year (or longer). If you are looking for a medication that can help you sleep without having the addictive problems associated with prescription sedatives (such as Restoril or Ambien), you may want to try trazodone, 25 to 100 mg, at bedtime.

6. *Hypoglycemia.* A common reason for high levels of cortisol during the night is nocturnal hypoglycemia. When there is a drop in blood glucose levels during the night, you release hormones that regulate glucose levels, such as adrenaline, glucagon, cortisol, and growth hormone. If too much of these hormones is released, it may wake you up. By following the recommendations listed in chapter 16 for hypoglycemia, you may help your sleep. If you wake up in the early morning hours feeling hungry, or feeling that your blood sugar level is down, try having a protein-carbohydrate snack, such as bread and nut butter or cheese and crackers.

7. *Irregular bedtimes.* A very common problem for people who suffer from insomnia is going to bed and getting up at irregular times. The body sleeps better when it has a routine, going to bed and getting up at approximately the same time every day. If you sleep in too late, you may find it hard to get to sleep the following night. That's why many people have difficulty sleeping Sunday night before Monday, having stayed up late on the two weekend nights. The extreme case of sleep disruption is working different shifts back to back. Unless you must, it's best to avoid jobs that require you to continually change your shift. Over time, you can lose a lot of sleep and compromise your health.

   The body has a sleep-wakefulness cycle, called the *circadian* cycle, which it goes through every day—ideally about sixteen to seventeen hours out of bed and seven to eight in bed. This cycle will function much more smoothly, ensuring better sleep, if you retire and get up at the same times every day.

8. *Inadequate sleep environment.* There may be problems with your sleep environment that subtly undermine your sleep without your realizing it. A common problem is a mattress that is either too soft or too firm. If at all possible, invest in a quality mattress that feels truly comfortable to you. The same applies for pillows (you want something more comfortable than what you'd find in the average motel). Room temperature is also an important variable; many people have problems sleeping if the temperature of their room is over 80 degrees. If you don't have air conditioning, use a fan to cool your room. The optimal temperature for sleep is about 70 degrees. Noise and light can also be problems. If you can't escape noise, get a fan or "white noise" machine to help mask it. In the case of excess light, dark curtains or eye shades will often help.

9. *Noisy partners.* One critical part of your sleep environment is your bed partner, if you have one. Loud snoring is a very common disrupter of sleep that affects millions of people who

simply lie there and put up with it. There are many solutions to snoring, including sprays and nose guards that you can get at your local drugstore. On the Internet, you'll find hundreds of devices that can help snoring. Or you may want to go to an otolaryngologist who specializes in the treatment of snoring. For more severe cases, laser surgery or surgical techniques using high-frequency radio waves have been used effectively. Snoring is not something you have to live with. For more information, see the books *Relief from Snoring and Sleep Apnea* by Tess Graham and *No More Sleepless Nights* by Peter Hauri and Shirley Linde.

10. *Sleeping pills.* Sleeping pills include benzodiazepine tranquilizers and sedatives, such as Xanax, Ativan, Klonopin, Valium, Librium, Restoril, and Dalmane, as well as nonbenzodiazepine sedatives, such as Ambien, Lunesta, and Sonata. Millions of people use sleeping pills, and they can be a lifesaver on certain occasions, such as night flights, or when negotiating highly stressful times. The problem comes when they are used on a long-term regular basis. They all have three major problems. One is that they can eventually lose their effectiveness when used nightly. If you take them every night, you'll find that sooner or later they don't work as well. Also, even though they put you to sleep, they may interfere with the quality of your sleep by reducing the amount of time you spend in deeper stages of sleep (or increasing your time in shallower sleep stages). Finally, they are all highly addictive unless used on only an occasional basis. Whether Xanax, Klonopin, Ambien, or Lunesta, if you take a prescription sedative for more than a few weeks, you're likely to become hooked on it. You may find you are unable to sleep without it.

So these are some of the more common problems that can interfere with sleep. Others, beyond the scope of this section, include specific sleep disorders such as sleep apnea and restless leg syndrome, or specific health conditions, such as asthma and allergies, acid reflux, or chronic pain. For an in-depth discussion of sleep, sleep problems, and measures for improving sleep, see the books *No More Sleepless Nights* by Peter Hauri and Shirley Linde or *The Promise of Sleep* by William Dement.

## General Guidelines for a Good Night's Sleep

Sleep is as integral to physical and mental well-being as proper nutrition and regular exercise. The guidelines below are designed to help you maintain a healthy sleep routine.

Do:

- Exercise during the day. Twenty minutes or more of aerobic exercise midday or in the late afternoon before dinner is optimal. At minimum, forty-five minutes of brisk walking daily will suffice. Many people find a short walk (twenty to thirty minutes) before bedtime to be helpful.

- Go to bed and get up at regular times. Even if you're tired in the morning, make an effort to stick to your scheduled wake-up time, and don't vary your nightly bedtime. The next day, you can resume whatever you're working on or doing. Your body prefers a regular cycle of sleep and wakefulness.

- Turn yourself down during the last hour or two of the day. Avoid vigorous physical or mental activity, emotional upsets, and so on.

- Try a hot shower or bath before bedtime.

- Develop a sleep ritual before bedtime. This is some activity you do nightly before turning in.

- Reduce noise. Use earplugs or a noise-masking machine, like a fan, if necessary.

- Block out excess light.

- Keep your room temperature between 65 and 70 degrees. Too warm or cold a room tends to interfere with sleep. Use fans for a hot room if air conditioning is unavailable. Your room should be ventilated, not stuffy.

- Purchase a quality mattress. Try varying the firmness of your mattress. Invest in a new one or insert a board underneath one that sags or is too soft. For a mattress that is too hard, place an egg-crate foam pad between the mattress surface and the mattress cover.

- Pillows should not be too high or too puffy. Feather pillows, which compress, are best.

- Have separate beds if your partner snores, kicks, or tosses and turns. Discuss this with him or her and decide on a mutually acceptable distance.

- See a psychotherapist if necessary. Anxiety and depressive disorders commonly produce insomnia. Talking to a competent psychotherapist can help. Getting more emotional support and expressing your feelings to someone you trust often helps sleep.

## Don't:

- Try to force yourself to sleep. If you're unable to fall asleep after twenty to thirty minutes in bed, leave your bed, engage in some relaxing activity (such as watching TV, sitting in a chair and listening to a relaxation recording or soothing music, meditating, or having a cup of herbal tea), and return to bed only when you're sleepy. The same applies for waking up in the middle of the night and having difficulty going back to sleep.

- Have a heavy meal before bedtime, or go to bed hungry. A small, healthy snack just before bedtime can be helpful.

- Indulge in heavy alcohol consumption before bedtime. For some people, a small glass of wine before bed may help, but your alcohol consumption should not exceed this.

- Consume too much caffeine. Try to limit caffeine intake to the mornings. If you're sensitive to caffeine, avoid it altogether and try decaf coffee or herbal teas.

- Smoke cigarettes. Nicotine is a mild stimulant, and apart from its more publicized health risks, it can interfere with sleep. If you are a smoker, talk to your doctor about the best ways to curtail this habit.

- Engage in nonsleep activities in bed. Unless they are part of your sleep ritual, avoid activities such as working or reading for extended times in bed. This will help to strengthen the association between bed and sleep.

- Nap during the day. Short catnaps (fifteen to twenty minutes) are okay, but long naps of an hour or more may interfere with sleep the following night.

- Let yourself be afraid of insomnia. Work on accepting those nights when you don't sleep so well. You can still function the next day, even if you had only a couple of hours of sleep. The less you fight, resist, or fear sleeplessness, the more it will tend to go away.

## In General:

- With your doctor's or health practitioner's approval, try natural supplements that can foster sleep. Herbs such as kava and valerian, in higher doses, can induce sleep. (See chapter 16 for more detailed information on these herbs.) Do not exceed recommended doses and be sure to discuss all herbs with your doctor before taking them.

- Some people find 0.5 to 3 mg of the hormone melatonin at bedtime to be helpful. Experiment with the dose to determine the amount that works best for you.

- The amino acid tryptophan is very helpful for many people in getting to sleep. You can obtain it at most health food stores either in the form of 5-hydroxytryptophan or in L-tryptophan. If you try 5-HTP, take 50 to 150 mg at bedtime; for tryptophan, try 500 to 1500 mg before going to bed. The effects of either form of tryptophan can be enhanced by taking it with a carbohydrate snack and 100 mg of vitamin $B_6$. You can take tryptophan every night if you need to. Finally, the amino acid GABA, 500 to 1000 mg before bedtime, may induce sleep for some people. Vary the dose, as some people find higher doses to cause agitation.

- For relaxing tense muscles or a racing mind, use deep relaxation techniques. Specifically, progressive muscle relaxation or recorded guided visualization exercises can be helpful (see chapter 4). Use a device that can play the recording in a continuous loop.

- If pain is causing sleeplessness, try an analgesic. In the case of pain, this is more appropriate than a sleeping pill.

- Avoid or minimize sleeping pills such as Restoril, Ambien, or Lunesta except for occasional emergencies. Prescription sedatives such as these can interfere with your sleep cycle and ultimately aggravate insomnia. If you must take a prescription medication for sleep, try trazodone at 25 to 100 mg.

- If you're dependent on a sleeping pill and feel that it's interfering with your sleep, consult a competent physician or psychiatrist experienced with helping people discontinue these medications. There are certain people who take prescription sedatives long term, but this is a method of last resort in severe cases of insomnia.

## Summary of Things to Do

1. If you suspect you are suffering from ongoing fatigue due to sustained stress—or after a very high-stress situation—you may be helped by reducing or eliminating caffeine and sugar from your diet as much as possible, as well as dealing with any food allergies (see chapter 16). Strive to have a higher-protein, lower-carbohydrate diet and reduce or eliminate processed or junk foods. It's important to simplify your life as much as possible in order to reduce stress, and make sure you get adequate sleep and exercise every day.

2. If you believe you have symptoms of either hypothyroidism or hyperthyroidism, have your doctor do a complete thyroid blood panel. Use the medications your doctor recommends and be sure to get adequate exercise.

3. Symptoms such as fatigue, headaches, "brain fog" or confusion, muscle aches and pains, chemical sensitivity, irritability, rashes, and allergies all suggest your body may be overly toxic. Follow all of the dietary and lifestyle recommendations listed in the section "Detoxifying Your Lifestyle." It's particularly important to reduce or eliminate caffeine, nicotine, alcohol and recreational drugs, refined sugar, and junk foods from your diet as much as possible. With your doctor's assistance, use only those prescription medications that you really need. Regular exercise accompanied by sweating is also very important. In consultation with your doctor or health care professional, you may want to try a four- or five-day "detoxification week" on raw foods or a vegan diet; take antioxidant supplements; work with detoxifying herbs such as milk thistle, dandelion, and burdock; and support colon detoxification by using psyllium seed products.

4. To relieve symptoms of PMS, reduce or eliminate sweets and refined carbohydrates from your diet as much as possible. You'll find reducing caffeine, alcohol, and salt also to be helpful. Increase vegetables and fresh fruits in your diet. Also increase your daily exercise. Take the supplements recommended in the section on PMS, including B-complex, $B_6$, vitamin A, calcium-magnesium, and fish oil capsules. Many women find the herb dong quai to be helpful. In consultation with your doctor or health care professional, use natural progesterone creams.

5. If you're dealing with menopause, discuss bioidentical hormones with a doctor or health professional who is knowledgeable about these alternatives to synthetic hormone replacement. Black cohosh is an herb that can be very helpful for menopause; you can use it alone or in combination with other herbs, such as dong quai and licorice. Eat a diet that is high in phytoestrogens and get regular exercise.

6.  For seasonal affective disorder (SAD), follow all of the suggestions listed in this chapter. Be sure to get exposure to the outdoors or to an indoor light box for at least one hour each day during the winter months. If the recommendations listed here are not enough, consider boosting your serotonin levels in the winter. This can be done either naturally, by taking tryptophan or Saint-John's-wort, or by consulting with your doctor about taking an SSRI medication such as Zoloft, Lexapro, Celexa, or Luvox (see chapter 18 for further information on SSRIs).

7.  The causes and cures for insomnia are complex. Review the section on insomnia carefully to determine the possible causes of your problem with sleep. Then try out all of the different suggestions listed in the general guidelines section. If you feel you aren't getting sufficient help, take a look at the books by Peter Hauri and Shirley Linde as well as William Dement below and/or consult a sleep specialist.

# Further Reading

Arem, Ridha. *The Thyroid Solution*. 3rd ed. New York: Ballantine Books, 2017.

Bourne, Edmund J., Arlen Brownstein, and Lorna Garano. *Natural Relief for Anxiety*. Oakland, CA: New Harbinger Publications, 2004.

Briden, Lara, and Jerilynn Prior. *Period Repair Manual: Natural Treatment for Better Hormones and Better Periods*. 2nd ed. Self-published: Amazon Digital Services, 2018.

Dement, William C. *The Promise of Sleep*. New York: Delacorte Press, 2000.

Graham, Tess. *Relief from Snoring and Sleep Apnea*. 2nd ed. Scotts Valley, CA: CreateSpace Independent Publishing, 2014.

Hauri, Peter, and Shirley Linde. *No More Sleepless Nights*. Rev. ed. New York: John Wiley and Sons, 1996.

Hoffstein, Victor, and Shirley Linde. *No More Snoring*. New York: John Wiley & Sons, 1999.

Lark, Susan M. *PMS: Premenstrual Syndrome Self-Help Book*. Berkeley, CA: Celestial Arts, 1989.

Murray, Michael, and Joseph Pizzorno. *Encyclopedia of Natural Medicine*. Rev. 3rd ed. New York: Atria Books, 2012.

Northrup, Christiane. *The Wisdom of Menopause*. Rev. ed. New York: Bantam, 2012.

Rosenthal, Norman. *Winter Blues: Everything You Need to Know to Beat Seasonal Affective Disorder*. 4th ed. New York: Guilford Press, 2012.

Selye, Hans. *The Stress of Life*. Rev. ed. New York: McGraw Hill, 1978.

Women's Health Initiative. 2002. "Risks and Benefits of Estrogen Plus Progestin in Healthy Postmenopausal Women." *Journal of the American Medical Association* 288: 321–33.

# 18

# Medication for Anxiety

The use of medication is a critical issue among those who struggle with anxiety on a daily basis, as well as for professionals treating anxiety disorders. For many people, medication is a positive turning point along the path to recovery. For others, medication can confuse and complicate the recovery process, when freedom from anxiety is purchased at the cost of long-term addiction to tranquilizers. For still other people—those who are either phobic of or philosophically opposed to all types of drugs—medication may not be an option, even when it's needed. One thing is clear: the pros and cons of relying on medication are unique and variable in each individual case.

As you will have gathered, this workbook offers a range of nonmedical strategies to help you overcome anxiety, panic, and phobias. My personal view is that natural methods should always be thoroughly explored before you develop a reliance on prescription drugs. Medications can induce unnatural changes in your body's physiology, with attendant short- and long-term side effects.

Quite a few people find that they can avoid drugs—or eliminate those they have been taking—by implementing a comprehensive personal health program that includes:

- Positive changes in nutrition and the use of appropriate supplements

- A program of daily, vigorous exercise

- A daily practice of deep relaxation or meditation

- Changes in self-talk and basic beliefs encouraging a less driven, more relaxed approach to life

- Human support from family and/or friends

- Simplifying your life and environment to reduce stress

Such approaches may be all you need if your anxiety symptoms are relatively mild to moderate in severity. "Mild to moderate" means that your problem does not significantly interfere with your ability to work or interfere with important personal relationships. Also, the problem does not cause you serious and/or constant distress.

If, on the other hand, you have a more severe problem with anxiety, *appropriate* use of medication may be an important part of your treatment. This is particularly true if you're dealing with panic disorder, agoraphobia, or obsessive-compulsive disorder. It's also true for social phobia and generalized anxiety disorder when these problems interfere with the quality of your life in a major way. Approximately 50 to 60 percent of my clients take medication. My impression is that for them, a *combination* of natural methods and medication provides the most helpful, effective, and compassionate approach to recovery.

Be aware that it's often unnecessary to take medications indefinitely. However, the use of the right medication for the right period of time can help you turn a corner toward improving your condition. This chapter presents some information about the various types of medication used to treat anxiety problems. Beyond this, you'll find a number of guidelines to help you decide whether medication is something you should consider.

## When to Consider Medication

In my experience, there are certain types of individuals, in certain types of situations, for whom medications are appropriate. What follows is a list of these types of situations, along with the types of medication that might appropriately be used.

1. You have panic attacks that are so frequent (for example, one or more per day) and severe that they impede your ability to work and earn a living, your primary personal relationships, and/or your sense of basic security and control over your life. It is particularly important to consider medication if you have *severe* symptoms of panic or anxiety that have not improved over a period of two or three weeks. "Severe" means that you have difficulty functioning and/or are suffering considerable distress. Enduring severe levels of anxiety for long periods of time can, unfortunately, predispose your nervous system to *stay* anxious much longer than it would if the anxiety were reduced by medication early on. Two types of medication are most frequently used to treat panic attacks. The first type is antidepressants. Though they're labeled "antidepressants," such medications also have a potent effect in reducing anxiety. The most commonly used antidepressants are *SSRIs*, or selective serotonin reuptake inhibitors, such as Paxil (paroxetine), Zoloft (sertraline), Luvox (fluvoxamine), Celexa (citalopram), and Lexapro (escitalopram). An additional related class of antidepressants, the *SNRIs* (serotonin-norepinephrine reuptake inhibitors), such as Effexor (venlafaxine), Pristiq (desvenlafaxine), or Cymbalta (duloxetine), are often tried when you have not responded to an initial trial of an SSRI. Yet another class of antidepressant medications sometimes used is the *tricyclics*, such as Tofranil (imipramine) or Pamelor (nortriptyline). These days, however, they are a second choice after SSRIs or SNRIs have been tried.

   The other type of medication used to treat panic (and other anxiety disorders) is the *benzodiazepine tranquilizers*. Among these, Xanax (alprazolam), Klonopin (clonazepam), or Ativan (lorazepam) are typically used. (Descriptions of the major types of drugs used to treat anxiety disorders follow this section.) Many doctors use tranquilizers on a short-term basis because extended use tends to be highly addictive. Withdrawal from extended use of benzodiazepines can be difficult. However, in severe cases these tranquilizers may be prescribed for a period of six months to two years at a high enough dose to significantly reduce the frequency and severity of panic, as well as anxiety about panic.

2. You are agoraphobic and have a difficult time undertaking real-life exposure to phobic situations (see chapter 7). That is, you've tried for some time without medication and not gotten very far. *Low* doses of a benzodiazepine tranquilizer, such as Klonopin (in the range of no more than 0.25 to 0.5 mg/day), may enable you to negotiate the first stages of exposure to your phobias. The benefits of exposure are likely to be retained even after the medication is discontinued, *if the dose has been sufficiently low.* This is less likely, however, for higher doses of tranquilizers (that is, more than 1 mg per day). You need to feel some anxiety while undertaking exposure for the technique to be effective. After exposure hierarchies have been completed with low doses of tranquilizers, it's important to rework them without medication, to ensure a full and permanent recovery from your phobias. The SSRI antidepressants (see the section of the same name later in the chapter) can also be highly effective in helping people undertake exposure. In fact, many psychiatrists consider SSRI medications to be an essential part of the treatment of panic disorder with or without agoraphobia.

3. You're dealing with acute anxiety in response to a crisis situation. You may benefit from relying on a benzodiazepine tranquilizer on a *short-term* basis to get you through a particularly stressful time (such as interviewing for a new job, dealing with a significant health crisis, the death of a close relative, or other such major life event). Alternatively, a sedative (Restoril or Ambien, for example) might be prescribed to help you sleep during such a time.

4. If you have chronic or severe depression accompanying panic disorder, agoraphobia, a specific phobia, generalized anxiety disorder, or any other anxiety disorder, you can often benefit from a prescription antidepressant medication. Milder cases of depression (that is, you do not lose your appetite, your ability to sleep, or your interest in simple pleasures, and/or you do not have suicidal thoughts) may respond to the herb Saint-John's-wort, the supplement S-adenosyl-L-methionine (SAMe), or amino acids such as tryptophan (L-tryptophan itself or the popular supplement 5-HTP), tyrosine, or DL-phenylalanine (see the section "The Use of Natural Supplements" at the end of this chapter). Moderate to severe cases of depression are often best treated with SSRIs, SNRIs, tricyclics, or other types of antidepressant medications. Such medications will help relieve depression, panic, and anxiety at the same time.

5. If you suffer from performance anxiety in public speaking or other performance situations—especially if the anxiety involves heart palpitations—you may be helped by short-term doses of beta-blocking drugs, such as Inderal (propranolol) or Lopressor (metoprolol). A benzodiazepine tranquilizer, such as Xanax or Klonopin, may also be used on occasion (not regularly) to help you negotiate high-performance situations.

6. Difficult cases of social phobia or generalized social anxiety (for example, you avoid a wide range of social situations or you are unable to attend important meetings at work) may be helped by SSRI antidepressant medications or sometimes by SNRI medications. Medications should be taken in conjunction with individual or, preferably, group cognitive behavioral therapy (see chapter 1, the treatment section on social phobia).

7.  Those with obsessive-compulsive disorder often benefit from the use of antidepressant medication, usually in combination with cognitive behavioral therapy, as well as exposure and response prevention. Medications such as Anafranil (clomipramine), Prozac (fluoxetine), Paxil (paroxetine), or Luvox (fluvoxamine) are frequently used in the treatment of this disorder. Between 60 and 70 percent of people with obsessive-compulsive disorder experience an improvement in their symptoms while taking one of these drugs. All of these medications appear to be helpful in treating obsessive-compulsive disorder itself, whether or not it is accompanied by depression. Anafranil, however, does have some potentially undesirable side effects.

For further information on various factors that can affect your decision to rely on medication, see the section "The Choice to Use Medication: What to Consider" later in this chapter.

# Types of Medication Used to Treat Anxiety Disorders

What follows is a description of the major classes of prescription medications used in the treatment of anxiety disorders. Potential advantages and drawbacks of each type of medication are considered.

## SSRI Antidepressant Medications

The SSRI (selective serotonin reuptake inhibitor) antidepressant medications include Prozac (fluoxetine), Zoloft (sertraline), Paxil (paroxetine), Luvox (fluvoxamine), Celexa (citalopram), and Lexapro (escitalopram). In the past twenty years, they have become the first-line medications used by most psychiatrists to treat anxiety disorders. The SSRIs tend to modulate levels of the neurotransmitter serotonin in the brain by preventing the reabsorption of serotonin at synapses (spaces between nerve cells). With more serotonin available at the synapse, the number of serotonin receptors on postsynaptic nerve cells in the brain can decrease (not as many are needed). The reduction in serotonin receptors takes place over the first month or two of taking an SSRI and is technically called *downregulation*.

Downregulation allows the millions of nerve cells in the serotonergic receptor system (particularly those in parts of the brain responsible for anxiety) to become less sensitive to changes in the neurochemical environment of the brain created by stress. That means less dramatic shifts in mood and less vulnerability to anxiety.

The SSRIs tend to be as effective—sometimes more effective—than the older tricyclic antidepressants that have been used to treat panic (for example, imipramine, amitryptilene, desipramine, or nortriptyline). They also have the distinct advantage of causing fewer side effects for most people than the older antidepressants. SSRIs are used most often to treat panic, panic with agoraphobia, generalized anxiety disorder, or obsessive-compulsive disorder. They have also found use with social phobia, particularly generalized social phobia, in which a person is phobic of most types of social situations and encounters. Sometimes they are used to treat post-traumatic stress disorder, especially when PTSD is accompanied by depression. People differ quite a lot in their response to the SSRIs. If you try one and experience no benefit, be willing to try another, or even go through trials of three different SSRIs. To gain full benefit from an SSRI, you may need to take it for *one to two years*. Relapse with SSRI medications appears to be low when the medication is taken for at least eighteen months; however, reliable data on the exact percentage of relapse is dependent on gender, age, ethnicity, and other factors. Typical effective daily doses for SSRIs are Prozac, 20 to 60 mg; Paxil, 20 to 40 mg; Zoloft, 50 to 100 mg; Luvox, 50 to 100 mg; Celexa, 20 to 40 mg; and Lexapro, 10 to 20 mg. Effective doses of these medications for OCD tend to be somewhat higher. However, some OCD clients find that they obtain good results from lower doses.

## Advantages

The SSRIs can be helpful for any of the anxiety disorders or depression. They have been particularly helpful for people with panic disorder, agoraphobia, generalized social anxiety, generalized anxiety disorder, or obsessive-compulsive disorder. SSRIs are easily tolerated and safe for medically ill or elderly persons. They are not addictive. They do not cause problems when taken long term. In most cases, they do not lead to weight gain.

## Drawbacks

Although SSRIs have fewer side effects than the older tricyclic antidepressants, they can cause side effects in some people, including jitteriness, agitation, restlessness, dizziness, drowsiness, headaches, nausea, gastrointestinal distress, and sexual dysfunction. These side effects tend to go away after two weeks, so it's important to try to ride them out during the early phase of treatment. *All of these side effects can be minimized by starting off with a very low dose of the medication and increasing it, over time, to therapeutic levels.* For example, doses might start at 5 mg per day for Prozac or Paxil and 10 mg for Zoloft or Luvox. To achieve such doses, you need to start with a quarter of a tablet per day in most cases, then gradually increase up to a tablet per day over a period of several weeks. If you doctor wants to start you at a high dose, be willing to educate him or her about the importance of gradually titrating the dose of an SSRI from a low dose upward. Be willing to take plenty of time in increasing your dose gradually. (You may notice side effects increase for a day or two after each dose increase.)

The one side effect that can be problematic over time is reduced sexual motivation and/or sexual dysfunction (for example, absent or delayed orgasm). This can be upsetting to many people and, in some cases, can lead them to discontinue the medication. For a certain percentage of people who take SSRIs, normal sexual functioning will resume after two or three months on the medication, so it's a good idea to stay with an SSRI even if at first you experience diminished sex drive. If the problem doesn't get better, it can be mitigated in one of four ways, under the supervision of your doctor: 1) reducing the dose of the SSRI by half on days you choose to be sexually active, 2) augmenting the use of the SSRI with 5 to 10 mg per day of Buspar, 3) supplementing the SSRI with the medications amantadine or cyproheptadine, or 4) trying the supplement DHEA, available at most health food stores, at 25 to 50 mg per day. Many people find that one or two of these interventions can help them restore more normal sexual activity while continuing to take an SSRI.

A third disadvantage is that SSRIs, while often effective, take as long as four to five weeks to produce any significant therapeutic benefit. Sometimes the full therapeutic potential is not achieved until the medication has been taken for twelve weeks or longer. There is some evidence that even further benefits occur over the course of one year. If you're suffering from severe and disabling panic or anxiety, your doctor may recommend you take a tranquilizer (most likely a high-potency benzodiazepine—see below) while waiting for the SSRI to take effect.

In recent times, many people have found the medication Paxil to be especially difficult to discontinue. Approximately 5 to 10 percent of people withdrawing from Paxil may experience severe symptoms such as panic attacks, mood swings, profuse sweating, depersonalization, and "electric shock"-like sensations. Before deciding to use Paxil, be sure to discuss this potential problem with your physician.

A final drawback of SSRIs is their expense. Without insurance, you can pay upward of $200 per month for some SSRIs. The optimal duration for taking an SSRI medication is one to two years. You increase your risk of a return of symptoms if you take the medication for a shorter time period.

**Note:** People with bipolar disorder (manic depression) should take SSRIs only under the supervision of a knowledgeable physician, as SSRIs can aggravate manic states.

## High-Potency Benzodiazepines

The high-potency benzodiazepine tranquilizers (BZs) Xanax (alprazolam), Ativan (lorazepam), and Klonopin (clonazepam) are commonly used to treat anxiety disorders. Older benzodiazepine drugs, such as Valium, Librium, or Tranxene, are occasionally tried when someone is sensitive to the side effects of the newer BZs. The benzodiazepines are often used in conjunction with SSRI antidepressants (or older tricyclic antidepressants) to treat severe cases of panic disorder, generalized social anxiety, generalized anxiety, OCD, and PTSD. Frequently, it's possible to very gradually withdraw from use of the BZ after the antidepressant medication has achieved its full antianxiety benefit (that is, from four to six weeks after starting the drug).

Benzodiazepine drugs generally depress the activity of the entire central nervous system and thus directly and efficiently decrease anxiety. They do so by binding with receptors in the brain that function to tone down or suppress activity in those parts of the brain responsible for anxiety—the amygdala, locus coeruleus, and limbic system, in general. In higher doses, BZ tranquilizers act like sedatives and may promote sleep. Lower doses tend to simply reduce anxiety without sedation. The main difference between various benzodiazepines is each medication's "half-life," or the length of time their chemical metabolites stay in your body. (For example, Xanax has a half-life of eight hours; Klonopin, eighteen to twenty-four hours; and Valium, forty-eight to seventy-two hours.)

Perhaps the most common tranquilizer used to treat anxiety disorders is Xanax (alprazolam). Alprazolam differs from other BZs in that it has an antidepressant effect, as well as the ability to relieve anxiety. It also tends to have a less sedating effect than other tranquilizers. Because Xanax has a short half-life, two or three doses per day are usually prescribed. If you take only one dose per day, you may experience "rebound anxiety"—the tendency to experience heightened levels of anxiety as the medication wears off. BZs with longer half-lives, such as Klonopin or Valium, tend to cause less rebound anxiety and can often be taken in a single dose per day. Research indicates that high doses of Xanax, 2 to 6 mg per day, are necessary to fully suppress panic attacks.

In clinical practice, however, it's common to administer low doses, in the range of 0.25 to 1 mg once or twice per day. An extended release form of Xanax, Xanax XR, has a longer half-life than ordinary Xanax and need not be taken as frequently as ordinary Xanax.

## Advantages

BZs work very quickly, reducing symptoms of anxiety within fifteen to twenty minutes. Unlike antidepressants, which need to be taken regularly, BZs can be taken on an as-needed basis. That is, you can take a small dose of Xanax, Ativan, or Klonopin only when you have to confront a challenging situation, such as an exposure task, going to a job interview, or taking a flight.

The BZs tend to have less bothersome side effects for many people than the antidepressant medications (especially the tricyclic antidepressants). Sometimes they are the only medication that can provide relief when a person is unable to take any of the antidepressant medications. Generic forms of BZs are available, reducing their cost.

## Drawbacks

BZs, unlike antidepressant medications, tend to be addictive. The higher the dose (that is, more than 1 mg per day for high-potency BZs) and the longer you take them (that is, more than two weeks), the more likely you are to become physically dependent. Physical dependency means that if you stop taking the medication abruptly, severe anxiety symptoms are likely to occur. Many people who have taken Xanax (or other BZs) in high doses for a month or low doses for several months report that it's very difficult getting off the medication. (There is some evidence that withdrawal from Klonopin, because of its longer half-life, may be slightly easier and less protracted than withdrawal from Xanax.) *Abrupt* withdrawal from these medications is *dangerous* and may produce panic attacks, severe anxiety, confusion, muscle tension, irritability, insomnia, and even seizures. A more gradual tapering of the dose, stretched out over many weeks or even months, is what makes discontinuation possible. The ease with which people can withdraw from Xanax varies, but as a general rule, it's best to taper off *very* gradually over a period of one to four months, under medical supervision. During this withdrawal period, you may suffer a recurrence of panic attacks or other anxiety symptoms for which the drug was originally prescribed.

If a BZ medication is tapered off too quickly, you can experience *rebound anxiety*. Rebound anxiety is the occurrence of anxiety symptoms *greater* than those you experienced prior to taking the drug in the first place. Rebound may lead to *relapse*, a return of your anxiety disorder at equal or greater severity than what you experienced before taking the medication. To minimize the risk of rebound, it is critical to withdraw from your dose of a BZ very gradually, preferably over several months. (For example, if you have been taking 1.5 mg of Xanax per day for six months, reduce your dose by 0.25 mg every two to three weeks.)

Another drawback of BZs is that they are effective only as long as you take them. When you stop taking them, your anxiety disorder has virtually a 100 percent chance of returning, unless you have learned coping skills (that is, abdominal breathing, relaxation, exercise, stress management, working with self-talk, assertiveness, and so on) and made lifestyle changes that will result in long-term anxiety relief. Taking a BZ only, without doing anything else, amounts to merely suppressing your symptoms without getting at the cause of your difficulty.

A final problem with benzodiazepines is that they tend to have a blunting effect, not only on anxiety but on feelings in general. Many people report that their emotional responses are muted while they are taking these drugs. For example, they may have trouble crying or getting angry, even at times when these reactions are appropriate. To the extent that anxiety is related to suppressed and unresolved feelings, taking these drugs will tend only to alleviate symptoms rather than relieve the cause of the problem. (Some people have a paradoxical reaction to benzodiazepines, during which they actually become *more* emotional or impulsive, although this tends to happen infrequently.) Emotional blunting is somewhat less likely with antidepressant medications, although it may occur.

Long-term use of BZs—that is, more than two years—is sometimes necessary in those cases of severe panic and anxiety that do not respond to any other type of medication. While it enables many people to function, long-term BZ use has several problems. Many long-term BZ users, especially at higher doses, report that they feel depressed and/or less vital and energetic than they would like. It is as though the medication tends to sap them of a certain degree of energy. Often, if they are able to switch to an antidepressant medication to help manage their anxiety, they regain a sense of vitality and enthusiasm for life. Many doctors currently regard the BZs as most appropriate for treating short-term, acute anxiety and stress rather than longer-lasting conditions such as agoraphobia, post-traumatic stress disorder, or obsessive-compulsive disorder. Wherever possible, chronic, long-term anxiety disorders are most appropriately treated with SSRI or SNRI antidepressants. There are, however, certain individuals who seem to need to take a low dose of a BZ over the long term in order to function. They accept the addiction and other side effects in exchange for protection from the anxiety that they have been unable to manage using solely natural techniques or other types of medication. If you are over fifty years old and have been taking a BZ medication for more than two years, you should periodically receive medical checkups, including an evaluation of your liver function.

## Serotonin-Norepinephrine Reuptake Inhibitor (SNRI) Antidepressants

SNRI antidepressants work by blocking the reuptake of two major neurotransmitters, serotonin and norepinephrine. At present, the three most commonly used SNRIs are Cymbalta (duloxetine), Effexor (venlafaxine), and Pristiq (desvenlafaxine). Desvenlafaxine is the mirror-image form of venlafaxine (what the venlafaxzine molecule would look like in a mirror), and is claimed by some to have fewer side effects than venlafaxine, though there is no systematic research on this. The SNRIs are potent medications and may be tried when response to SSRIs is insufficient. They are most commonly used to treat depression, panic disorder, and/or generalized anxiety disorder but may be used to treat other anxiety disorders such as generalized social anxiety disorder or OCD.

The main advantage of SNRIs over the SSRIs is that they can stabilize both the noradrenergic and the serotonergic receptor systems, instead of just the serotonin system alone. So for certain people, SNRIs can have a more potent anxiety-reducing effect than the SSRIs. However, this is far from always being the case, and many studies show roughly equal efficacy between the SSRIs and SNRIs. They have the same disadvantages as the SSRIs, with side effects including dizziness, nausea, weakness, dry mouth, insomnia, and sexual dysfunction. Like the SSRIs, the dose needs to be tapered off gradually when SNRIs are discontinued. Abrupt discontinuation is associated with serious withdrawal symptoms.

## Serotonin Modulator and Stimulator (SMS) Antidepressants

SMS antidepressants are a relatively newer class of medications that, in addition to promoting serotonin reuptake inhibition like SSRIs, also stimulate transmission at one or more serotonin receptor sites.

Viibryd (vilazodone), with a normal dose range of 10 to 40 mg per day, acts both as a serotonin reuptake inhibitor and also facilitates activation of the serotonin receptor 5-HT1A, a mechanism of action it shares with the anxiety-reducing medication Buspar (buspirone) as well as the atypical antipsychotic medication Abilify (aripiprazole).

Viibryd was approved in early 2011 for use in the United States. In September 2011, the FDA raised questions about whether Viibryd showed any advantage over previously and commonly available SSRIs. Some users have reported good results with Viibryd, with respect to both anxiety and depression, while others have reported side effects such as nausea, diarrhea, sleeplessness, and weight gain, leading them to discontinue the drug. Viibryd was marketed as having fewer sexual side effects than other SSRIs, though results so far have shown that this benefit is not invariably reported.

Trintellix (vortioxetine), with a normal dose range of 5 to 20 mg per day, was introduced in the United States in late 2013. It is described as a multimodal antidepressant because it has a differential action on different types of serotonin receptors. Specifically, it has an antagonistic (inhibitory) reaction toward serotonin receptors 5-HT3A and 5-HT7, while it tends to facilitate neurotransmission at 5-HT1A and 5-HT1B receptors. It's also a potent serotonin reuptake inhibitor like typical SSRIs.

Preliminary research indicates that these multiple effects on several different serotonin receptors may result in increased noradrenaline (as in SNRIs) and dopamine (as in mood stabilizers) as well as increased glutamate transmission. So the drug appears to have a variety of effects beyond that of simple serotonin reuptake inhibition.

Trintellix is currently being studied for potentially beneficial cognitive effects, apart from its antidepressant effects, in elderly persons.

Fetzima (levomilnacipran) was approved in the US in 2013 to treat major depression. It also appears to have beneficial effects for anxiety disorders. It is closely related to the drug milnacipran (a medication often used for pain management, especially with fibromyalgia), which is not used in the US. Its primary action is similar to SNRIs, although it also has an ability to block NMDA receptors similar to some anesthetics as well as ketamine, which will be described later in this chapter. An NMDA (N-methyl-D-aspartate) receptor is a type of *glutamate receptor* in the brain. Like serotonin, norepinephrine, and dopamine receptors (sites on nerve cells that bind with chemical neurotransmitters), glutamate receptors are another receptor type that have been found to play an important role in anxiety and mood disorders.

## Tricyclic Antidepressants

Tricyclic antidepressants include Tofranil (imipramine), Pamelor (nortriptyline), Norpramin (desipramine), Anafranil (clomipramine), Elavil (amitriptyline), and Sinequan (doxepin), among others. These medications (especially imipramine) are sometimes used to treat panic attacks, whether such attacks occur by themselves or in conjunction with agoraphobia. Tricyclic antidepressants seem to reduce both the frequency and the intensity of panic reactions for many people. They are also effective in reducing the depression that often accompanies panic disorder and agoraphobia. While it used to be believed that Tofranil was the most effective antidepressant for treating panic, more recent evidence indicates that any of the tricyclic antidepressant medications can be helpful, depending on the individual. Anafranil tends to be specifically helpful in treating OCD, though it is associated with a number of side effects.

The tricyclic antidepressants have been used less since the 1990s than SSRI antidepressants because they tend to have more troublesome side effects. For example, in studies of imipramine, usually about one-third of the subjects drop out because they cannot tolerate side effects (only about 10 percent do in studies using SSRIs). On the other hand, tricyclic antidepressants are sometimes a better choice than SSRIs for certain people because most of them (other than Anafranil) modify a different receptor system in the brain (the noradrenergic system instead of the serotonergic system, though some of the tricylics affect both serotoneregic and noradrenergic systems). As with SSRIs, tricyclic antidepressants are best tolerated by starting with a very low dose (for example, 5 mg per day of imipramine) and gradually working up to a therapeutic dose level (approximately 100 to 200 mg per day).

### Advantages

Tricyclic antidepressants, like the SSRIs, do not lead to physical dependence. They have a beneficial effect on depression as well as on panic and anxiety. They block panic attacks, even if you are not depressed. Because generic forms are available, they are inexpensive.

### Drawbacks

Tricyclic antidepressants (unlike SSRIs) tend to produce anticholinergic side effects, including dry mouth, blurred vision, dizziness or disorientation, and postural hypotension (causing dizziness). Weight gain and sexual dysfunction can also occur. With imipramine, in particular, anxiety may *increase* during the first few days of administration. With clomipramine (effective for OCD), side effects can be particularly bothersome.

Although these side effects tend to diminish after one or two weeks, they persist for 25 to 30 percent of people who take tricyclic antidepressants after the initial adjustment period.

Like the SSRIs, tricyclic antidepressants take about three to four weeks to offer therapeutic benefits. While able to block panic attacks, these medications may not be as effective as SSRIs and benzodiazepine tranquilizers in reducing anticipatory anxiety about the possibility of having a panic attack or having to face a phobic situation.

Finally, about 30 to 50 percent of people will relapse (experience a return of panic or anxiety symptoms) after discontinuing tricyclic antidepressant medications. This is, however, a much lower relapse rate than occurs when benzodiazepines are discontinued.

## MAO Inhibitor Antidepressants

If you have given SSRIs, SNRIs, SMS modulators, and tricyclic antidepressants a fair trial and still have obtained no benefit, your doctor may try the oldest class of antidepressant medications—the

MAO inhibitors (MAOIs). Nardil (phenelzine) is the MAOI most commonly used to treat panic, although Parnate (tranylcypromine) is sometimes used. While MAOIs are potent medications, they are frequently last in line to be tried because they can cause serious or even fatal rises in blood pressure when combined with 1) foods that contain the amino acid tyramine, such as wine, aged cheeses, and certain meats, and 2) certain medications, including some over-the-counter analgesics. If you are taking an MAOI, you should be under strict supervision by your doctor.

### Advantages

MAOIs have a potent panic-blocking effect and are sometimes effective when other types of antidepressants have failed. There is also some research indicating that they are helpful in treating social phobia, especially generalized social phobia (a tendency to be phobic toward a wide range of interpersonal situations). They may also help severe depression that has been unresponsive to other classes of antidepressants.

### Drawbacks

Side effects include weight gain, hypotension (low blood pressure), sexual dysfunction, headache, fatigue, and insomnia. These side effects may be most pronounced during the third and fourth weeks of treatment and then are likely to diminish.

Dietary restrictions are critical. When taking an MAOI, you need to avoid foods containing tyramine, including most cheeses, homemade yogurt, most alcoholic beverages, aged meats and fish, liver, ripe bananas, and certain vegetables. Over-the-counter cold medicines, diet pills, and certain antihistamines also need to be avoided. Prescription amphetamines and SSRI or tricyclic antidepressants should be avoided as well.

## *Other Antidepressants*

Other antidepressant medications occasionally used with anxiety disorders include Remeron (mirtazapine), Wellbutrin (bupropion), and Desyrel (trazodone). Remeron is classified as a noradrenergic and specific serotonergic antidepressant (NaSSA), and, like Effexor, it has a dual action, increasing the levels of both norepinephrine and serotonin at the synapse. Remeron is very sedating at lower doses and may be used to promote sleep. At higher doses, it is an effective antidepressant, and may be used when Effexor is not well tolerated. Psychiatrists sometimes use it in combination with an SSRI, like Paxil or Celexa, to enhance the antianxiety and/or antidepressant effects of the SSRI, a strategy called *augmentation*.

Wellbutrin (bupropion) is often helpful for depression but can be difficult for people with anxiety disorders to tolerate, since its side effects can include anxiety and insomnia. On the positive side, Wellbutrin is one of the small number of antidepressants that does not have sexual side effects.

Trazodone (brand name Desyrel) is an older antidepressant medication that has been around since the early 1980s. While not frequently prescribed for anxiety, it can be a highly effective sedative for many people. It has the advantage of being less addictive (unlike sedatives such as Restoril, Ambien, or Lunesta), and may be more potent for some people than natural sedatives like melatonin and tryptophan. Its side effects are similar to those listed for the tricylic antidepressants.

## Beta Blockers

Although there are several different beta-adrenergic blocking drugs (popularly called *beta blockers*), the three most commonly used with anxiety disorders are Inderal (propranolol), Tenormin (atenolol), and Lopressor (metoprolol). These medications can be helpful for anxiety conditions with marked body symptoms, especially heart palpitations (rapid or irregular heartbeat) and sweating. Beta blockers are quite effective in blocking these peripheral manifestations of anxiety, but are less effective in reducing the internal experience of anxiety mediated by the central nervous system. Inderal or Lopressor may be used in conjunction with a benzodiazepine tranquilizer, such as Xanax, in treating panic disorder when heart palpitations are prominent. By themselves, beta blockers are often given in a single dose (for example, 20 to 40 mg Inderal; 25 to 50 mg metoprolol) to relieve body symptoms of anxiety (rapid heartbeat, shaking, or blushing) prior to a high-performance situation, such as public speaking, a job interview, final examinations, or a musical recital. Beta blockers are also often used to treat mitral valve prolapse, a benign heart arrhythmia that sometimes accompanies panic disorder.

Although these medications are relatively safe, they can, at higher doses, produce side effects, such as the excessive lowering of blood pressure (causing dizziness or light-headedness), fatigue, and drowsiness. In some people, they can also cause mild depression. Unlike tranquilizers, these medications do not tend to be physically addictive. Still, if you've been taking them for a while, it's preferable to taper your dose gradually to avoid rebound elevations of blood pressure. Beta blockers are not recommended for people with asthma or other respiratory illnesses that cause wheezing, or for diabetics.

## Buspar

Buspar (buspirone) has been available for over thirty years. To date, it has been found useful in diminishing generalized anxiety but is less effective in reducing the frequency or intensity of panic attacks. Some research indicates that Buspar can be helpful in treating social phobia or in augmenting the effects of SSRI medications used to treat anxiety disorders. Some practitioners prefer it over Xanax (and other benzodiazepines) for treating generalized anxiety because it is less prone to cause drowsiness and is nonaddictive. There is little risk of your becoming physically dependent on Buspar or requiring a protracted period of time to withdraw from it. Research in recent years, however, has not found Buspar to be any more effective than SSRIs in treating anxiety disorders.

An ordinary starting dose for Buspar is 5 mg two or three times per day. It takes from two to three weeks before the full antianxiety effect of this medication is achieved. Some people with generalized anxiety respond well to Buspar, while others report side effects (lethargy, nausea, dizziness, or paradoxical anxiety).

## Other Medications Used to Treat Anxiety

When antidepressant medications and/or BZ tranquilizers are ineffective or not fully effective in treating panic disorder, psychiatrists may try other medications such as Depakote (valproic acid), Neurontin (gabapentin), Gabitril (tiagabine), or Lyrica (pregabalin). Although such medications are often used to treat seizure disorders or bipolar disorder, they also have an anti-anxiety effect. It's thought that they work by increasing the activity of the neurotransmitter GABA (gamma-aminobutyric acid) in the brain. (Tiagabine is actually a selective GABA reuptake inhibitor.) Certain people, most often those with generalized anxiety disorder, seem to benefit from one or another of these medications, taken either alone or with an SSRI antidepressant. Effective dose ranges for Depakote are 700 to 1500 mg per day; Neurontin, 300 to 1800 mg per day; Gabitril, 4 to 10 mg per day; and Lyrica, 150 to 300 mg per day.

The advantage of these medications is that they work rapidly, are nonaddictive, and are not associated with sexual side effects. Numerous people receive genuine help from these drugs. On the downside, some people report that Neurontin or Gabitril makes them feel tired, lethargic, or occasionally nauseated. Depakote is generally well tolerated but has been associated with liver problems in certain people (so it needs monitoring). If you have not had a good response to antidepressants and want to avoid the addictive problems associated with benzodiazepines, these medications are worth trying.

## Cannabidiol

Cannabidiol (CBD) is a compound that can be derived from the cannabis plant, one of over 104 chemical compounds known as cannabinoids found in the cannabis plant. It is important to distinguish cannabidiol from THC (tetrahydrocannabinol), which is the *psychoactive* ingredient of a particular strain of the cannabis plant associated with the "high" people experience from smoking marijuana. Cannabidiol and marijuana are derived from *different strains* of the same species of cannabis, *Cannabis sativa*. The strain of the plant that produces marijuana has high concentrations of THC, and can be sold as the active ingredient in other products, such as cookies, quite independent of the dried leaves used in marijuana cigarettes (in the popular vernacular called "joints," among other terms).

All of the cannabinoid chemicals, including THC, bind with a set of specific, *cannabinoid receptors* in the brain. While there is over a decade of research on THC and its psychoactive properties, more recent research since 2011 on the nonpsychoactive cannabidiol compounds has shown promising results both for relief of pain as well as help for anxiety and mood disorders.

CBD oil is made by extracting cannabidiol from the cannabis plant, then diluting it with a carrier oil like coconut or hemp seed oil.

CBD has recently been gaining more attention in the medical and health world, with some studies confirming it may help treat a variety of ailments like chronic pain and anxiety. It has also been more widely available without prescription in recent years—considerably more so, in fact, than marijuana or THC-containing products.

### Pain Relief

Certain components of the marijuana plant, including CBD, appear to demonstrate pain-relieving effects. Studies have shown that CBD may help reduce chronic pain and inflammation by increasing endocannabinoid receptor activity.

As mentioned, the brain has its own built-in *cannabinoid receptor system*. This is sometimes referred to as the endocannabinoid system (ECS), and it serves a variety of functions including helping to regulate pain, anxiety, sleep, appetite, and even immune system activities. *Endocannabinoids* are brain-produced neurotransmitters that help bind ingested cannabidiol compounds to specific receptor sites, where they have a pain-reduction and antianxiety action. Many of the cannabidiol-specific receptors are concentrated in parts of the brain that activate both pain and anxiety, such as the amygdala, hippocampus, caudate, and cingulate areas.

Preliminary studies with rodents have demonstrated efficacy for cannabidiols in reducing pain. When rats received CBD injections to reduce pain from surgical incisions, they showed decreased pain sensitivity. Rats with sciatic nerve pain also showed decreased pain sensitivity in response to CBD injections. Human studies have also shown that CBD can be effective in managing pain related to multiple sclerosis and even arthritis.

## Treatment of Anxiety and Depression

Anxiety and mood disorders affect a very wide proportion of the global population. As mentioned in the preface to this book, yearly incidence of anxiety and mood disorders worldwide is at least 18 percent, approaching one in five people.

Historically, anxiety and depression have been treated by a combination of cognitive behavioral therapy and/or psychoactive medications, frequently SSRIs or SNRIs, as described earlier in this chapter. While often helpful, these medications can also cause a number of side effects, including drowsiness, agitation, insomnia, sexual dysfunction, and headache (see the previous section on SSRIs). Apart from SSRIs and SNRIs, it's well known that tranquilizers like benzodiazepines are quickly effective in reducing anxiety with minimal side effects. Their downside is that they can become addictive and may lead to dependency or abuse.

In the past few years, CBD oil has shown increasing popularity as a natural treatment for both depression and anxiety. It has become an increasingly available natural alternative to prescription medication. A few of the author's clients have found benefit from cannabidiol oil in helping to mitigate their anxiety symptoms. Placebo-controlled studies of CBD oil have shown a reduction in anxiety, cognitive impairment, and overall discomfort with repeated use of the oil.

CBD oil has also been used to treat insomnia and anxiety in children with post-traumatic stress disorder. Antidepressant effects of CBD have been demonstrated to date mostly in animal studies. It appears, in addition, that CBD is able to modify serotonin receptor activity in the brain, an effect long recognized in helping reduce depression and mood disorders.

To sum up, CBD oil shows promise in both animal and human studies in alleviating symptoms of anxiety and depression. Individuals will tend to vary as to how much benefit they obtain from use of standardized extracts of CBD oil.

One caveat to keep in mind is that efficacy in treating anxiety and depression has been shown for CBD over the *short term*. Ongoing research is examining the benefits of *long-term* use of CBD.

Finally, keep in mind two important considerations before using cannabidiol. First, as already mentioned, even though CBD is available online, different states in the United States vary in their permissiveness with regard to its use, mostly because of its association with THC, which is much more heavily regulated, particularly in certain states. Second, be aware of the dose you obtain and the recommended frequency of dosing. Also be aware that, like most supplements, different CBD products may vary in their purity (perhaps depending on which carrier oil is used). The amount of CBD displayed on a product's label may vary from the actual amount contained in the product. It's recommended that you speak with a health practitioner who is knowledgeable and well versed in the use of CBD oil and its proper dosing before you begin to use it. The field of CBD use is rapidly evolving, so improvements in the availability, quality, purity, and variety of CBD oil products will change rapidly in the next few years. As mentioned, the author has clients who have reported help with their anxiety issues through the use of CBD oil.

## Recreational and Medical Marijuana

Recreational marijuana has been used for seventy years to seek a "high" many users claim to be satisfying. This high is produced by a psychoactive compound in marijuana called THC (tetrahydrocannabinol). At present, recreational marijuana is legal in ten states when obtained from a registered dispensary. Medical marijuana—that is, marijuana obtained by prescription at a medical marijuana dispensary—is currently legal in thirty states and in Washington, DC. These numbers will have likely changed by the time you read this chapter. There is considerable support among the American population for medical uses of THC- based products as well as recreational marijuana. Recreational marijuana was legalized in Canada in late 2018, though regulations and availability vary by province. In the US, a state-federal conflict exists in that marijuana remains a Schedule I drug according to the FDA, lumped into the same category with opiates. Thus, while recreational use is currently legal in ten states, and medical use by prescription is legal in about thirty states, it is still illegal at the federal level to use marijuana or THC-containing products, leading to conflicts for some people between state and federal regulations. Many recreational users overlook the conflict because possession and use of small amounts of recreational marijuana is currently (as of 2019) very rarely prosecuted, unlike the situation a decade or two ago. The situation with both recreational and medical marijuana is rapidly changing and varies by state; the numbers reported in this chapter will likely be outdated by 2020 or 2021.

### Marijuana and Anxiety

Most important for this chapter's discussion, based on preliminary research and much anecdotal information, use of marijuana or THC-containing products for anxiety has resulted in quite mixed reviews. Some people with anxiety disorders report a temporary calming, relaxing effect. Others report just the opposite. Marijuana increases their anxiety directly, or increases their tendency to react with anxiety to the altered state of consciousness marijuana often produces. Some anxious people have even reported highly distressing "acid trip"–like experiences, leading to panic attacks and an adverse higher level of generalized anxiety that can last for weeks.

Research on marijuana and anxiety has begun, but, based on reports the author has received from clients, cannabidiol (free of THC) seems to be a much safer alternative for anxiety and anxiety disorders than marijuana or THC-containing products. Along with potential adverse effects on anxiety, long-term use of marijuana is associated with a number of side effects. These include development of tolerance (necessitating higher or more frequent doses), reversible cognitive deficits (reasoning deficits that diminish with cessation of use), *amotivational syndrome* (a recurrent reduction in motivation), and, with use of very potent doses (often unidentified in recreational sources), occurrence of hallucinations or brief psychotic reactions. Even if obtained from a dispensary, THC levels in marijuana today *range from 12 to 25 percent*, whereas average

THC levels in marijuana were about 4 percent twenty years ago. Street sources of THC should particularly be avoided, since they may be combined with other substances that are potentially very anxiety provoking or toxic.

To sum up, here are a few important facts regarding marijuana and anxiety:

- Marijuana can provide short-term relief from anxiety symptoms for some people, but for other people, it can cause increased anxiety and even panic attacks.

- For some people, withdrawal from marijuana (just as in the case of alcohol) can result in serious anxiety. If you've used marijuana for a long time and you suddenly stop, you may have a severe anxiety reaction.

- Yet another issue is that people with anxiety who are calmed by marijuana may tend to overindulge in it as a way to self-medicate, ultimately leading to dependence and substance abuse.

- Finally, just as with alcohol, marijuana intoxication and driving do not mix.

## Ketamine Treatment of Depression

Ketamine has been around for a long time, usually administered by IV infusion. It was approved by the FDA in the 1970s for use as a veterinary anesthetic, especially at higher doses. Ketamine has had a variety of uses, including treatment-resistant depression (TRD) and especially suicidality. It is definitely relevant to people struggling with anxiety disorders. A number of studies have found about 50 percent (or in some studies more than 50 percent) of people dealing with anxiety disorders also struggle with depression. In the case of more severe cases of OCD and PTSD, comorbidity with depression approaches 70 to 80 percent.

Ketamine is also available on the illicit drug market as a recreational drug. At higher doses, it produces a feeling of dissociation or depersonalization that certain users view as a "high."

Currently ketamine, administered by intravenous infusion, is being used as an off-label treatment for major depression and treatment-resistant depression (TRD) at over two hundred hospitals and medical clinics in the United States. At the time of this writing, it's in an experimental phase for the treatment of anxiety and anxiety disorders, but is relevant, as mentioned, because many people with anxiety disorders also struggle with depression. Currently, the degree of standardization and quality of care offered at ketamine clinics is variable and not well monitored.

Many practitioners view ketamine as a second-line treatment to be used after a client has had nominal response or excessive side effects in response to standard antidepressant medications such as SSRIs, SNRIs, or SMS modulator drugs such as Trintellix. There are two widely recognized advantages of ketamine. First, it has a more rapid onset of efficacy relative to most antidepressant medications. Improvement in depressive symptoms can appear within twenty-four hours of dosing rather than two to three weeks, as with most traditional antidepressant medications. Second, ketamine is considered superior to ECT (electroconvulsive treatment). While ECT also has a rapid onset of efficacy, it often has significant side effects, especially temporary memory loss of events up to a day or longer prior to ECT administration, for many patients who receive it.

Common SSRI and SNRI antidepressant medications have a long onset of efficacy because they downregulate serotonin and norepinephrine receptors quite gradually in areas of the brain where such receptors are common, such as the limbic system and prefrontal cortex. Ketamine works quite differently. Although its action is not yet fully understood, it appears to act by blocking N-methyl-D-aspartate (NMDA) receptors in the brain, thus increasing access to the neurotransmitter *glutamate.*

In animal studies, it is well known that stress contributes to loss of glutamate release and glutamate reuptake in the prefrontal cortex and hippocampus. Long-term stress, in turn, can lead to *loss of interconnectivity of neurons* in the prefrontal cortex. It has been shown that continuous ketamine dosing tends to *reverse* these effects, leading to neurogenesis and increased connectivity within the prefrontal cortex. More important, it appears one of the many brain biomarkers of major depressive disorder is decreased prefrontal neuron connectivity. Ketamine helps reverse this.

## Recent Use of Ketamine

At the time of this writing, intravenous infusions of ketamine for depression are still considered experimental, and its use for treating major depression is off-label. Its major advantages include its ability to improve outcome in treatment-resistant depression that has not responded to multiple courses of standard antidepressant medication, including SSRIs, SNRIs, and other atypical antidepressants such as Trintellix. Its rapid onset of action is especially important in providing quick relief from debilitating depression symptoms and, *of particular importance, decreasing both suicidal ideation and suicide risk in patients who are overtly suicidal.*

Pharmaceutical companies have recognized the potential of fast-acting antidepressants and are experimenting with different routes of administration, including intranasal, oral, intramuscular, and sublingual. They are also working on ketamine-derivative drugs that might avoid the dissociative side effects of standard ketamine.

Currently, *two main types* of ketamine are used to treat major depression that hasn't responded to two or more SSRI, SNRI, or other antidepressant medications (a syndrome known as "treatment-resistant depression").

1. The IV infusions of ketamine previously described are used in a large number of medical clinics as a fast-acting remedy for treatment-resistant depression. IV ketamine is a mixture of two mirror-image molecules: R-ketamine and S-ketamine. While it was approved decades ago as an anesthetic, the FDA continues to view intravenous treatments for *depression* as an "off-label" use.

2. Esketamine (Spravato), a different form of ketamine, is given as a nasal spray. It contains only the S-ketamine molecule.

People who want to use esketamine nasal spray are required to do so in a doctor's office under medical supervision. The health care provider is mandated to monitor a person using esketamine spray for two hours after each use. This is mainly because of the possibility of side effects such as feelings of dizziness, dissociation, or depersonalization, which can be quite uncomfortable for some people and also can interfere with attention and judgment. Users are not allowed to take the spray home and are advised not to drive for twenty-four hours following administration of the esketamine nasal spray.

In many cases, use of ketamine infusions or esketamine nasal sprays can be quite expensive. Insurance coverage for ketamine is at the present time quite spotty, with differences in coverage depending on the state as well as the duration of treatment.

### Side Effects of Ketamine and Esketamine

There are, to date, a number of *downsides* to ketamine use that have been reported:

- About 60 percent of clients who receive ketamine experience a rapid but often only temporary remission of severe depression. This may be due to insufficient duration of ketamine treatment. Ongoing research utilizing a number of treatments over several months has demonstrated a greater likelihood (though not certainty) of long-term positive response, without the need to continue receiving ketamine doses indefinitely.

- During or following administration, ketamine may cause dissociative responses where the recipient suddenly has a disconcerting "out-of-body" or depersonalization-type experiences. (For people using street-based ketamine recreationally, it appears that these types of depersonalization experiences are actually sought as a type of "high.") One important caution is that use of street-based ketamine as well as the dangerous street drug fentanyl can lead to very serious, if not life-threatening, problems.

- While dissociative experiences can be quite uncomfortable for people, it appears that occurrence of dissociative symptoms is, in fact, positively correlated with good treatment outcome in response to ketamine. Severity of dissociative experiences is also dose dependent.

- At the time of this writing, not all ketamine clinics are equal. Some have practitioners who are not fully trained in ketamine administration. So it is up to the consumer to evaluate quality of any given clinic. Hopefully the FDA will set up at least a voluntary reporting system so that outcome data and reports of adverse reactions will be available to all practitioners who administer ketamine.

- Some animal studies show repeated, long-term administration of ketamine can cause excitotoxicity effects, that is, adverse effects to neurons due to excessive stimulation. Research on effects of repeated ketamine treatments is still ongoing at the present time.

- Infusion or nasal spray doses and frequency seem to vary from one clinic to another, and there does not, at the time of this writing, seem to be a fully standardized model of "best practices" for use of ketamine.

## Conclusion

In recent years, the use of ketamine for treatment of major depression and treatment-resistant depression has become widespread in both the United States and Europe. Ketamine has the upside of rapid onset of action in comparison with most standard antidepressant medications. This is an important benefit for people who are actively suicidal. However, at the time of this writing, ketamine infusions remain largely an experimental treatment for depression. As of 2019, the FDA has approved the use of esketamine nasal sprays under strict medical supervision. As mentioned, the nasal spray of esketamine contains only one of two ketamine molecules, that is, only the S-ketamine, and not both S-ketamine and R-ketamine forms of the molecule, as in the intravenous infusions. People and families who wish to use ketamine for treatment of depression should carefully evaluate the quality of training and experience of practitioners at their ketamine clinic of choice.

# The Choice to Use Medication: What to Consider

The decision to include medication in your effort to recover from anxiety involves many considerations. First and foremost, it's always a decision to be made in consultation with your physician. Your doctor, preferably a psychiatrist, should be knowledgeable and experienced in treating anxiety disorders and should work with you in a collaborative (not authoritarian) way. Second, your decision depends on a number of personal factors, including 1) the severity of your problem with anxiety, 2) your personal outlook and values regarding medication, and 3) your patience, which may be tested in those situations where several medications need to be consecutively tried before the right one for you can be found.

Be wary of pat answers and simple generalizations when you consider undertaking a course of medication or newer substances to treat anxiety and depression, such as cannabidiol or ketamine. The following twelve vignettes illustrate the complex range of situations that might lead a person to decide for or against taking medication.

1. A busy physician has numerous duties at work, at home, and in his community. He takes time to meditate, jog, express feelings, and work with self-talk, but still has debilitating panic attacks. He finds that an SSRI antidepressant helps him sleep better and carry out his round of daily responsibilities with less anxiety.

2. A mother who has been housebound with agoraphobia for a long time has a difficult time beginning exposure therapy. She finds that taking an SSRI medication helps her get started. After one year of exposure, she is confident enough to continue without medication.

3. A secretary who has been taking medication for mixed anxiety and depression for a year discovers she is pregnant. She stops her medication and puts up with intensified symptoms for nine months in order to have a healthy baby.

4.  A man going through a divorce has a heart attack followed by mixed anxiety and depression. Although he has been opposed to taking medication up to this time, he decides to rely on a benzodiazepine medication to help him negotiate this severe crisis.

5.  A woman who has just been promoted to a more demanding job learns her mother has died. She elects to take medication for a period of several months to handle her stressful life circumstances.

6.  A chiropractor who teaches classes in nutrition and is heavily involved in alternative health practices has obsessive-compulsive disorder. He finds that he needs to take an SSRI antidepressant at a higher dose in order to handle his work.

7.  A student who decides to enroll in a certificate program to be an acupuncturist has a strong desire, despite her panic attacks, to embrace only natural methods (such as herbs, nutrition, tai chi, and meditation) to handle her anxiety. She decides to refrain from using prescription medications but is able to obtain some relief from her anxiety through use of cannabidiol (CBD).

8.  A man who has been taking various SSRI antidepressants for panic disorder over five years wants to evaluate how he might do without medication. He discontinues it over a period of two months and does well.

9.  A long-term user of benzodiazepines feels they are causing her to be depressed and decides she would rather have some anxiety and emotional intensity in her life than feel numbed or de-energized by a tranquilizer. She gradually tapers her use of BZs over an extended period of time of six months.

10. A minister with panic disorder is unable to tolerate any antidepressant medication. He finds he is best able to function taking a low dose of a tranquilizer every day over the long term.

11. A woman who feels suicidal after the sudden death of her husband obtains relatively fast relief from her suicidal thoughts and depression by receiving ketamine infusions at a registered ketamine clinic.

12. A recovering alcoholic with two years' sobriety begins taking Xanax to manage his anxiety. Within two months, he starts escalating the dose. Both his doctor and his 12-step program friends advise him to discontinue the medication. In the interest of maintaining a commitment to a substance-free lifestyle, he does so.

Whether you're considering starting prescription medication or trying a nonprescription medicine like cannabidiol, the two most important factors to look at in making a decision for yourself are your own *personal values* and the *severity of your condition*. Each of these is considered below.

## Personal Values

What are your personal values about medication? Are you open to including medication as a part of your recovery program, or do you feel strongly about adhering to natural methods alone? While your symptoms may warrant trying medication and while your doctor might encourage you to do so, the decision is ultimately your own. If you happen to be committed to the ideal of natural healing without the aid of medication, that is a perfectly legitimate option. At the opposite extreme, there are people who lack sufficient interest or motivation to put in the time and effort involved in practicing relaxation, exercise, exposure, and cognitive skills on a daily basis. They seek immediate relief of symptoms through taking a drug. In many cases, this is also a viable choice. It is not for anyone to judge a person's decision to seek relief from anxiety disorders through medication. Medications certainly do provide a great deal of relief for many people.

In making a choice about whether to rely on prescription medication, it's important to have all the information that you need to make the most informed and enlightened decision possible. Such a decision should not be based solely on impulse—for example, a desire to take a high dose of medication to eliminate all symptoms of anxiety as soon as possible. Nor should it be based upon fear or avoidance of medication because you have a phobia of it. The purpose of this chapter is to give you as much information as possible so that you can make the optimal decision for yourself.

## Severity of Your Condition

Apart from your personal values, the next thing to look at in considering medication is the severity of your symptoms. As a general rule, the more severe your problem, the more likely you will benefit from a trial of medication. Severity can be defined in two ways: your ability to function and your level of distress. Use the following questions to evaluate the severity of your own condition.

- Does your problem with anxiety significantly interfere with your ability to function in your everyday life? Are you having a hard time working, or are you unable to work at all? Is your ability to raise your children or be responsive to your spouse impaired by your anxiety? Do you have a hard time organizing your thoughts to complete basic tasks, such as cooking or paying bills?

- Does your problem with anxiety cause you considerable distress, to the point that you have two or more hours every day during which you feel *very uncomfortable*? Is it hard for you just to make it through each day? Do you wake up each morning in a state of dread? If your answer to *any* of these questions is yes, you may want to consider medication.

- Are you dealing with significant depression? Significant depression accompanies anxiety disorders in up to about 50 percent of cases. The highest association is with generalized anxiety disorder (GAD) and obsessive-compulsive disorder (OCD), while the lowest association is with specific phobias. There is also a syndrome—"mixed anxiety and depression"—that has received attention in recent years. Symptoms of depression include lack of energy, continuous low mood or apathy, loss of appetite, disturbed sleep, frequent self-criticism, difficulty concentrating, and possibly suicidal thoughts. If you are depressed, antidepressant medication can be especially helpful because it tends to restore the motivation and energy you need to practice the skills promoted in this bòok (such as abdominal breathing, exercise, exposure, and cognitive behavioral therapy). If you are having suicidal thoughts, you and your doctor may want to consider ketamine infusions or treatments with esketamine nasal spray to achieve more rapid remission of both your depression and your suicidal thoughts.

### Chronicity of Your Anxiety Disorder

In addition to severity of symptoms, *chronicity*—how long you've had your problem—is another important factor to consider. If your anxiety is of recent origin and a response to stressful circumstances, it may pass when you learn stress management techniques and work through whatever problem instigated the stress. On the other hand, if you've been suffering for more than a year—and especially if you've tried cognitive behavioral therapy and have not yet received the benefit you wanted—a trial of medication may be helpful. *To conclude, the more severe and/or the more chronic (long-standing) your condition, the more likely you may be to respond favorably to medication.*

## *Genotypic Testing*

Antidepressant medications such as SSRIs, SNRIs, and other more recent types such as SMS (serotonin modulator and stimulator) medications have been used as first-line drugs to treat both anxiety disorders and mood disorders such as major depression. For some fortunate individuals, the first antidepressant tried relieves symptoms and has minimal side effects, even if it takes three or four weeks to show efficacy. For many people, however, the first antidepressant medication tried is either ineffective or causes undesirable side effects.

Finding the right medication may involve several trials (each lasting at least three weeks) of different antidepressants until a person finds a medicine that *both* helps and has tolerable side effects (significant side effects often subside after about two weeks into a trial). This process of trial and error with different medications can take two or more months, and requires considerable persistence and patience on the part of both the treating health care provider as well as the client seeking help. In some cases, if you have tried several medications to no avail, and particularly if you have suicidal thoughts, you may want to consider ketamine infusions or receive esketamine nasal spray treatments at an approved medical facility. Typically, you may experience a remission from your symptoms within twenty-four hours.

*Genotypic testing* can speed up identification of medications that are more likely to be suitable for your particular brain and body. This type of testing is indicated *after* you have had two or three trials on various antidepressant medications without much success. The testing has not been clinically perfected, and thus is considered a second-line approach to treating anxiety and mood disorders.

Genotypic testing is currently used outside the field of psychiatry in other fields of medicine, to show whether certain medicines (such as, for example, tamoxifen) can be effective in treating breast cancer.

The crux of genotypic testing is to establish whether your body has appropriate enzymes for metabolizing various types of drugs. Your body has different enzymes, made in your liver, called P450 (or CYP450) enzymes, to process different types of medications. Because inherited traits, established by specific genes, can lead to variations in these enzymes, antidepressant medications can affect you differently according to whether you have the right enzyme(s) for metabolizing the drug.

Genotypic testing has enabled doctors to identify one particular CYP450 enzyme with a significant variation in a majority of humans, which has been designated CYP2D6. To date, it appears that having this enzyme enables you to better process several different types of SSRI or SNRI antidepressants, including Prozac, Paxil, Luvox (fluvoxamine), Effexor, and Cymbalta, among others. It also predicts potentially good response to some of the older tricyclic antidepressants such as Pamelor, Elavil, Tofranil, Sinequan, and Anafranil.

A separate gene test can help identify the presence of a different enzyme, CYP2C19, which enables your body to metabolize a different set of antidepressants, such as Celexa, Pristiq, Lexapro, and Zoloft. Other nonantidepressant psychotropic medications metabolized by the CYP2C19 enzyme include the atypical antipsychotic medications Abilify and Zyprexa.

Note that both the CYP2D6 and the CYP2C19 enzymes metabolize a number of other medications outside the realm of psychiatric application.

There are other genotypic tests for a variety of other drug-metabolizing enzymes, including CYP2C9, CYP3A4, and CYP3A5. So you may need to have more than one genotypic test done to provide sufficient evidence for making an informed choice of the "right" antidepressant medication for you. These tests can also be used to predict metabolism of a variety of nonpsychiatric medications.

Any given genotypic test you receive will classify you into one of four categories: 1) *normal metabolizer*, meaning you have the necessary enzyme(s) for metabolizing the drugs associated with that test normally, with relatively few side effects; 2) *intermediate metabolizer*, meaning you may not be able to process the medications associated with the test as well as normal metabolizers do, so you have an increased risk of initial side effects and need closer observation and management if you take one of the drugs; and 3) *poor metabolizer*, meaning you have insufficient amounts of the enzyme associated with the test to process test-specific medications, with the downside that the medication can build up in your system and likely cause more lasting side effects. In this situation, it may still, in some cases, be possible to take the medication at a lower dose and taper up to therapeutic dose very gradually; 4) *ultrarapid metabolizer* (the enzymes associated with this test metabolize their associated drugs too quickly, causing the drug to leave your body before it has a chance to work properly).

To sum up, genotypic testing may be useful to do *after* you've been through a process of trial and error with *at least two or three different antidepressant medications* without positive outcome, either because 1) the medications aren't fully effective after a monthlong trial with each one, or 2) the side effects are unacceptable to you and don't subside after the first week or two on the drug. In the days before genotypic testing, some psychiatrists persisted in trying four or five different antidepressant medications and ultimately succeeded in finding one with a good fit for a client. So, in principle, genomic testing *is an option rather than a necessity.* It offers an attempt to speed up medication selection over the lengthy process of trying out up to half a dozen different antidepressant medications, including not only SSRIs and SNRIs but also SMS (serotonin modulator and stimulator) medications such as Trintellix, as well as older tricyclic antidepressants such as Tofranil, Pamelor, Elavil, and others.

## Current Limitations of Genotypic Tests

Genotypic testing is still in the early stages of development. Some of its limitations include the following:

- One genotypic test may be insufficient to determine the optimal medication for you. It is often necessary to have two or more different tests to find a medication that best fits your particular brain and body. Such tests can often be quite expensive.

- Genotypic tests are not yet available for the complete array of all antidepressant medications. The tests may be worth trying after you have failed trials on at least two or three different medications. But if genotypic testing itself fails to establish an "optimal" medication for you, don't give up. You and your doctor may want to continue trying out additional drugs by trial and error to see if there is one that could be effective. For example, for certain individuals with social anxiety disorder, the first generation MAO inhibitor antidepressants, such as Nardil and Parnate, can be effective when all other antidepressant medications have failed. With these medications, however, you have issues of potential weight gain as well as a critical list of dietary restrictions.

- Tests only focus on how your body metabolizes different medications; they provide no information on how the drug physiologically affects the brain or might affect brain receptors to improve symptoms.

- The cost of testing can vary depending on which test is ordered, the number of tests ordered, and the coverage offered by your health insurance carrier. Call your health provider insurance company in advance to evaluate their coverage for any genotyping tests you wish to receive.

## Conclusion

The material in this section has been based primarily on research and clinical testing procedures available at the Mayo Clinic (Rochester, Minnesota) and its satellite campuses in Jacksonville, Florida, and Phoenix, Arizona. Many other clinics offer genotypic testing. Perhaps the best known and best researched test outside of Mayo Clinic's work is the GeneSight Psychotropic test, available through Assurex Health. GeneSight offers a number of different genomic tests that evaluate the same CP450 enzymes as the Mayo Clinic, plus several other groups of enzymes that may be less relevant to psychiatric conditions. The company's genotypic tests classify a list of thirty-eight psychiatric drugs into three categories: 1) green bin (use the drug as directed), 2) yellow bin (use the drug with caution and monitoring), or 3) red bin (avoid the drug unless you take a low dose and have extensive monitoring).

**Note:** The field of genotypic testing to predict antidepressant medication response is currently highly competitive and consists of various proprietary companies and facilities that offer the tests. So, unlike a majority of self-help approaches, genotypic testing has been recommended by mentioning only two of the better-known providers of the tests.

Finally, a few caveats should be offered for genotypic testing in general. The testing is still considered an experimental procedure pending full approval by the FDA. The FDA, in fact, points out that some associations between enzyme types and a proclivity for certain antidepressant medications have not been proven by rigorous research but based only on observational evidence. People should be aware that the testing can be costly and that they only provide *one avenue* for improving treatment of anxiety and mood disorders. While having genotypic testing done *may* help you better select an appropriate antidepressant medication, that is *all* that it can offer. Testing does not address the multiplicity of other factors that affect anxiety and mood disorders. So readers need to be aware that genotypic testing is a relatively new technology that may have *some* benefit for *some* people who have failed multiple trials of antidepressant medications.

# How Long to Continue Medication

For anyone who is considering trying or is presently taking a prescription medication, how long to take it is a very important issue. Unfortunately, there is no simple answer. The length of time you need to take medication depends on at least three different factors:

- *What type of medication* (for example, tranquilizer or antidepressant)

- *What type of anxiety disorder* (for example, panic, social phobia, or obsessive-compulsive disorder)

- *Your motivation and commitment to utilize natural approaches* (as a committed program of nonmedication approaches may help you stop relying on medication or else reduce your dose)

## What Type of Medication

Some types of medication, such as tranquilizers or beta blockers, are often used on an as-needed basis only. That is, you only use the medication when dealing with an acute, anxiety-provoking situation, such as confronting a phobia or giving a presentation. Tranquilizers can also be used over a period of a few weeks to help you get through a particularly difficult situation, such as the death of a loved one or taking the bar exam. For a period of one to two years, tranquilizers may be useful if you are unable to take any type of antidepressant medication for anxiety. Long-term use of tranquilizers (more than a year), while having certain problems, may even be justified in some cases (see the previous section on benzodiazepine tranquilizers).

Antidepressant medications are usually taken on a daily basis for a minimum of six months to one year. In my experience, they are *most effective in treating anxiety disorders when taken for a period of one to two years*. Risk of relapse once you discontinue the antidepressants is lower if you've taken them for this length of time and then taper off of them gradually. For some people, long-term use of antidepressant medication (that is, more than two years), at a *maintenance dose* level (usually at the lowest end of the therapeutic dose range), offers an optimal quality of life.

## What Type of Anxiety Disorder

If you have a fairly mild case of agoraphobia, or a specific phobia, you may need to take a low dose of a tranquilizer—such as 0.25 to 0.5 mg of Ativan (lorazepam)—only up to and during the early stages of exposure to your phobic situation. Then, during later stages, you may wean yourself off the medication and work through your exposure hierarchies on your own. Being able to do so without the use of any tranquilizer will enhance your mastery over your phobia. On the other hand, if you are having frequent panic attacks and are practically (or completely) housebound, you may benefit from taking medication for a longer time. For SSRI antidepressant medications, the one- to two-year period mentioned above is optimal. Long-term maintenance on a low dose of antidepressant medication may be necessary in some cases.

For social phobia, you may take an antidepressant (SSRI or SNRI antidepressant) or, if you don't respond to antidepressants, a benzodiazepine, especially if you suffer from generalized social phobia (anxiety in a wide variety of social situations). One to two years on the medication will likely optimize your treatment. Long-term maintenance at a low dose, as with agoraphobia, may be necessary in some cases.

With obsessive-compulsive disorder, long-term use of an SSRI medication at a higher dose is often the best strategy. After two years, you can try lowering the dose to see what is the minimum dose you need to correct the neurobiological problems associated with OCD. On the other hand, some people with OCD are able to manage their problem with cognitive therapy and exposure and response prevention (ERP) alone—sometimes from the outset and sometimes after a year or two on medication. (See the book *Brain Lock* by Jeffrey Schwartz, listed at the end of this chapter.)

Generalized anxiety disorder will require medication only in moderate to severe cases, especially if accompanied by significant depression, or in situations where you are unmotivated or unwilling to make the behavioral and lifestyle modifications that can help.

Finally, post-traumatic stress disorder may frequently be helped by antidepressant medication in conjunction with cognitive behavioral therapy; severe cases may need a long-term maintenance dose.

## Your Motivation and Commitment to Utilize Natural Approaches

In many cases, it's possible to eliminate or at least reduce your need for medication over the long term, if you maintain a committed program of natural approaches. *The brain has an inherent ability to heal from the stress-induced imbalances that may have led to your original need for medication.* While it may take your brain somewhat longer to recover than would be the case for a broken bone or a torn ligament, the brain can regain, with proper cognitive, behavioral, and lifestyle modifications, much or all of its natural integrity over time. Your very belief that you can recover from anxiety and eventually wean yourself off medication will help make it more likely that you do. The popular idea of "mind over matter" is not an idle notion. Any of the approaches suggested in this book will help you heal yourself naturally. The more of these approaches you are able to implement on a regular basis, the sooner and more powerfully you will be able to foster a state of natural health in body and mind.

# Discontinuing Medication

If you've decided that you want to stop relying on prescription medications, observe the following guidelines:

1. *Be sure you've gained some level of mastery of the basic strategies for overcoming anxiety and panic presented in this book.* In particular, it would be a good idea to have established a daily practice of deep relaxation and exercise, along with skills countering fearful self-talk, to overcome anxiety symptoms. If you plan to withdraw from Xanax or a BZ tranquilizer, these skills will serve you well in dealing with possible recurrences of anxiety during the often extended withdrawal period, as well as over the long run. Be assured that any resurgence of high anxiety during withdrawal from a tranquilizer is temporary and should not persist if you proceed through your withdrawal in a sufficiently *gradual* manner.

2. *Consult with your doctor to set up a program for gradually tapering off the dosage of your medication.* This is especially important if you've been taking a BZ tranquilizer (the tapering-off period is dose-dependent but may need to be as long as six months, a year, or, in some cases, even longer). A tapering-off period (usually a month or two) also needs to be observed if you're curtailing your use of an antidepressant medication like Paxil or a beta blocker such as Inderal. Generally, the longer you've taken a medication, the longer and more gradual the tapering period should be.

3. *For many people, benzodiazepine tapering can be difficult.* The nervous system adapts to these drugs, and it may take you quite some time to readapt to living without them, especially if you have taken them for more than a month or two. Often psychiatrists prescribe an SSRI antidepressant, or other nonaddictive antianxiety medication such as Neurontin, during and after the BZ tapering-off process in order to ease withdrawal symptoms. For people unable to tolerate these prescription medications, sometimes high doses of the amino acids tryptophan, theanine, GABA, taurine, and glycine—administered either intravenously or orally—can be helpful both during and for some time after the tapering-off period.

   There are two approaches to withdrawing from the benzodiazepines. One is to reduce the dose *very slowly* over a period of several to many months—preferably with the aid of a nonaddictive antianxiety medication, as previously described. Alternatively, drug rehabilitation programs do a more rapid tapering off over a period of two to three weeks and use an alternative (long half-life) benzodiazepine, such as Valium, or else phenobarbital, in lieu of the high-potency benzodiazepine (such as Xanax or Klonopin) that is being withdrawn. After withdrawal from the secondary drug, an antidepressant or other nonaddictive antianxiety medication may be used to assist adjustment for several months after the tapering off is finished. For more detailed information on benzodiazepine tapering, see the resources by C. Heather Ashton listed at the end of this chapter.

4.  *Be prepared to increase your reliance on the strategies described in this workbook during your tapering-off period.* Especially important are abdominal breathing, relaxation, exercise, coping strategies for anxiety, and countering negative self-talk. Your withdrawal from medication is an opportunity to practice and improve your skills at using these strategies. You'll gain increased self-confidence by learning to use self-activated strategies to master anxiety and panic without having to rely on medication.

5.  *Don't be disappointed if you need to rely on medication during future periods of acute anxiety or stress.* Stopping regular use of a medication doesn't necessarily mean that you might not benefit from the *short-term* use of that medication in the future. For example, using a tranquilizer or sleep medication for two weeks during a time of acute stress due to a traumatic experience is appropriate and unlikely to lead to dependence. If you're subject to seasonal affective disorder, you may stand to benefit from taking an antidepressant medication during the winter months. Don't consider it a sign of weakness or a lack of self-control if you occasionally need to rely on prescription medications for a limited period of time. Given the stress and pressures of modern life, there are quite a few people who occasionally use prescription medications to help them cope.

## Working with Your Doctor

The purpose of this chapter has been to provide a balanced view of the role of medications in treating anxiety. There are certainly a variety of situations where the benefits of prescription drugs outweigh their associated risks and drawbacks. It's important, however, that before taking *any* medication you become fully aware of all of its potential side effects and limitations. It is your doctor's responsibility to 1) obtain a complete history of your symptoms, 2) inform you of the possible side effects and limitations of any particular drug, and 3) obtain your *informed consent* to try out a medication. It's your responsibility not to withhold information your doctor requests in taking your medical history, as well as to let him or her know, should he or she fail to ask, whether 1) you have any allergic reactions to any drugs, 2) you are pregnant, 3) you are taking any other prescription or over-the-counter medications, or 4) you are taking any natural supplements.

Once this exchange of information has taken place between you and your physician, both of you will be in a position to make a *fully informed and mutual decision* about whether taking a particular prescription medication is in your best interest. If your doctor is unwilling to take a collaborative rather than authoritarian stance, or to allow for your informed consent, seek out another doctor who will. Medications may enable you to turn the corner in recovering from your particular problem, but it is essential that they be used with the utmost care and responsibility.

**Note:** The Internet offers websites that distribute various antianxiety medications, especially tranquilizers, without a prescription. It's best to avoid these sites, as they may take your money without sending you anything, send you the wrong medication, or send you an inferior or toxic version of the medication you ordered. It is worth your time and money to consult with an experienced physician or psychiatrist when you are in need of medication, and to utilize reputable pharmacies that require a prescription.

# In Conclusion

*Appropriate* use of medication does not conflict with holistic values or a natural lifestyle. There is a time and place for the use of medication in treating anxiety disorders, and not to use them at those times is equivalent to not taking good care of yourself. The real question to ask is this: *What is the most compassionate thing you can do for yourself?* In some cases, the answer may be to wean yourself off medication—especially if you have become overly dependent on or addicted to a drug for several years without having evaluated how you might fare without it. In some cases, the answer may be to use medication for a period of several months (up to a year) to get through a difficult time or to jump-start your motivation to utilize cognitive behavioral and other natural approaches. In other cases, long-term maintenance use of medication (particularly the SSRIs), *in conjunction with the full spectrum of cognitive behavioral therapy, natural, and lifestyle changes suggested in this book*, may be the most compassionate response you can have for yourself.

There are few set answers when it comes to the subject of medication. Getting all the information you can, working with a competent physician (preferably a psychiatrist) skilled with treating anxiety disorders whom you can trust, and then listening to your own intuition is the best you can do.

# The Use of Natural Supplements

Since this chapter is about prescription medications, it doesn't include detailed information on natural substances that can be useful in the treatment of anxiety problems. Full descriptions of all of the natural supplements used to treat anxiety and depression may be found in the section "Supplements for Anxiety" in chapter 16.

There are two classes of such substances. *Natural tranquilizers* include herbs such as kava, valerian, passionflower, and chamomile, as well as amino acids such as theanine and GABA. *Natural antidepressants*, which can have an anxiety-reducing effect as well, include the herb Saint-John's-wort, S-adenosyl-L-methionine (abbreviated as SAMe), and the amino acids tryptophan and tyrosine. You may find any of these supplements at your local health food store or online. Any one or a combination of them may be quite helpful as an alternative to prescription drugs in treating your problem with anxiety and/or depression. The key consideration in deciding to try natural supplements is whether you consider your anxiety problem to be in the *mild to moderate* range of severity. *If anxiety is more of a nuisance—a discomfort or an inconvenience in your life*—and not a debilitating or highly distressing condition, you might want to consider natural supplements first before consulting with a psychiatrist about prescription drugs. If you are already taking an SSRI antidepressant or BZ tranquilizer, do not try natural supplements without first consulting with a doctor well versed in combining prescription medications with supplements.

A more extensive discussion of natural supplements for anxiety and depression can be found at the end of chapter 16, Nutrition.

## Summary of Things to Do

1. Review this chapter to provide yourself with an overview of the various types of medications used to treat anxiety disorders. Be familiar with the benefits and limitations of those medications that may have relevance for your particular issue.

   If you are not currently taking medication but wonder whether you could benefit from doing so, contact a psychiatrist who is experienced in treating anxiety disorders to discuss your options. The Anxiety and Depression Association of America offers a "Find a Therapist" link on their website, adaa.org, that may assist you in finding a specialist in your local area (see appendix 1).

   If you are currently taking a medication and would like to stop, consult your prescribing physician to discuss the appropriateness of doing so. If you and your physician jointly decide that you are ready to discontinue the medication, follow the guidelines in the section "Discontinuing Medication." Remember, it's preferable to stop medication only after you've gained some mastery of the skills discussed in chapters 4 through 15 of this book. If you wish to withdraw from a benzodiazepine medication that you have been taking for more than a month, prepare to take some time tapering off the dose very gradually, possibly over a period of several months or, in some cases, even up to a year. Consult the website benzo.org.uk and *The Ashton Manual*, still considered one of the most authoritative sources for negotiating withdrawal from benzodiazepine medications. Though Dr. Ashton has retired, her important manual on benzodiazepine withdrawal can be obtained online by doing a Google search of "The Ashton Manual." It is also available through Amazon Kindle.

2. If you feel your problem with anxiety is relatively mild (if it's more of an inconvenience or a nuisance than a debilitating or highly distressing condition), consider trying natural supplements, as described at the end of chapter 16, Nutrition, before resorting to drugs. You may also want to take a look at the books *Healing Anxiety Naturally* by Harold Bloomfield or my book *Natural Relief for Anxiety*.

## Further Reading

Bergamaschi, Muteus M., Regina Helena Costa Queiroz, Marcos Hortes Nishara Chagas, Danielle Chaves Gomes de Oliveira, Bruno Spinosa De Martinis, Flávio Kapczinski, et al. 2011. "Cannabidiol Reduces the Anxiety Induced by Simulated Public Speaking in Treatment-Naïve Social Phobia Patients." *Neuropsychopharmacology* 36(6): 1219–26.

Bloomfield, Harold. *Healing Anxiety Naturally.* New York: HarperPerennial, 1998.

Bourne, Edmund, Arlen Brownstein, and Lorna Garano. *Natural Relief for Anxiety.* Oakland, CA: New Harbinger Publications, 2004.

Mayo Clinic. Cytochrome P450 tests, mayoclinic.org/tests-procedures/cyp450test/about.

"New Warning Against Use of Marijuana for Two Groups." *New York Times,* national edition. August 30, 2019, A22.

Norden, Michael. *Beyond Prozac.* Rev. ed. New York: ReganBooks/HarperPerennial, 1996.

Preston, John, John H. O'Neal, and Mary C. Talaga. *Handbook of Clinical Psychopharmacology for Therapists.* 8th ed. Oakland, CA: New Harbinger Publications, 2017.

Schwartz, Jeffrey, and Beverly Beyette. *Brain Lock: Free Yourself from Obsessive-Compulsive Behavior.* 20th anniversary ed. New York: ReganBooks/HarperPerennial, 2016.

Serafini, Gianluca, Robert H. Howland, Fabiana Rovedi, Paolo Girandi, and Mario Amone. 2014. "The Role of Ketamine in Treatment-Resistant Depression: A Systematic Review." *Current Neuropharmacology* 12(5): 444–46.

Shannon, Scott. 2016. "Effectiveness of Cannabidiol for Pediatric Anxiety and Insomnia as Part of Posttraumatic Stress Disorder: A Case Report." *Permanente Journal* 20(4): 108–11.

Thielking, Megan. 2018. "Ketamine Gives Hope to Patients with Severe Depression. But Some Clinics Stray from the Science and Hype Its Benefits." statnews.com/2018/09/24/ketamine-clincis-severe-depression-treatment/.

Zanelati, T. V., C. Biojone, F. A. Moreira, F. S. Guimarães, and S. R. L. Joca. 2010. "Antidepressant-like Effects of Cannabidiol in Mice: Possible Involvement of 5-HT1A Receptors." *British Journal of Pharmacology* 159(1): 122–28.

# 19

# Meditation

Meditation has been practiced for over three thousand years for the purpose of training and calming the mind. As you may know, it originated as a spiritual practice within ancient Hinduism and Buddhism, though it was later practiced in various forms in many other religions. Eastern philosophy has taught that the origin of human suffering is in our automatic, conditioned thoughts (the term "automatic thoughts" in cognitive therapy is similar to this notion). Nothing in life is inherently bad except that we think about it or react to it as such. The purpose of meditation practice is to learn to step back and simply witness your automatic thoughts and reactive patterns without judgment. If you are caught up in your mind's automatic patterns, regular meditation practice can help you become gradually freer of them.

How does meditation help achieve this freedom? In a word, you can say that it is by the enlargement or "expansion" of *awareness*. Awareness can be defined as a pure, unconditioned state of consciousness that you can experience deep within yourself. It exists "beneath" or prior to the conditioned patterns of thinking and emotional reactivity you've learned over a lifetime. This unconditioned awareness is always available to you, but most of the time it's clouded over by the incessant stream of mental chatter and emotional reactions that make up your ordinary, moment-to-moment experience. Only when you become very quiet and still, willing to "just be," observing your inner experience in the present moment without judgment and without striving to do anything, can this uncluttered awareness that underlies your thoughts and feelings begin to reemerge.

When you experience this unconditioned state of awareness, you simply feel a deep sense of peace. Out of this place of inner peace can arise other unconditioned states, such as unconditional love, wisdom, deep insight, and joy. In itself, this state of inner peace is nothing you need to develop. You were born with it. It's always there, deep inside of you. You can discover it if you simply become still and quiet long enough to allow it to emerge. The practice of meditation is one of the most direct, straightforward ways to do this.

Meditation practice allows you to expand your awareness to the point where it's larger—or more "spacious"—than your fearful thoughts or emotional reactions. As soon as your awareness is larger than your fear, you are no longer claimed by the fear but can stand outside of it (in your mind) and merely witness it. It's as though you're identified with a part of your inner being that's larger than the part that's constricted by fearful thoughts. As you continue to practice meditation and enlarge your awareness, it becomes easier on an ongoing basis to observe the stream of thoughts and feelings that make up your experience. You are less prone to get "stuck" or lost in them.

You might be concerned that increasing your ability to observe your inner thoughts and feelings sounds like becoming internally divided rather than more connected with yourself. In fact, the opposite is true. It's your reactive thoughts and conditioned emotional patterns that tend to pull you away from your own center—to lead you away from your deeper inner self and into what has been popularly termed "mind trips" or "personal dramas." To practice meditation is to cultivate greater self-integration and wholeness. As you deepen and enlarge your awareness, you begin to be in touch with more of yourself. Your reactive thoughts and feelings still occur, but you're not so strongly swept up by them. You're more free to truly enjoy your life because you don't get quite as stuck—or stuck as long—in any particular state of anxiety, worry, anger, guilt, shame, grief, and so on. Rather, you're able to simply acknowledge your reaction, allow it to move through your experience, and let it go. Your inner consciousness becomes spacious enough that you can observe a worried thought, then choose to let the thought go if it's unreasonable. You begin to have more choice over what you think and experience. You are not quite so scattered by your mind's endless cascade of reactive thoughts and feelings. While these thoughts and feelings still occur, your relationship to them is different. Your inner awareness becomes spacious enough that you can more easily step back and witness your thoughts and feelings rather than be carried away by them.

## Benefits of Meditation

Meditation was first popularized in the United States in the mid-1960s in the form of Transcendental Meditation, or TM. In Transcendental Meditation, an instructor selects a Sanskrit mantra (a word, phrase, or sound) for you. You are then instructed to repeat the sound mentally while sitting upright in a quiet place. You need to concentrate completely—but unforcefully—on the mantra while letting any distractions just pass through your mind.

In the 1970s, Herbert Benson did research on Transcendental Meditation, which he published in his well-known book *The Relaxation Response*. Benson developed his own version of meditation, which involved mentally repeating the word "one" on each exhalation of the breath. He documented a number of physiological effects of meditation, including:

- A decrease in heart rate

- A decrease in blood pressure

- A decrease in oxygen consumption

- A decrease in metabolic rate

- A decrease in the concentration of lactic acid in the blood (associated with anxiety reduction)

- An increase in forearm blood flow and hand temperature

- An increase in electrical resistance of the skin (associated with deep relaxation)

- An increase in alpha brain wave activity (also associated with relaxation)

Benson established that the positive benefits of meditation are not exclusive to TM, and that an individually selected mantra is unnecessary. His own "respiratory-one" method achieved the same physiological effects as Transcendental Meditation. He referred to the deep state of physiological relaxation induced by meditation as the "relaxation response."

Since the time of Benson's work, considerable research on the long-term benefits of meditation has established that it can alter personality traits, behaviors, and attitudes. If you suffer from an anxiety disorder, meditation can break up obsessional mental patterns and help you restructure your thoughts more productively. (Regular meditation has an even greater impact on repetitive mental patterns than the practice of progressive muscle relaxation, which is directed more toward relieving muscle tension.)

Meditation has repeatedly been found to reduce chronic anxiety and worry. Often the dosage of tranquilizers or other medications you are taking can be reduced if you are meditating daily. Other long-range benefits include:

- Sharpened alertness

- Increased energy level and productivity

- Decreased self-criticism

- Increased objectivity (the capacity to view situations nonjudgmentally)

- Decreased dependence on alcohol, recreational drugs, and prescription drugs

- Increased accessibility of emotions

- Heightened self-esteem and sense of identity

In the 1980s and 1990s, Jon Kabat-Zinn did extensive research on meditation as a method of stress management. Utilizing an approach to meditation that he referred to as "mindfulness," Kabat-Zinn developed a comprehensive program for stress management known as "mindfulness-based stress reduction" (MBSR), which has been taught at universities and clinics throughout the United States. The term "mindfulness" refers to the basic stance of all forms of meditation: silently witnessing the ongoing stream of your inner experience with complete acceptance and without judgment. Some people prefer this term because it is a purely psychological concept without the "Eastern" overtones of the word "meditation." Two of Kabat-Zinn's books, *Full Catastrophe Living* and *Wherever You Go, There You Are*, have been widely influential in bringing meditation or mindfulness practice into mainstream society.

More recently meditation practice has been shown to prevent relapse among people who have had three or more episodes of major depression (Segal, Williams, and Teasdale 2013). It is one of the few interventions, apart from medication, that has been empirically demonstrated to help prevent recurrence of depression. At present, meditation and mindfulness practice are being used by many physicians and psychotherapists as an adjunct to treatment of a wide variety of physical and psychological problems. In short, meditation/mindfulness practice is a powerful psychological technique for calming the mind. Although it has origins in spiritual traditions, you do not have to adopt any particular spiritual perspective in order to practice and benefit from meditation.

# Types of Meditation

There are two broad types of meditation: *concentrative* and *nonconcentrative*. Sometimes these are referred to as structured and unstructured meditation. The concentrative approach emphasizes concentrating your attention during meditation by maintaining a specific focus on a particular object. Every time your mind starts to wander during a meditation session, you bring your attention back to a particular object of focus. For example, you might focus on a particular word that you repeat over and over, such as "one," "now," or "relax." Another popular and widely practiced form of concentrative meditation involves focusing on your respiration. As you meditate, you simply keep bringing your attention back to the cycle of your breath, experiencing the rising and falling of your breath, preferably from your abdomen.

The nonconcentrative, unstructured approach to meditation does not narrow attention to a particular object. Instead, the total content of experience—whatever comes up in awareness—becomes the object of focus. You simply witness whatever thoughts, feelings, desires, or physical sensations arise in your experience without resisting them or judging them in any way. You carefully pay attention in such a way that you are aware of the present moment, and all that is contained in your present experience, without any judgment.

The term "mindfulness" is sometimes used to refer to the nonconcentrative type of meditation, since mindfulness means to pay attention on purpose to whatever arises in the present moment, without judgment (Kabat-Zinn 2005). For the purpose of this chapter, mindfulness is understood more as an attitude, stance, or approach that you can take in any form of meditation, whether concentrative or nonconcentrative. In concentrative meditation, you can maintain a mindful stance toward the thoughts, feelings, and sensations that arise in your experience while focusing on whatever object of meditation you choose. Mindfulness is a nonjudgmental, accepting stance toward the stream of your experience that you can assume in any type of meditation, and, in fact, even at any time in your ongoing daily experience outside of meditation. Meditation is a deliberate, time-limited process for which you set aside a specific time. Mindfulness is a stance, approach, or attitude that you can take during meditation practice as well as toward all of your waking experience.

# Learning to Meditate

Learning to meditate is a process that involves at least three distinct stages:

- Right attitude

- Right technique

- Cultivating mindfulness

*Right attitude* is a mind-set or mental stance that you bring to meditation. Such an attitude takes time and commitment to develop. Fortunately, the practice of meditation itself helps you learn right attitude. *Right technique* involves learning specific methods of sitting and focusing your awareness that facilitate meditation. *Cultivating mindfulness* is the process of making a fundamental shift in your relationship with your own inner experience. It is developing a nonjudgmental "inner observer" within yourself that enables you to simply witness rather than react to the ups and downs of everyday existence.

## Right Attitude

The attitude that you bring to the practice of meditation is critical. In fact, cultivating right attitude is a part of the practice. Your success and ability to persevere with meditation practice will in large part be determined by the way you approach it. The following eight aspects of right attitude are based on the writings of Jon Kabat-Zinn. His books (see "Further Reading and Resources" at the end of the chapter) are highly recommended if you're serious about undertaking a regular meditation practice.

### Beginner's Mind

To observe your immediate, ongoing experience without any judgments, preconceptions, or projections is often referred to as "beginner's mind." In essence, with beginner's mind you perceive something with the freshness you would bring to it if you were seeing it for the very first time. It's seeing—and accepting—things as they actually are in the present moment, without the veil of your own assumptions or judgments about them. For example, next time you're in the presence of familiar people, consider seeing them as much as possible as they actually are, apart from your feelings, thoughts, projections, or judgments. How would you see them if you were meeting them for the first time?

### Nonstriving

Almost everything you do during your day is likely to be goal directed. Meditation is one thing that is not. Although meditation takes effort to practice, it has no aim other than to allow you to "just be." When you sit down to meditate, it's best to clear your mind of any goals. You are not trying to relax, blank your mind, relieve stress, or reach enlightenment. You don't need to evaluate the quality of your meditation according to whether you reach such goals. The only intention you bring to meditation is simply to be—to observe your "here and now" experience just as it is. If you are tense, anxious, or in pain, you don't strive to get rid of these sensations; instead, you simply observe them and be with them as best you can. You let them remain simply as they are. In so doing, you cease resisting or struggling with them.

### Acceptance

Acceptance is the opposite of striving. As you learn to simply be with whatever you experience in the moment, you cultivate acceptance. Acceptance does not mean that you have to like whatever comes up (such as tension, irritation, frustration, or pain, for example); it simply means you're willing to be with it without trying to push it away. You may be familiar with the saying "What you resist persists." As long as you resist or struggle with something, whether in meditation or life in general, you actually energize and magnify it. Acceptance allows the discomfort or problem to just be. While it may not go away, it becomes easier to deal with because you cease to struggle with and/or avoid it.

In meditation practice, acceptance develops as you learn to embrace each moment as it comes, without moving away from it. As you learn to do this, you discover that whatever was there for a given moment will soon change—more quickly, in fact, than if you tried to resist it.

In life, acceptance does not mean that you resign yourself to the way things are and cease trying to change and grow. On the contrary, acceptance can clear a space in your life for you to reflect clearly and act appropriately. Energy is freed up to act when you are no longer reacting to or struggling with the difficulty. Sometimes, of course, it's necessary to go through a range of emotional reactions around a problem first before you can get to acceptance.

## Nonjudgment

An important prerequisite for acceptance is nonjudgment. When you pay attention to your ongoing experience through the day, you'll notice that you frequently judge things—both outer circumstances as well as inner circumstances (your own moods and feelings). These judgments are based on your personal values and standards of what is "good" and "bad." If you doubt this, try taking just five minutes to notice how many things you judge during that short time interval. To practice meditation, it's important to learn not so much to stop judging but to gain some distance from the process. You can simply observe your inner judgments without reacting to them, least of all judging them! Instead, you cultivate a suspension of any judgment, watching whatever comes up, including your own judging thoughts. You allow such thoughts to come and go, while continuing to observe whatever object you have selected as a focus for meditation.

## Patience

Patience is a close cousin to acceptance and nonstriving. It means allowing things to unfold in their own natural time. It is letting your meditation practice be whatever it is without rushing it.

Patience is needed to make time to meditate for a half hour every day. Patience is also required to persist with your meditation practice through the days or weeks when nothing particularly interesting happens. To be patient is to stop hurrying. This often means going against the grain of a fast-paced society where rushing from one destination to another is the norm.

The patience you can bring to your meditation practice will help assure its success and permanence. Sitting in meditation regularly will help you develop patience, as it will help you cultivate all of the characteristics described in this section. The attitudes that help you develop your meditation practice are the very same attitudes that are deepened by the practice itself.

## Letting Go

Our minds are often like monkeys. We grab on to a particular thought or emotional state— sometimes one that is actually painful—and then we don't let go. Cultivating the ability to let go is crucial to meditation practice, not to mention a less anxious life. When you hold on to any experience, whether pleasant or painful, you impede your ability to simply be present in the here and now without judgment or striving. Learning to let go of things is assisted by learning to accept them. Letting go is a natural consequence of a willingness to accept things as they are.

If you find that, prior to meditation, you have a hard time letting go of some concern, you can actually use your meditation as a means to witness the thoughts and feelings you're creating around the concern—including the process of "holding on" itself. The more minutely you observe the specific thoughts and feelings you have created around a problem, the more quickly you'll be able to expand your awareness around that problem and let it go. When the concern is intensely charged emotionally, it's probably best to release your feelings by talking them out or writing them out in a journal before you sit down to meditate. Cultivating all of the attitudes described in this section will help with letting go.

## Commitment and Self-Discipline

A strong commitment to work on yourself, along with the discipline to persevere and follow through with the process, are two more aspects essential to establishing a meditation practice. While meditation is very simple in nature, it's not always easy in practice. Learning to value and make time for "just being" on a regular basis requires a commitment in the midst of a society that is strongly oriented toward doing. Few of us have grown up with values that cherished non-striving, and so learning to stop goal-directed activity, even for just twenty to thirty minutes per day, requires commitment and discipline. The commitment is similar to that which is required in athletic training. An athlete in training doesn't practice only when he or she just feels like it, when there is time enough to fit it in, or when there are other people around to keep him or her company. The training requires the athlete to practice every day, regardless of how he or she feels or whether there is any immediate sense of accomplishment.

To establish a meditation practice, it's best to sit quietly for at least twenty minutes whether you feel like it or not—whether it's convenient or not—five to seven days per week, for at least two months. (If you find you're unable to sit that often at first, don't chastise yourself—just do your best.) You will likely find it easier if you set aside a particular time of day to do your practice, such as first thing in the morning or before dinner in the evening. At the end of two months, if you've practiced regularly, the process will likely have become enough of a habit (and sufficiently self-reinforcing) for you to continue. The experience of meditation varies from session to session: sometimes it feels good, sometimes it seems ordinary, and other times you will find it difficult to meditate at all.

Although the point is not to strive for anything, a long-term commitment to regular meditation practice will transform your life fundamentally. Without changing anything that might happen in your life, meditation will change your relationship to everything you experience, on a deep level.

## *Right Technique: Guidelines for Practicing Meditation*

There is a technique to proper meditation. Probably the most important aspect is to sit in the right fashion, which means sitting upright with your back straight either on the floor in a cross-legged position or in a chair with your feet flat on the floor. There seems to be a certain energetic alignment within the body that occurs from sitting up straight. It's not as likely to happen when you're lying down, although lying down is fine for other forms of relaxation. It's also helpful to relax tight muscles before you meditate. One way to do this is through practicing yoga. In historic times, the main purpose of yoga postures was to relax and energetically balance the body prior to meditating. The guidelines that follow are intended to help make your meditation practice easier and more effective:

- *Find a quiet environment.* Do what you can do to reduce external noises and distractions. If this is not completely possible, play a recording of soft, instrumental sounds or sounds from nature. The sound of ocean waves can also make a good background. Or you can use a white noise generator to mask external noise.

- *Reduce muscle tension.* If you're feeling tense, take some time (no more than ten minutes) to relax your muscles. Yoga postures, if you're familiar with them, are an excellent way to unwind. Progressive muscle relaxation of the upper body—your head, neck, shoulders, arms, chest, and abdomen—is often helpful (see chapter 4). If you feel too much energy or your mind is racing, doing some physical exercise first can make it easier to meditate afterward.

- *Sit properly.* Eastern style: Sit cross-legged on the floor with a cushion or pillow supporting your buttocks. Rest your hands on your thighs. Lean slightly forward so that some of your weight is supported by your thighs as well as your buttocks. Western style (preferred by most Americans): Sit in a comfortable, straight-backed chair with your feet on the floor and legs uncrossed, hands on your thighs (palms down or up, whichever you prefer). In either position, keep your back and neck straight without straining to do so. Do not assume a tight, inflexible posture. If you need to scratch or move, do so. In general, do not lie down or support your head; this will tend to promote sleep.

- *Set aside twenty to thirty minutes for meditation.* (Beginners might wish to start out with ten minutes.) You may wish to set a timer within reach or run a background recording that is twenty to thirty minutes long so that you'll know when you're done. If having a clock or watch available to look at makes you more comfortable, that's okay. After you have practiced twenty to thirty minutes per day for several weeks, you may wish to try longer periods of meditation up to forty-five minutes to an hour.

- *Make it a regular practice to meditate most or all days every week.* Even if you meditate for only five minutes, it's important to do it every day. It's ideal if you can find a set time to practice meditating. Twice a day is excellent; once per day is a minimum.

- *Don't meditate on a full stomach.* Meditation is easier if you don't practice on a full stomach or when you're tired. If you are unable to meditate prior to a meal, wait at least a half hour after eating to do so.

- *Select a focus for your attention.* The most common devices are your own respiration cycle or a mantra. The structured meditation exercises below use both of these techniques. Other common objects of meditation are external and include pictures, recorded repetitive music or chants, or a sacred object. If you are practicing unstructured meditation or mindfulness, simply relax and *witness* any thoughts and feelings passing through your stream of consciousness. Embrace all of the guidelines described in the previous section, "Right Attitude."

- *During meditation, it can be helpful to close (or almost close) your eyes in order to reduce outside distractions.* Some people, however, find they prefer to keep their eyes slightly open—just enough to see external objects indistinctly. This can reduce the tendency to be distracted by inner thoughts, feelings, and daydreams. Try this if you are having difficulty with distractibility.

- *During meditation, you will find you are often distracted by extraneous thoughts, feelings, and bodily sensations.* When this happens, don't judge yourself. Just gently bring your attention back to whatever you have selected as your focus. If an unpleasant thought or feeling tries to capture your attention, try reminding yourself, "This is just a thought" or "This is just a feeling." Just be present with the thought or feeling without going into it. Eventually, it will shift and pass. Good questions to ask yourself occasionally are "Can I just be in a space for whatever comes up?" and "Can I just be fully present with this?"

- *Distraction, boredom, restlessness, sleepiness, and impatience are common reactions during meditation.* When these states come up, just notice them, allow them to be as they are, and then return to being fully present in the moment.

- *When you've finished with your practice for the day, open your eyes gently (if they've been closed) and stretch your body.* Notice how you are feeling, but whether the feeling is positive or negative, don't judge it. If you feel good after your practice, refrain from setting any expectation that your next practice should be the same way. Let each practice session be a unique experience unto itself.

Ultimately, meditation practice has no goal other than for you to *just be*—to be fully aware in the present moment. However, an important benefit of regular meditation is the cultivation of mindfulness: the capacity to stand back and observe the ongoing stream of your experience without getting caught up in it.

You are unlikely to be aware of just how distractible your mind is until you first sit down to meditate. Using structured meditation techniques will build your capacity to concentrate in the beginning. Later you may want to drop these forms and focus more directly on simply observing the ongoing stream of your experience.

## Cultivating Mindfulness: Meditation Exercises

Mindfulness is paying attention without judgment to whatever comes up in the present moment of your experience. It is witnessing your immediate experience just as it is, without trying to change, react to, or interfere with it. A good way to appreciate mindfulness is to realize that it encompasses all of the attitudes described in the section on right attitude: nonstriving, acceptance, nonjudgment, beginner's mind, patience, letting go, commitment, and self-discipline.

Mindfulness is not something that you have to strive hard to attain. If you strive for it, it will tend to elude your grasp. By relaxing, letting go, and simply observing the ongoing stream of your experience without judgment, you will begin to experience what mindfulness actually is. Words cannot teach the meaning of mindfulness nearly so well as direct experience.

Ultimately, mindfulness can change the way you deal with fear and pain in a profound way. As your practice strengthens, you can learn to relax and stay present even when fear and pain move through the present moment.

The following meditation exercises were inspired by Jon Kabat-Zinn, Jack Kornfield, and other teachers of meditation. (Several are available for download on the website associated with this book; see the very end of the book for more information.) They derive from basic practices that have been used by students of meditation for many centuries. Several of the exercises described here emphasize maintaining a focus on your breathing cycle—continually bringing your attention back to your breath each time you become distracted. It is probably best to do the exercises in sequence. Once you've gained some experience with meditation, you can choose which exercise you prefer. The walking meditation can be used by itself, or as a break from a long period of sitting meditation.

## Basic Meditation Exercise

1. Sit in a comfortable yet upright position. Focus on your breathing cycle as you breathe slowly from your abdomen for ten minutes. Let the sensations of inhaling and exhaling be the object of your focus.

2. If your mind wanders from the focus on your respiration, let it do so without judging it. Then gently bring your attention back to your breathing cycle. Do this as many times as you need to during the course of your meditation. Just keep a gentle focus without forcing your mind.

3. If you find yourself getting frequently distracted, use the *Calming Breath Exercise* (described in chapter 4 of this book). When you feel you've relaxed enough to stay relatively well focused on your breathing cycle, try dropping the count.

4. Begin practicing this exercise for ten minutes, and gradually work up to thirty minutes. You may find it useful to set a timer or play a thirty-minute recording of meditative music so that you'll know when you're done.

## Sensing Your Body During Meditation

1. Begin this exercise by focusing on your respiration. Then expand your attention to include an awareness of your entire body. Focus in particular on your arms and legs, along with your breath cycle. You can extend your focus to your hands and feet. When your attention wanders, bring it back to focus on your arms and legs.

2. As in the preceding exercise, don't judge yourself when your mind wanders. Each time you find yourself distracted, gently bring your attention back to a focus on your arms,

legs, and respiration. You may need to do this many times at first. With practice, your concentration should improve.

3.   Start with practicing this exercise for ten minutes per day, and gradually work up to thirty minutes.

## Witnessing Thoughts and Feelings

1.   When you've become comfortable with the first two exercises above, let your awareness expand to include all of your thoughts and feelings.

2.   Simply observe your thoughts and feelings as they come and go, just as you would watch cars going by or leaves floating down a river. Let each new thought or feeling be a new object to witness.

3.   If you become "stuck" in feelings or reactions during this process, simply *observe* that you are feeling stuck, and allow time for it to pass.

4.   Note the impermanence of your thoughts and feelings. They tend to come and go quickly unless you prolong a particular one by "holding on" to it.

5.   If certain thoughts keep coming back, let them do so. Just keep observing them until they eventually move on.

6.   If you notice particular feelings of restlessness, impatience, irritability, or "wanting to get through this," simply observe those feelings without judgment, and then allow them to pass.

7.   If feelings of fear, anxiety, anger, sadness, or depression arise, don't go into them. Just be with the feelings and simply witness or observe them until they pass. You may find that bringing your attention back to your chosen object of meditation, whatever it may be, helps you move through such feelings.

8.   When you first begin to practice witnessing thoughts and feelings, start with shorter periods of practice, then work up to thirty minutes per day.

## Observing Whatever Comes into Awareness

1.   Let yourself observe, without judgment, whatever passes through your awareness: thoughts, reactions, physical sensations of discomfort, impatience, restlessness, sleepiness, comfort, relaxation. Let each aspect of your experience arise and move on without giving any one aspect special attention. Whenever you get stuck in a particular thought or reaction, go back to a chosen meditation object—whether it's a mantra, a single word, or just your respiration cycle. Stay with this through any momentary periods of feeling stuck. Practice acceptance and nonjudgment toward whatever occurs in your experience while you sit, for up to thirty minutes each day.

## Walking Meditation

1. In the privacy of your home, take five minutes to walk slowly, with awareness. You can walk back and forth or in a loop.

2. Keep in mind as you walk that you're not trying to get anywhere. Instead, you are being mindful of the process of walking itself.

3. Be fully present with each step that you take. Focus on the sensations you feel in your feet, ankles, calves, knees, and thighs as your legs move slowly through each step. Go as slowly as you wish in order to stay focused.

4. If your attention wanders into thoughts, reactions, or other distractions, allow it to do so without judgment. Then bring your focus back to the sensations in your legs and feet as you slowly walk.

5. Start practicing walking meditation daily for five minutes, and work up to fifteen minutes.

Practicing any of these exercises regularly will help you establish a foundation for developing mindfulness as a way of life. Beginning a meditation practice is straightforward. Maintaining it takes additional commitment, as described in the following section.

# Maintaining a Meditation Practice

The motivation, commitment, and self-discipline necessary to establish a meditation practice has been mentioned already in the section on right attitude. Learning to meditate can be compared with learning a sport like baseball, racquetball, or golf. A significant amount of time in training is necessary before you become proficient. This involves a commitment to keep sitting on those days when you don't feel like it or find it inconvenient to do so. Setting aside a regular time to practice for twenty to thirty minutes each day makes this easier. The best times are generally first thing in the morning upon awakening or in the late afternoon before dinner. Other good times would be before lunch or on a break at work. By setting aside a regular time, you build a place for meditation into your life.

Besides your own personal commitment and self-discipline, there are several things that can greatly support your practice. It can be quite helpful to find a local class or group that meditates regularly. You may find such a class at some local hospitals or colleges (adult education programs) in your area. Or there may be a free-standing meditation group within driving distance. Programs in Transcendental Meditation, or TM (a specific form of mantra meditation that has been around for many years), are offered in certain areas. Having the support of a group with whom you meditate regularly will help motivate you at those times when it seems hard to keep up with your daily practice.

In some places, you may be fortunate to be close to a teacher thoroughly grounded and skilled in the practice of meditation. If you are interested in finding a group or teacher in your area, you can contact the Insight Meditation Society or Spirit Rock Meditation Center, listed in the resources at the end of this chapter, and request a referral for a teacher in your area.

The Insight Meditation Society offers meditation retreats in various places throughout the United States. A meditation retreat generally involves being in meditation for up to eight hours per day (with hourly breaks), alternating between sitting and walking forms of meditation. Retreats can go from one to ten consecutive days, although a few go even longer. Doing a retreat is a powerful way to deepen your ongoing meditation practice. It is generally not recommended for beginners.

Finally, there are a number of excellent books that can support your practice. One meditation book specifically designed for people with anxiety disorders is *Calming Your Anxious Mind* by Jeffrey Brantley.

## Common Concerns That May Come Up

As you undertake to meditate regularly, you may have many questions and concerns. The following is based on a list compiled in the book *Calming Your Anxious Mind*.

- *There isn't enough time to meditate.* Usually when you say you don't have time for something, it means that it doesn't have enough priority for you to give it time. It's likely that meditation and mindfulness, practiced regularly, will gradually transform your life and your ability to handle your anxiety. The question you have to answer is how much of a priority are you willing to give to meditation. How committed are you to giving it a regular place in your life?

- *Meditation is too boring.* Sometimes meditation can be boring. This is to be expected. The question in this case is whether you have unreasonable expectations about what meditation ought to be. If you are being mindful, the solution to boredom is to carefully witness your state of boredom when it comes up. By carefully investigating it, you may learn some things about the boredom. For example, boredom often contains specific negative self-talk and judgments. By carefully investigating your thoughts and reactions around your state of boredom to see what's there—instead of just reacting—you may find yourself less bored.

- *When I sit still and meditate, it makes me more anxious.* Does meditation really make you more anxious? Or is it possible that by stopping and sitting still, you begin to become more aware of anxiety that was already present? When you're not distracted, any anxiety that was covered up by distraction is likely to come forward. Now you have the opportunity to work with your anxiety instead of running from it or otherwise trying to avoid it. By accepting your anxiety as much as possible—and making it the object of your attention and awareness—you have the opportunity to change the way you relate to it. You have the opportunity to just be with it until it shifts. One of the most important ways in which meditation practice can help you better deal with anxiety is by training you to simply accept anxiety states instead of trying to run from them. The more you learn to accept and work with your anxiety as it arises, the less it becomes an "enemy" that you're trying to combat. Ultimately, the less you struggle against anxiety, the easier it will be to deal with. So if you feel more anxious during meditation, just stay with it and allow it to be to the greatest extent possible. You will learn a whole new way to deal with anxiety and worry by doing so.

- *It's difficult to meditate because I'm too anxious or agitated.* What if mindfulness practice does not seem to help you quiet down? What if you continue to feel highly agitated and distracted after ten or more minutes of meditation? If this happens, your body may indeed be too charged up to sit still. The best thing to do is to get physical. Try doing some form of aerobic exercise (see chapter 5) or take twenty minutes to do a sequence of yoga postures. After you've discharged the energy from your body, try sitting in meditation again.

- *It's difficult to discipline myself to meditate regularly.* While the goal is to meditate seven days per week, you may find yourself unable to do this at first. Don't try to be perfect, just do the best you can. As you continue to practice, you'll begin to experience some of the benefits of meditation and perhaps find yourself motivated to keep it up every day. It's true that meditation practice takes discipline, just like learning to play the piano or mastering a sport. You need to make a commitment to yourself to practice regularly in order to keep meditating over the long term. However, don't chastise yourself if you can't do it every day at first. Do the best you can. Read books, listen to recordings, or, best of all, find a local group that sits regularly. All of these things will help you sustain your motivation to practice regularly.

## Meditation and Compassion

An important aspect of developing a capacity to observe your mind is to bring compassion into your observation. It may not be enough to learn merely to observe your reactive thoughts and feelings. Without cultivating compassion toward your reactivity, you may remain at war with it. To bring compassion and heart into your self-observation is to begin to make peace with yourself.

Many people, especially if they are perfectionistic, treat themselves as though they were a harsh drill sergeant disciplining a new recruit. If this seems hard to imagine, watch yourself to see how much time you spend criticizing yourself, putting yourself down, or pushing and driving yourself to do what you don't really want to do. When you're not pushing or criticizing yourself, you may fall into a more passive stance of fear. Out of fear, your mind constantly scares you with "What if this…" or "What if that…" When you fall into a victim stance, you may depress yourself with "It's no use…" "It's hopeless…" "It's a lost cause…" As soon as you start to feel less depressed, a tendency toward perfectionism may kick in and keep you on a treadmill with "I should…" "I must…" "I have to…" Notice how much you criticize, scare, depress, or push yourself, and you'll learn quite a bit about your own mind. For more information on the various types of unhelpful self-talk, see the sections on the Worrier, the Critic, the Victim, and the Perfectionist in chapter 8, Self-Talk.

Cultivating compassion in self-observation is fundamental to changing your relationship with yourself. Compassion allows you to move away from judgment, criticism, and even contempt and toward tolerance, acceptance, and love. Compassion depends on accepting yourself—and the rest of the world—*as it is*, an attitude that can be cultivated through meditation practice. Living with your limitations and embracing your humanness is something you can learn. For a more in-depth statement about the role of compassion in meditation, see Jack Kornfield's book *A Path with Heart*.

## Meditation and Medication

Few, if any, books on meditation address the question of how prescription medications affect the experience of meditation. Some formal meditation training programs, such as Transcendental Meditation, request that beginners get off all nonessential prescription drugs before learning to meditate. My personal observation is that different medications affect people in different ways.

Two generalizations, however, might be made:

1.  Benzodiazepine medications such as Xanax, Ativan, or Klonopin seem to increase distractibility, making it more difficult to focus during meditation. It has been found that the benzodiazepines tend to increase beta wave activity in the brain (rapid, nonsynchronous brain waves associated with thinking) and reduce the ability to enter into alpha brain wave states (synchronous brain waves associated with relaxed states of mind as well as meditation). While it's certainly not impossible to meditate while taking a benzodiazepine medication, you may find it somewhat more difficult.

2.  SSRI antidepressant medications (such as Prozac, Zoloft, Paxil, or Celexa) do not seem to impede meditation for most people. There are certain people who report that meditation is more difficult while taking an SSRI or SNRI medication. On the other hand, some people find it easier to meditate after taking SSRIs because they feel calmer and less subject to intrusive thoughts and feelings. In general, it seems that SSRI medications do not pose a significant impediment to cultivating a meditation practice.

Information on the effects of tricyclic antidepressants (such as imipramine or nortriptyline) or other antianxiety medications such as Neurontin, Gabitril, or Buspar on meditation is difficult to find. It's possible to evaluate the effects of such medications if you reduce your dose for a few days while meditating and then resume taking your normal dose. Please consult with your prescribing physician before you try this.

## Conclusion

The purpose of this chapter has been to present meditation practice as one additional strategy you can use to help better deal with anxiety, fear, and worry. Though meditation is a powerful coping strategy, it in no way supersedes any of the other methods for dealing with anxiety and fear presented in this book. Abdominal breathing, exercise, working with fearful self-talk, facing fears through exposure, utilizing good nutrition, dealing with conditions that can aggravate anxiety, working on assertiveness and self-esteem, and, finally, relying on medication, if needed, can all be very helpful to your recovery from your anxiety difficulties, just as meditation can be. Ultimately, you will discover for yourself what role meditation can play in your journey to overcome anxiety by making time to practice it daily, if possible. You may find it to be quite a powerful tool, if you stick with it over the long run.

Keep in mind that "success" in meditation is just doing it. The more often you do it, the more quickly you will train your mind to be less reactive, more stable, and better able to observe. You will be training it to be able to take each moment as it comes, without valuing any one above any other. Working regularly with the resistance of your mind builds inner strength. Regular meditation practice will foster the development of the very attitudes that help facilitate the practice in the beginning: acceptance, patience, nonjudgment, letting go, and trust.

## Summary of Things to Do

1.  To begin a meditation practice, follow the guidelines in the section "Right Technique" for the first week or two. You may want to begin with ten-minute meditation periods and gradually increase the duration up to thirty minutes. Make a commitment to yourself to practice every day. It's best to find a specific time of day and a specific place for your practice where you're free of distractions. Review the section on "Right Attitude" to help cultivate the proper approach to take toward your practice.

2.  After a week or two—or when you feel you have gained some familiarity and comfort with meditation—try out the various meditation exercises in the section "Cultivating Mindfulness." Practice them one at a time and work through the sequence to determine which exercise or exercises you prefer. After you've spent time working with these exercises, you will begin to work out your own preferred style of practice.

3.  To support your practice, find a class or group that meditates regularly. If this is unavailable, you may want to work with recordings relevant to meditation and read some of the books on meditation listed below, perhaps starting with those by Brantley, Kabat-Zinn, Kornfield, and Goldstein.

## Further Reading and Resources

### Books

Brantley, Jeffrey. *Calming Your Anxious Mind*. 2nd ed. Oakland, CA: New Harbinger Publications, 2007. (Directly examines how meditation practice can help deal with anxiety and worry.)

Goldstein, Joseph. *Insight Meditation*. Boston: Shambhala, 2003.

Kabat-Zinn, Jon. *Full Catastrophe Living*. Rev. ed. New York: Bantam, 2013.

———. *Wherever You Go, There You Are*. 10th anniversary ed. New York:Hatchette, 2005. (Kabat-Zinn's books provide a good introduction to meditation and mindfulness practice.)

Kornfield, Jack. *A Path with Heart*. New York: Bantam Books, 1993.

Levine, Stephen. *A Gradual Awakening*. New York: Anchor Books, 1989.

Nhat Hanh, Thich. *The Art of Living*. New York: HarperOne, 2017.

Salzberg, Sharon. *Loving-Kindness*. Boston: Shambhala, 2002.

Segal, Zindel V., J. Mark G. Williams, and John D. Teasdale. *Mindfulness-Based Cognitive Therapy for Depression*. 2nd ed. New York: Guilford Press, 2013.

## Meditation CDs and Programs

A good collection of meditation CDs is available through Sounds True in Boulder, Colorado, (soundstrue.com). Meditation programs with CDs or downloadable files by Jon Kabat-Zinn can be ordered by going to mindfulnesscds.com.

## Meditation Retreats

Two major centers for meditation retreats are the Insight Meditation Society in Barre, Massachusetts (dharma.org), and Spirit Rock Meditation Center in Woodacre, California (spiritrock.org). Contact either of these centers to find out about meditation centers and retreats in other parts of the country.

# 20

# Relapse Prevention

Approximately 30 to 40 percent of people who receive state-of-the art treatment for their anxiety problems have limited recovery. They do not experience the relief they were hoping to find. Of those people who do initially derive benefit from treatment, a significant percentage relapses after a period of time. In some cases, the relapse is caused by a temporary increase in personal stress and may be overcome. In other, less fortunate cases, relapse tends to be more enduring.

## Setbacks vs. Relapse

It is critical to understand that progress in recovery from an anxiety disorder is *nonlinear*. Temporary setbacks—where you might experience the recurrence of a panic attack, a sudden feeling of resistance to entering a phobic situation you had previously mastered, or outright intolerance of unpleasant sensations during exposure—*are an entirely normal and expected part of the recovery process.*

You may have gone a month or two entirely free of panic attacks and all of a sudden, the right constellation of stressors may again evoke an unexpected surge of panic. Or you may believe you've conquered your fear of flying and actually have taken two successful flights. Then you decide to take a longer distance flight, and the flying phobia stubbornly reasserts itself. You are having a setback.

Setbacks are one thing; relapse is quite another.

The fundamental characteristic of a *setback* is that it is a *temporary disruption* of your progress toward recovery that doesn't last. Having a bad day—or even a bad week—where your anxiety returns, but you proactively cope with it and move on, *is a normal part of recovery.*

The primary purpose of this chapter is to provide you with skills and strategies for handling setbacks. Then you can effectively stop the temporary disruption of a setback from moving on into relapse.

*Relapse* is a series of setbacks over time. Relapse occurs when you fail to recognize the most common *reasons for relapse* described in the following section, "Reasons for Failing to Get Better After Treatment." If you are unaware of potential reasons why you might relapse, you may also fail to utilize strategies suggested for handling/overcoming each common cause for relapse.

Relapse also can occur when you consistently turn a blind eye to typical *warning signs* that predict you could be heading toward relapse. These warning signs are often hidden, and the second section of this chapter, "Watching for Hidden Signs of Potential Relapse," enumerates some of the most common warning signs.

Briefly again, setbacks during the course of recovery from an anxiety disorder—whether panic attacks, phobias, or excessive worry—are *temporary, normal, and inevitable*. Responding to setbacks by perceiving the common warning signs of potential relapse, as well as drawing on a variety of skills to *stop* the setback, enables you to move forward with your recovery without any risk of relapse. As you continue to work through temporary setbacks, they are likely to become less frequent and intense. Ultimately, you can reach a point where setbacks are quite rare, and the potential for relapse is negligible. Your anxiety condition becomes a memory: a thing of the past.

## Reasons for Failing to Get Better After Treatment

Why do people fail to get better in spite of good treatment? Why do others relapse? Assuming they have received a well-administered course of cognitive behavioral therapy (CBT) and, in some cases, additional medication appropriate for anxiety disorders, what happens?

The present section of this chapter describes five possible reasons for not fully recovering after receiving CBT and/or medication. The second part of the chapter enumerates a number of "warning signs" that suggest the potential possibility of relapsing.

If you've not recovered because you did not receive appropriate treatment (that is, your therapist sat and just talked with you or tried some other form of treatment instead of cognitive behavioral therapy), you need to keep looking until you find effective help. Keep in mind that the reasons for not fully recovering that follow assume you've already had proper, CBT-oriented treatment and yet have not improved as much as you would like.

### You Don't Continue to Practice the Basic Techniques and Strategies of Cognitive Behavioral Therapy

Recovery from panic, phobias, excess worry, or obsessions and compulsions requires consistent effort over a period of time. You need to make time each day (or at least three or four days per week) to practice abdominal breathing, do deep muscle relaxation, engage in aerobic exercise, challenge and counter anxiety-provoking self-talk, and incrementally face either internal anxiety sensations (especially with panic disorder) or avoided external situations (phobias). If you're unable or unwilling to make such an effort during the course of cognitive behavioral therapy, you will probably not benefit as much from it. If you cease to keep up with the basic practices of relaxation, exercise, and countering anxiety-provoking self-talk *after the completion of therapy*, you can also increase your risk of relapse. Recovery from an anxiety disorder requires a permanent change in your lifestyle, with time allocated each day (or close to daily) for practicing the skills that keep anxiety and phobias from recurring.

If you find you're having difficulty maintaining a commitment to the daily practices that can ensure your long-term recovery, there are a couple of things you might do. First, you might arrange with your therapist to have periodic "booster sessions" (after you've finished therapy) to help you stay on track with your recovery program. Second, if you live in a large metropolitan area, you can attend an anxiety disorders support group. Such a group needs to be a place where the focus is on what everybody is doing to maintain or embrace recovery—not just venting about their problems. If you can't find a local support group, you can do an Amazon search for books specific to your particular anxiety disorder (see the bibliography of books listed at the end of chapter 1 for recommendations of books specific to each type of anxiety disorder). Or you can look for YouTube videos or podcasts relevant to your particular issue with anxiety.

### *You Do Not Take Medication When It's Needed, or Do Not Take the Proper Dose, or Stop Taking It Before It Has Offered Its Full Benefit*

Often prescription medication is unnecessary. However, if your problem is relatively severe, you may well need to combine CBT with medication to obtain the best results. "Severe" means that your problem meets at least one of the following criteria:

- Your anxiety is disruptive enough that it's difficult for you to get to work and/or function in your job (or it has caused you to cease working).

- Your anxiety interferes with your ability to maintain fulfilling and close relationships with family members and/or significant others (or it prevents you from establishing a relationship with any significant other).

- Your anxiety causes you significant distress at least 50 percent of the time you're awake. It's not just a nuisance or an irritation—you often feel overwhelmed and find it hard to get through the day.

If you believe your anxiety disorder meets one or more of these criteria, it's likely you could benefit from a trial of medication such as an SSRI like Lexapro, Zoloft, Celexa, or Paxil; an SNRI medication such as Cymbalta or Pristiq; or perhaps the medication Buspar or an SMS modulator antidepressant such as Trintellix. Not to try medications because you're afraid of them or philosophically opposed to them may hamper your recovery, if your situation is severe. Some of my own clients have remained stuck for years until they finally decided to try medication.

Detailed guidelines for when to use medication and which ones to use can be found in chapter 18, Medication for Anxiety. You might also obtain a referral to a psychiatrist skilled in the treatment of anxiety disorders. In general, psychiatrists have more knowledge about medications for anxiety than does your primary care physician. Another way to find a referral to therapists or psychiatrists who specialize in anxiety in your area is to visit the website of the Anxiety and Depression Association of America (ADAA) at adaa.org. On the homepage of the site, there is a link "Find a Therapist." If you click on this link and enter your zip code, you can bring up a list of anxiety specialists in your particular area.

Another problem with medication is the failure to take it long enough. Research has found, for example, that the most effective period of time to take SSRI antidepressant medications such as Lexapro, Celexa, Zoloft, or Paxil (or SNRIs such as Pristiq or Cymbalta) is approximately one year to eighteen months. Rates of relapse have been found to range from 50 to 70 percent for a group who took these kinds of medications for only six months, whereas the relapse rate dropped to 30 percent for a group who took the medications for eighteen months. Often you can downsize an initially high dose of the medication to a lower "maintenance" dose. Again, see chapter 18, Medication for Anxiety, for further information.

Staying on an SSRI, SNRI, or SMS modulator/stimulator antidepressant medication longer enables your brain to recover and regenerate from the initial trauma caused by severe anxiety symptoms—that is, the initial trauma, say, of severe panic disorder or a severe social anxiety disorder *may* have had physical effects on the brain. Unfortunately, the longer severe anxiety symptoms persist untreated, the greater potential for trauma to the brain, and thus the greater risk of long-term anxiety symptoms. Beginning medication sooner rather than later can mitigate such traumatic effects. Then staying on the medication for a period of a year to eighteen months—or in some cases even longer—allows the brain the opportunity to rest and regenerate. While the information in this paragraph is based largely on the author's thirty years of treating anxiety disorders, there is some research to back it up. See the book *Handbook of Clinical Psychopharmacology for Therapists* by John Preston, John O'Neal, and Mary Talaga.

A final issue with medications, especially SSRIs or SNRIs, is that you may have excessive side effects to the drug because your doctor started you at the therapeutic dose level, the recommended dose range for clinical efficacy of the drug, according to the *Physician's Desk Reference*. Many people with anxiety disorders cannot tolerate a medication that is initially administered at a therapeutic dose level, so they discontinue the drug immediately or after a few days due to side effects. It's very important to start any SSRI or SNRI medication at a fractional dose, perhaps a fourth of fifth of the low end of the normal therapeutic dose range. Then you gradually titrate the dose upward over a period of two weeks to a month, until you reach the low end of the therapeutic dose range. More details about the gradual titration of antidepressant medications in the treatment of anxiety disorders can be found in chapter 18, Medication for Anxiety. Some doctors who are unaccustomed to working with anxiety disorders may be unaware of this issue.

The above observations apply primarily to antidepressant medications used to treat anxiety, such as the SSRIs, SNRIs, and SMS modulators. Relapse rates following the use and discontinuation of high-potency tranquilizers, such as Xanax, Ativan, or Klonopin, tend to be high—even after taking them for as short a time as a month—if you haven't learned any other skills or made lifestyle changes to help overcome your problem (again, see chapter 18, Medication for Anxiety).

## You Don't Modify Your Lifestyle in a Way That Supports Greater Peace and Ease in Your Life

Even if you've received cognitive behavioral therapy and have taken the proper medication(s), your recovery may still be limited if your lifestyle is so complicated and busy that you continually keep yourself at a high level of stress. Anxiety disorders are caused by three sets of factors, as described in chapter 2: heredity, personality factors (based on childhood experiences), and cumulative stress. You can't do much about your genetic makeup or your early childhood experiences, but you can do a lot to mitigate stress in your life. If you reduce and manage your stress, you will reduce your vulnerability to anxiety. External stress factors include things like work demands, rush-hour commutes, smog, food additives, negative family members and relatives, or noise pollution, to name just a few. These types of stressors usually require external solutions: taking direct action to mitigate a stressful circumstance in your life, such as altering the time of day you commute to work, upgrading to a healthier diet, or seeking out couples therapy if you have ongoing issues with your spouse or partner.

Internal stress factors have to do with your own attitudes, such as overemphasizing success at the cost of everything else, or a tendency to cram too many things into too short a time. Internal sources of stress require internal solutions—basically shifting your attitudes and priorities. Many people do not recover from panic, phobias, or excessive worry until they are willing to place as much importance on their peace of mind and health as they do on career success and material accomplishments.

Learning to simplify your life is one of the *most* important interventions you can take to reduce your level of stress. While page limits precluded a chapter on this topic in this book, please consult chapters 7 and 8 on nourishing yourself and simplifying your life in the author's more compact book on anxiety, *Coping with Anxiety: Ten Simple Ways to Relieve Anxiety, Fear & Worry*, second edition.

## You Fail to Address Personality and Interpersonal Issues That Perpetuate Anxiety

Cognitive behavioral therapy and exposure may help you change panic/worry-provoking thoughts and face your fears. However, they may not modify core personality traits that predispose you to be anxious in the first place. If you grew up with perfectionistic, overly controlling parents, for example, you're likely to be perfectionistic yourself. Nothing in yourself or your life ever quite meets your overdrawn standards, and so you set yourself up for continuous stress. Or if your parents were highly critical of you, you may have grown up with an excessive need to please and win approval. If you spend your life trying to please others at the expense of your own personal needs, you're likely to harbor a lot of unexpressed resentment and thus be more prone to anxiety. Insecurity, overdependency, overcautiousness, and excessive need for control are additional personality issues common to people with anxiety disorders. Such core personality traits are often associated with interpersonal problems—for example, perhaps you expect too much of your spouse or significant other (perfectionism) or you don't ask enough (excessive need to please). Or you may resent your parents' attempts to control you, but you don't assert your own needs with them.

Chapter 11, "Personality Styles That Perpetuate Anxiety," examines four major personality issues that not only predispose people to anxiety but can also contribute to relapse after effective treatment:

- Perfectionism

- Excessive need for approval

- Tendency to ignore physical and psychological signs of stress

- Excessive need for control

For each personality issue, the chapter lists a variety of constructive strategies for overcoming the adverse effects of that particular personality trait.

### You Are Confronted with Existential Issues

The problem at the root of your anxiety may lie still deeper than personality. Anxiety may persist in spite of therapy and medication because you experience a sense of emptiness or meaninglessness about your life. In the present time, with so many conflicting values and a loss of traditional authorities such as the church or consistent social norms, it's easy to feel adrift and confused. The very pace of modern life, including its emphasis on virtual rather than face-to-face communication, can lead to feelings of confusion, if not outright chaos. What has been called "existential anxiety" does not respond to cognitive behavioral therapy and demands a different kind of approach.

If your life feels meaningless and without direction, perhaps you need to discover your own unique gifts and creativity, and then find a way to meaningfully express them in the world. Each of us has a unique gift to offer—a unique contribution to make.

The first section of chapter 21, Personal Meaning, "Finding and Fulfilling Your Unique Purpose," contains a series of guidelines and exercises for identifying and pursuing your own unique purpose. First, there is a detailed questionnaire for identifying your most important personal *values*. Second, the values questionnaire is followed by exercises that enable you to identify your most important *goals*, based on your principal values. There you can list both your short-term and your long-term goals, as well as identify any possible obstacles you might encounter in the process of achieving your goals. Finally, the section takes you through a series of steps to create a *plan of action* to achieve your most important goals. A series of guidelines for carrying out your plan of action, plus a final section on making a genuine commitment to your plan, wraps up the section.

### Conclusion

Of the five different potential reasons described above for not maintaining your gains from anxiety treatment, which ones do you think might apply to you? If you perceive that you haven't fully recovered from treatment—and might be headed toward a relapse—what can you do about it? When you figure out what is needed to assure your continued recovery following anxiety treatment, your *whole life* begins to work better and you start to feel better. Your problem with panic, phobias, excessive worry, or obsessions will certainly get better, as will your depression, headaches, insomnia, or tendency to be short-tempered or irritable. *All of you gets better.*

# Watching for Hidden Signs of Potential Relapse

Relapse after partial or complete recovery from an anxiety disorder is usually unexpected. You feel confident you are doing better, that the panic attacks or phobias you might have struggled with for years seem to be receding into the background. But then you encounter a sudden, unexpected cascade of stressors. Or you unconsciously slip back into old patterns of behavior or avoidance that long ago led to the very problem with anxiety you thought you'd overcome. In this type of circumstance, you may experience a temporary setback, handle it well, and move on. However, if you don't fully move through the temporary setback, you may be headed for the possibility of a more lasting return of your anxiety problem. There are a number of *warning signs* that suggest the potential of more than just a temporary setback—that is, a more lasting relapse and return of the original anxiety problem you'd thought you had overcome.

## Cognitive Warning Signs

Certain mental tendencies or thinking patterns can signal the onset of a setback or even a potential relapse in the aftermath of recovering from anxiety.

- *You are prone to excessive or prolonged worrying.* You find that you begin to start anticipating danger or threat as you return to situations that previously evoked strong anxiety prior to effective treatment.

- *You find yourself beginning to overestimate the risk of threat or danger* of situations that therapy helped you appraise more realistically. You fail to reassess the risk realistically.

- *You try to suppress or fight against your worrying.* Rather than just accepting worry with an attitude of "Okay, it's here again, so I'll let it be there and just go about my business," you resist and try to either bury or flee from the worry.

### Constructive Response

One of the best ways to deal with cognitive warning signs, and virtually the oldest and most iconic strategy for dealing with any surge of anxiety, is Claire Weekes's famous four-step approach for accepting rather than resisting anxious thoughts: 1) accept the thoughts—don't run from them; 2) accept what your body is doing (that is, your physical anxiety sensations)—don't fight against it; 3) float with the waves of anxiety/anxious thoughts and feelings rather than trying to force your way through them; and 4) allow time to pass.

Please see chapter 6 in this book for a more complete description of these four steps. If you want to go further, you can even read one of Claire Weekes's classic books, *Hope and Help for Your Nerves* or *Peace from Nervous Suffering*.

An alternative way to handle cognitive warning signs of potential relapse is to draw on helpful coping statements, such as "This feeling isn't comfortable, but I can accept it," "This isn't the worst thing that could happen," or "This is a good opportunity to learn to cope with my fears." A list of twenty-three coping statements can be found in the section "Coping Statements" in chapter 6. When practicing coping statements, follow the guidelines in the section "Ways to Work with Coping Statements," also in chapter 6. The three most common ways to work with coping statements are 1) to write down your preferred list of coping statements every day, 2) to recite, *slowly with feeling*, your preferred list of coping statements from your written list, or 3) to record and play back your preferred list of coping statements from your smartphone. Rehearsing your coping statements frequently helps you internalize them. If you've utilized all of the above strategies for dealing with cognitive warning signs of relapse but still experience excessive worry, you may wish to consult with a therapist who specializes in working with anxiety disorders. If you previously worked with an anxiety therapist, and they are still available, you may want to see them for a few "booster sessions."

## *Physical Warning Signs of Being Overstressed*

Excess stress can lead to physical sensations that tell you that you are overdoing or overpacing your life. These physical warning signs of excessive stress can include:

- Feeling overly tired or exhausted

- Feeling sweaty

- Queasiness in your stomach

- Shaking

- Dizziness or light-headedness

- A feeling of remoteness, as if "you're not all there," often referred to as "depersonalization"

Please see the *Panic Attack Worksheet 1: Bodily Symptoms* in chapter 6 for a complete list of the types of physical sensations that could indicate at least a setback and possibly the potential for relapse toward your original anxiety disorder.

### Constructive Response

A variety of strategies for diminishing warning signs of excessive stress are described in chapter 4, Relaxation, including abdominal breathing, muscle relaxation exercises, guided visualizations for anxiety (see appendix 2 for further resources), and the regular practice of meditation (see chapter 19). Physical exercise is one of the most potent strategies for relieving symptoms of excessive stress. Chapter 5, Physical Exercise, provides detailed information and guidelines for utilizing exercise to mitigate stress.

Finally, good time management and allowing yourself sufficient downtime can go a long way toward relieving symptoms of excessive stress. See the sections "Downtime" and "Time Management" near the end of chapter 4 for a detailed discussion of both of the these major remedies for stress.

## *Safety Behaviors*

In contrast to cognitive warning signs of relapse or physical sensations of being overstressed, *safety behaviors* are self-protective behaviors you engage in to try to thwart a recurrence of anxiety. They often have a tendency to backfire. In your attempt to dodge or escape anxiety through such behaviors, you end up bringing on more anxiety.

Some common types of safety behaviors follow:

- *Excessive reassurance seeking.* For example, you have a mild headache that seems to last more than a day. You fear you might have a serious problem such as a brain tumor or subdural hematoma, so you keep calling doctors or even make appointments to see doctors to obtain reassurance for what is essentially a very common symptom (most likely a simple tension headache).

- *Procrastination.* For example, you have an upcoming exam or perhaps a performance before a group of people. Instead of giving yourself ample time to prepare, you wait to the last minute and then stress yourself out trying to adequately prepare in much too short a time.

- *Overpreparation.* Again, using the example of an upcoming exam or live performance, you spend excessive time overpreparing for it, leading to significant "anticipatory anxiety" (anxiety ahead of a somewhat demanding situation) that makes you miserable for several days before the actual event.

- *Overchecking or double-checking.* Let's say you are worrying about high blood pressure because you had a single high reading at the doctor's office (a not uncommon occurrence). So you purchase a home blood pressure cuff and repeatedly check your blood pressure at home. Even if most of your readings are in a normal range, you keep checking to make sure you are okay.

  Or, as another example of overchecking, your husband is late in getting home (perhaps due to an extended work schedule or excessive traffic), and you become worried and keep calling him, despite the fact that he provides an adequate explanation for being late. A single phone call is not enough. Of course, the situation can get much worse if your husband decides to turn off his phone in order to stop receiving repeated calls.

- *Perfectionism.* Striving for perfection is a warning sign not just for potential return of anxiety (and even relapse) but for disillusionment and even depression as well. Perfectionism often rears its head in advance of performance situations, whether speaking up in a group, making a presentation, or perhaps a live musical performance. Striving for complete perfection usually turns out to be an exercise in futility. You typically set your standards at a level that is just not realistically attainable. Then you feel self-critical or even ashamed if you don't meet your excessive expectations. For more information about perfectionism and how to deal with it, see the section on perfectionism in chapter 11, Personality Styles That Perpetuate Anxiety.

- *Overreliance on a support person.* In working on facing a long-standing phobia, it often helps to have a support person go with you. For example, if you're making your first flight after many years of avoiding flying, having someone accompany you can provide both distraction and reassurance that helps mitigate your anxiety. Or perhaps you have a phobia of going to the dentist, and you've let dental problems amass because your dental phobia has kept you away from dealing with your issues for a few years. It may be quite helpful to have someone accompany you when you make your first visit to the dentist in a long time. Just having the support person sit in the waiting room while you're having the checkup may be sufficient.

Support people are a kind of "crutch" that can help you when you first face a phobic situation you've avoided for years. However, if you keep taking your support person with you whenever you face the phobia, you will never *master* the phobia because you'll never gain the confidence that you can deal with it on your own. In order to *complete* exposure to most phobias, it eventually becomes necessary to relinquish the safety behavior of having a support person go with you. Only then can you feel fully confident about having overcome the fear. This is especially important in situations where you *really need to be able to enter a situation without needing someone to be with you* all the time, such as driving far away from home or driving on freeways.

## Constructive Response

1.  *Notice* you are engaging in safety behavior(s) in order to protect yourself from anxiety.

2.  *Expose rather than oppose.* Desist from fighting or fleeing an uncomfortable exposure situation (facing what you fear). The key to overcoming safety behaviors is *full acceptance* of the situation and an ability to *tolerate discomfort* (as long as discomfort doesn't soar to an overwhelming degree, which is very often unlikely).

3.  *Cope.* Your goal is simply to deal with an anxiety-provoking situation without falling back on safety behaviors that can undermine your progress. You can still rely on your most helpful *coping strategies* to move through exposure to an uncomfortable situation and tolerate the discomfort. Two common coping strategies are relying on abdominal breathing (see chapter 4) or utilizing coping statements, such as "I can be anxious and still deal with this situation" or "I've handled this before and I can handle it again, in spite of anxiety." (See the section "Coping Statements" in chapter 6 for a full list of possible coping statements.) A complete list of *coping strategies* can be found in the section "Coping Strategies to Counteract Panic at an Early Stage" in chapter 6. If you are merely dealing with high anxiety rather than panic attacks, you can substitute the word "anxiety" for "panic" in the heading, that is, "Coping Strategies to Counteract *Anxiety* at an Early Stage."

    **Note:** There is a very important difference between a coping strategy and a safety behavior. A coping strategy is a proactive skill you utilize to negotiate an anxiety-provoking situation. A safety behavior, on the other hand, is something you do to avoid or bypass any anxiety that might come up in facing an anxiety-provoking situation. It is an escape tactic. The attempt to escape anxiety usually backfires and only brings on more anxiety.

4.  *Consider obtaining help from a therapist* who specializes in the treatment of anxiety disorders, if you are encountering consistent difficulty in relinquishing safety behaviors in the process of dealing with panic attacks, phobias, or excessive worry.

# Summary of Things to Do

1.  Understand the difference between temporary setbacks and full relapse, as described at the beginning of this chapter.

2. Be aware of reasons why relapse might occur after effective treatment. (See "Reasons for Failing to Get Better After Treatment" above.)

3. Be cognizant of "warning signs" that can suggest the possibility of a setback or even relapse. (See "Watching for Hidden Signs of Potential Relapse" above.)

4. Embrace an attitude of *acceptance toward the discomfort of anxiety* rather than trying to escape from it.

5. Rely on your preferred coping strategies to negotiate and fulfill an attitude of approach and acceptance toward anxiety-provoking situations rather than escape. For detailed information on these coping strategies, see the "Constructive Response" sections at the end of "Cognitive Warning Signs," "Physical Warning Signs," and "Safety Behaviors" (above).

## Further Reading

McKay, Matthew, Michelle Skeen, and Patrick Fanning. *The CBT Anxiety Solution Workbook: A Breakthrough Treatment for Overcoming Fear, Worry, and Panic.* Oakland, CA: New Harbinger Publications, 2017 (see especially chapter 11).

———, Martha Davis, and Patrick Fanning. *Thoughts and Feelings: Taking Control of Your Moods and Your Life.* 4th ed. Oakland, CA: New Harbinger Publications, 2011.

Preston, John, John O'Neal, and Mary Talaga. *Handbook of Clinical Psychopharmacology for Therapists.* 8th ed. Oakland, CA: New Harbinger Publications, 2017.

# 21

# Personal Meaning

The chapters of this book up to this point have considered the physical, emotional, behavioral, and mental aspects of anxiety disorders. Guidelines have been offered for dealing with these various levels of the problem. On a bodily level, anxiety, panic, and phobias can be helped through abdominal breathing, relaxation, exercise, and/or medication. Emotionally, learning to identify and express feelings can relieve the tension that lies behind anxiety. Behaviorally, exposure can overcome phobic avoidance. On a mental level, replacing fearful self-talk and mistaken beliefs with realistic thoughts and assumptions can help reduce anxiety in all of its diverse forms.

For many people, the wide range of approaches presented up to this point will be enough to ensure recovery. Making a commitment to follow through with the program outlined in this book, whether on your own or with a therapist, will help you take back your life from anxiety. You may require a bit more, however. All the techniques described so far can help a great deal, yet for certain people they aren't quite enough. An underlying level of anxiety remains—an anxiety that comes from not having answered basic questions about the meaning and purpose of your life.

Existential psychologists such as Rollo May have used the term "existential anxiety" to refer to the type of anxiety that arises from having been unable to reach your full potential in life. This anxiety consists of a vague sense of tension, boredom, and perhaps even "quiet desperation" that arises from feeling held back, for one reason or another, from being all that you can be. You live with a feeling of incompleteness—a sense that something vital is missing—although you may not consciously recognize what it is. If someone were to ask you, "Where is your life going?" or "What do you think your life is about?" you would tend to have trouble answering. Or you might think of things that, on further reflection, don't seem "quite enough" to make your life as meaningful as you would like it to be.

For some people, a lack of purpose or meaning in life can provide fertile ground for the development of panic attacks and phobias. Although panic may be caused by a number of factors, it sometimes reflects a sudden revelation (and desperation) that your life has no obvious direction. Similarly, the fear of being trapped or confined, or "unable to escape," that underlies so many phobias *may* reflect a deeper fear of being trapped by your current circumstances in life, whether involving a dead-end career, a relationship, or any other situation that feels confining yet would require substantial risks to move beyond. Phobic avoidance, in turn, *may* reflect a deeper avoidance of the very risks that are necessary to realize your full potential and life purpose. It has been my experience with a number of clients that their anxiety disorders (it doesn't seem to matter which particular type) did not fully resolve until they found something that could give their life a greater sense of meaning *along with taking the necessary risks to embrace it*. In one case, this involved a career change, and in still another it meant cultivating a creative talent with music.

This chapter gives you the opportunity to reflect on the question of your life's meaning, purpose, and goals, as well as to explore whether spirituality might provide at least one direction in which to find answers. Spirituality is a universal concept. It refers not to any particular religion but to a basic sense of there being a larger purpose to life, as well as a larger power—a "Higher Power," if you will—that transcends the human order of things. Not only may spirituality provide life with greater meaning, but it can help overcome anxiety directly because it leads to qualities such as inner peace, serenity, faith, and unconditional love.

If you feel that meaning and spirituality are important, you may want to take a look at my book *Beyond Anxiety & Phobia: A Step-by-Step Guide to Lifetime Recovery*, which explores these topics in considerably more depth. In fact, this book presents a wide range of approaches intended to go beyond what is presented in *The Anxiety & Phobia Workbook*. It was written as a supplement or companion to the workbook. See the book listed in the "Further Reading" section at the end of this chapter.

## Finding and Fulfilling Your Unique Purpose

Each of us has one or more special purposes to fulfill that can give our life a sense of completeness. People who fulfill their special purpose often say, by the time they reach their senior years, that they feel satisfied with their life—that they did as much as they could to accomplish what they set out to do. Common examples of life purposes might include raising a family, succeeding in a fulfilling career, making a contribution to your community, developing and expressing an artistic talent, completing an educational goal and using what you've learned to serve others, overcoming an addiction or the problems of a dysfunctional childhood, and conveying what you've learned to others. Life purposes appear to have a twofold function: 1) allowing you to feel more complete and whole, and 2) allowing you in some way to serve or contribute to the betterment of others. Realizing what truly gives your life meaning and purpose is likely to carry you beyond your own personal needs and to have a beneficial impact on someone else—whether that someone is a child, the people you work for, your community, or anyone to whom you convey what you've learned from your experience. In discovering your true purpose and potential, you move beyond immediate concerns for personal security and satisfaction toward making a meaningful contribution.

If you currently feel out of touch with your life purpose, how do you go about discovering what it is? The questionnaire that follows is designed to stimulate your thinking in ways that can help you formulate your own unique values. Your answers to the questions may give you some insights into what is most important for you to do with your life. Give yourself at least one full day to reflect on these questions and write out your answers. You may even want to ponder these questions for a week or longer. After you've arrived at the answers for yourself, continue on through the sections of this chapter describing how to set goals, break each goal into a sequence of steps, and finally take committed action on each goal. Then you might want to share your answers to these questions (your personal values, goals, and timelines) with a close personal friend or counselor and get that person's input and feedback. If realizing your purpose involves making a career change, it might be helpful to work with a career counselor. If it involves going back to school, you'll want to talk to an academic guidance counselor at the school you're considering.

# *Personal Values Inventory*

1. Does the work you're presently doing express what you truly want to be doing? If not, how can you begin to take steps toward discovering and doing work that would be more personally fulfilling?

2. Are you satisfied with the education you've obtained? Would you like to go back to school and increase your education and training? If so, how can you begin to move in that direction?

3. Do you have creative outlets? Are there any areas of your life where you feel you can be creative? If not, what creative activities could you develop?

4. What kinds of interests or activities spark your enthusiasm? What do you naturally enjoy doing alone, with friends or family, outdoors or indoors?

5. What would you like to do with your life if you could do what you truly wanted? (Assume, for the purpose of this question, that money and the responsibilities of your current job and family are not a limitation.)

6. What would you like to accomplish with your life? What would you like to have accomplished by the time you reach seventy in order to feel that your life has been productive and meaningful?

7. What are your most important values? What values give your life the greatest meaning? Some examples of values include:

   - Happy family life
   - Good health

   - Peace of mind
   - Serving others

   - Material success
   - Intimacy

   - Career achievement
   - Creative expression

   - Personal growth
   - Spiritual awareness

   - Dedication to a social cause

8. Is there anything that you deeply value and yet feel you haven't fully experienced or realized in your life? What changes do you need to make—or what risks do you need to take—to more fully realize your most important values?

9. Do you have any special talents or skills that you haven't fully developed or expressed? What changes do you need to make—or what risks do you need to take—in order to develop and express your special talents and skills?

10. In light of the above questions, your most important life purposes would include the following (list):

# From Personal Values to Goals

Identifying your most important personal values is a critical first step. The next step is planning goals for your life based on your values. How do you specifically plan to embody and realize what you most value?

## *Setting and Moving Forward with Goals*

Give yourself some time—up to several days if necessary—to clarify what your most important goals are, based on the values/purposes you identified from the *Personal Values Inventory.* Think about the probable time frame for reaching these goals and write down your most important goals for each time period, using the chart below.

### *My Most Important Personal Goals*

For the next month: _____

For the next six months: _____

For the next year: _____

For the next three years: _____

Be sure your goals are realistic. Review the section "Work on Goals That Are Realistic" in the section on perfectionism in chapter 11. If you wonder whether a particular goal might be reaching too far, do a reality check by speaking about it with friends or a counselor. At the same time, don't underestimate yourself. Many goals that look difficult at the outset are attainable when broken down into a sequence of incremental steps.

## *Dealing with Obstacles Toward Goals*

Are you genuinely working toward the goals you want for your life? Or are you making excuses and setting up obstacles to the attainment of these goals? The popular phrase "taking responsibility for your life" simply means that you take full responsibility for working toward your own goals. To avoid self-responsibility is to do little or nothing about what you want and/or to expect someone else to do it for you. Avoiding self-responsibility will ensure that you'll have feelings of powerlessness, inadequacy, or even hopelessness.

What are some of the obstacles you might be putting in the way of going after what you want? *Fear* is the greatest impediment to doing something about your goals, just as it is in the case of overcoming phobias. If you don't see yourself moving toward what you want, ask whether you're letting any of the following fears get in your way:

- Fear of losing present security—for example, you can't do what you want and still make a living

- Fear of failure

- Fear of personal rejection or the disapproval of others

- Fear of succeeding (then what would you have to deal with!)

- Fear of your goal involving too much work

- Fear of your goal involving too much time

- Fear of your goal involving too much energy

- Fear that your goal is too unrealistic—for example, that others will discourage you

- Fear of change itself

The solution to such fears about taking action on your life goals is the same as the solution to dealing with a phobia: *face the fear and go forward in steps.* There is no way to eliminate some risk and discomfort in achieving a major goal, but breaking the goal down into sufficiently small steps (much like you would for exposure to a phobia, see chapter 7) will enable you to go forward.

While fear can be a major obstacle in moving forward on your goals, guilt can also be an impediment. You may wish to consider whether any of the following beliefs are keeping you from seeking what you want:

"I'm not good enough to have _____."

"I don't deserve to have _____."

"No one in my family has ever done something like that before."

"Others won't approve if I go after _____."

"No one will accept this idea if I try to put it into practice."

The first two beliefs really could have been listed under fears, but they also involve guilt. To overcome the feeling of not deserving to achieve your goal, you might want to work intensively with the simple affirmation "I deserve" or "I deserve to have _____." Don't be sparing in the use of repetition with this particular affirmation. Continue to work with it until you develop an emotional conviction that it is true. Developing the conviction that you deserve what you truly want will add significantly to your self-esteem.

## Develop a Plan of Action

After you've worked through specific obstacles to taking action on your goals, it's time to develop a plan of action. Break each of your goals down into a sequence of steps. Remember that this is a long-range plan. As an option, you may wish to specify a time frame for accomplishing each step. Be sure that you reward yourself after the accomplishment of each step, just as you would working through the steps of exposure to a phobia. You might ask family members or friends for their support in your undertaking.

Use the worksheet below to list specific steps you might take to progress toward an important personal goal. If you want to pursue more than one goal, make photocopies of the sheet—or download the version on the website associated with this book (see the last page of this book for more details). You may find that you can clarify specific steps more easily by talking about them with a friend or counselor.

A plan of action gives you a map to follow in going after what you want. You can refer to it as you monitor your progress or if you get stuck at any time along the way. If you have trouble with any particular step, you may need to investigate once again whether fears or feelings of guilt are getting in your way.

## *Plan of Action: Steps Toward Your Goal*

1.  Your goal (be as specific as possible):

    _____

    _____

2.  What small step can you take right now to make some progress toward achieving this goal?

    _____

    _____

3.  What other steps will you need to take to achieve this goal? (Estimate the time required to complete each step.)

    _____

    _____

### *Example*

You might be feeling increasingly dissatisfied with your present line of work and would like to do something else. Yet you're not quite sure about what you want to do, let alone how to go about training for it. The broad goal of "getting into another line of work" might seem a bit overwhelming, taken as a whole. But if you break it down into its component parts, it becomes more manageable:

1. Find a career counselor you respect (or take a course in exploring career options at a local college).

2. Explore different options by:

   - *Working with the counselor or taking an appropriate course.*

   - *Reading about different vocations* in such books as *What Color Is Your Parachute?* and the *Occupational Outlook Handbook.*

   - *Talking to people who hold positions in vocations you feel drawn to.*

3. Narrow down vocational options to one particular type of work. (Obtain whatever help you need to do this.) Focus is extremely important in achieving goals.

4. Obtain education or training for the line of work you've chosen.
   Find out where training is available in your area through internet research or by speaking directly to people already involved in the type of work.

   - *Apply to appropriate schools or training programs.*

   - *Apply for an educational grant or loan if your education or training will require a full-time commitment.*

5. Complete your education or training (if possible while maintaining your current job).

6. Search for an entry-level position in your new career.

   - *Obtain resources that tell you where jobs are available* (professional or trade newsletters, journals, alumni organizations, newspapers, and job hotlines and websites are all good resources).

   - *Prepare a professional-looking resume.*

   - *Apply for jobs.*

   - *Go for interviews.*

7. Begin your new career.

## Take Committed Action

You've identified your most important values and developed specific step-by-step goals to fulfill them. The final step is to make a genuine commitment to carry out the action plan you've devised for each goal.

Taking action is work. It involves making time in your schedule—or your entire life—to focus on moving forward with goal-related steps you've planned out in advance. It also involves courage, a willingness to work through any anxiety that may come up in confronting certain steps along your path (such as interviewing for a job, completing final exams, or taking incremental steps in facing a phobia). A critical ingredient is perseverance. Make your best effort to follow through on all of the steps toward attaining a goal. When obstacles and setbacks interrupt your progress, accept these as part of the process, work through any temporary fear or frustration that comes up, and then continue forward until you've reached your goal. The ultimate reward is the knowledge that you are acting upon your genuine values and realizing your unique purpose(s)—what you came into the world to do.

In sum, finding and fulfilling your unique life purpose is a three-part process: 1) *identifying your most important values*, 2) *setting specific goals*, with a specific sequence of incremental steps to achieve each goal, and 3) *taking committed action* to achieve each goal.

You may be interested to know that there is a branch of therapy called acceptance and commitment therapy (ACT for short) that provides a technology for conducting these three steps. Before working with values and goals, ACT places special emphasis on *acceptance*—dropping the struggle with or resistance to whatever current limitations exist in your life. The other key aspect of ACT is *commitment*—making a genuine commitment to change what you want to change in your life. Readers interested in exploring ACT, which also includes a component of mindfulness practice, might take a look at some of the basic ACT primers, such as *ACT Made Simple* by Russ Harris and *The Mindfulness & Acceptance Workbook for Anxiety* by John Forsyth and Georg Eifert.

### Life Purpose Visualization

To assist you in your journey toward finding personal meaning, write a scenario on a sheet of paper of what your life would look like if you were to fully realize your unique life purpose(s). You can design separate visualizations for each purpose or incorporate the realization of all of your life purposes into a single description. Be sure to make your scenario sufficiently detailed to include where you're living and working, whom you are with, what activities make up your day, and what a typical day would look like. Once you've completed a detailed description, read it over thoughtfully on a regular basis. You might also want to record it, preferably in your own voice. You may want to begin your recording with a few minutes of preliminary instructions to relax. Visualizing the fulfillment of your life purpose on a regular, consistent basis can go a long way toward accelerating the process of actually realizing your goals.

# Spirituality

This section on spirituality is included because many clients of mine have achieved breakthroughs in their condition as the result of developing their spiritual life. If this section speaks to you, then it may serve to motivate you to cultivate your spirituality. If you already have a deep spiritual commitment, what follows may simply reinforce what you know rather than teach you anything new. Conversely, if this section seems repellent or inapplicable, you need not feel compelled to read it or incorporate it into your recovery program. You can entirely overcome your particular problem with anxiety by relying on the strategies and guidelines presented in previous chapters of this workbook.

Spirituality involves the recognition and acceptance of a Higher Power beyond your own intelligence and will, with whom you can have a relationship. This Higher Power can provide you with an experience of inspiration, awe, joy, security, peace of mind, and guidance that goes beyond what is possible in the absence of the conviction that such a power exists.

For our purposes here, spirituality can be seen as being distinct from religion. Different world religions have proposed various doctrines and belief systems about the nature of a Higher Power and humanity's relationship with it. Spirituality, on the other hand, refers to the *common experience* behind these various points of view—an experience involving an awareness of and a relationship with something that transcends your personal self as well as the human order of things. This "something" has been given various names ("God" being the most popular in Western society) and defined in ways that are too numerous to count. For the purposes of this chapter, it can be referred to as a (or "your") *Higher Power.* You can choose to define what that means for yourself in whatever way feels most appropriate. Your own sense of a Higher Power can be as abstract as "cosmic consciousness" or "cosmic intelligence" or as down-to-earth as the beauty of the ocean or mountains. It can be quite personal, as in the case of Jesus, Mohammed, or Krishna. Even if you regard yourself as an agnostic or atheist, you may get a sense of inspiration from taking a walk in the forest or contemplating a beautiful sunset. Or a small child's smile may give you a special sense of joy. Whatever inspires you, fills you with awe, or takes you beyond yourself into a larger perspective points in the direction of what is referred to here as your Higher Power.

The purpose of this section is to emphasize that there is much healing and benefit to be obtained by cultivating your spiritual life (if that is something you feel drawn to or feels right for you). Of all the methods and guidelines suggested in this workbook, a personal spiritual commitment is likely to reach the deepest in helping you overcome the basic sense of fear or insecurity that underlies the various types of anxiety disorders. Whereas other methods described in previous chapters work at different levels—body, feelings, mind, or behavior—spiritual awareness and growth can effect a transformation in your whole being. It can help you develop a basic trust and faith that is unshakable. Of course, the other methods described in previous chapters are still important and necessary. Please keep in mind that the ideas and exercises presented in this chapter are not a substitute for working with all of the other strategies and skills in this book.

A number of my clients have experienced major turnarounds in their condition as a result of cultivating their spirituality. Developing a relationship with their Higher Power did not necessarily cure a specific phobia or obsession, but it provided the moral support, courage, hope, and faith for them to follow through with their personal recovery program. It provided them with a sense that they are not alone in the universe and that there is a source of guidance and support that is available at times of confusion and discouragement.

## The Impact of Spirituality

Beyond cognitive behavioral therapy, spirituality has a special role to play in recovery from anxiety:

- It can increase your belief and hope that recovery is possible.

- It can provide a way to handle more severe and chronic anxiety disorders.

- It can lead to distinct changes in personality, attitude, and behavior that increase your ability to cope with an anxiety disorder.

- It can provide a more positive frame of reference for perceiving your difficulties with anxiety (or life in general). An attitude of focusing on what seems to be an arbitrary hardship that is insurmountable can shift to one of seeing it as an opportunity to grow and evolve as a human being.

What are some of the specific benefits to be gained by developing your spirituality? Before enumerating several of these, it is important to understand that no one pursues spiritual growth in order to "get" such benefits. You choose to develop yourself spiritually only because you feel a deep, inner prompting to do so. The benefits are simply consequences that follow from choosing to cultivate a relationship with your Higher Power. If you have already developed your spiritual life, you will understand the benefits listed below.

## Security and Safety

A sense of inner security and safety is especially important if you frequently deal with anxiety, worries, panic attacks, or phobias. Through developing a connection with your Higher Power, you gain security through the conviction that you are not all alone in the universe, even at those times when you feel temporarily separated from other people. You feel increasingly safe as you come to believe that there is a source you can always turn to in times of difficulty. There is much security to be gained through the understanding that there is no problem or difficulty, however great, that cannot be resolved through the help of your Higher Power.

## Peace of Mind

Peace of mind is the result of feeling a deep, abiding sense of security and safety. The more reliance and trust you develop in your Higher Power, the easier it becomes to deal, without fear or worry, with the inevitable challenges life brings. It's not that you give up your self or your will to such a power; rather, you simply learn that you can "let go" and turn to your Higher Power when you feel stuck with a problem in life and don't know how to proceed. Learning how to let go when solutions to problems aren't immediately apparent can help reduce worry and anxiety in your life. Peace of mind is what develops in the absence of such anxiety.

## Self-Confidence

As you develop a relationship with your Higher Power, you come to remember that you did not create yourself. You are reminded that you are a part of the universe of creation, as much so as the mountains, stars, and all wildlife. If this is a benign and supportive universe we live in—and developing a relationship with your Higher Power will help you believe that it is—then in essence you're good, lovable, and worthy of respect just by virtue of the fact that you're here. However you behave—whatever choices you make—you are still inherently good and worthwhile. Your own judgments of yourself, however negative, do not ultimately count if you are a creation of the universe like everything else. As one person humorously put it, "God doesn't make junk." (It is, of course, a mistake to assume that this type of reasoning can be used to justify ignorant or unethical behavior. It's important to keep in mind the distinction between how a person behaves and what a person is in essence.)

## Relinquishing an Excessive Need for Control

Worry has to do with predicting unfavorable outcomes associated with situations you can't fully control. By worrying, you provide yourself with an illusion of control. If you worry about something enough, you feel that somehow you might prevent it. Somehow you won't be caught unexpectedly off guard. If you were to stop worrying, you imagine that you would give up control.

Spiritual growth, regardless of the tradition or approach you follow, encourages the cultivation of a willingness to surrender control. Without relinquishing self-responsibility, you allow your Higher Power (however defined) to have some influence in determining the outcome of situations you feel you can't fully control. Being able, at times, to just turn over your worries to a Higher Power can relieve some of the burden you think you have to carry in order to solve your problems. For further information on dealing with worry, see chapter 10, Overcoming Worry.

## Ability to Gain Distance from Conditioned Emotional Reaction Patterns

Spiritual practices, particularly mindfulness meditation (see chapter 19, Meditation) can help you become more in touch with your *unconditioned inner self*. This is a deep, inner state of consciousness, beyond ego, that is always still and at peace no matter what melodramas you may be caught up with in your mind. Moving into your unconditioned self is like reaching a calm oasis beyond anything you might be anxious about. Such a state can be deliberately cultivated if you're willing to make the time for it.

Some ways to do so include meditation, quiet time devoted to inspirational reading, inspirational music, guided visualizations, or physical disciplines such as yoga or tai chi.

## The Capacity to Give and Receive Unconditional Love

The most fundamental characteristic of your Higher Power is that it offers you an experience of unconditional love. This is a kind of love that differs from romantic love or even ordinary friendship. It involves an absolute caring for the welfare of another, without any conditions. That is, no matter how another person appears or acts, you have compassion and care for him or her without judgment. As you develop a deeper connection with your Higher Power, you come to experience greater degrees of unconditional love in your life. You feel your heart opening more easily to people and their concerns. You feel freer of judgment toward them or of making comparisons among them. Unconditional love shows up in your increased capacity both to give love to others and to experience more of it coming into your life. You begin to experience less fear and more joy in your life and help inspire others to experience their own capacity for unconditional love. This kind of love also manifests itself through the experience of having everything you need in your life to get on with what you want to do. This is spoken of in the Bible by the saying "Seek ye first the Kingdom, and all will be added unto you."

## Guidance

Developing a relationship with your Higher Power will provide you with guidance for making decisions and solving problems. Your Higher Power has a universal wisdom that goes beyond what you can accomplish through your own intellect. In traditional religions, this has been referred to as the "all-knowingness of God" or "divine intelligence." Through connecting with your Higher Power, you can draw upon this greater wisdom to help you resolve all kinds of difficulties. You have probably already experienced this aspect of your Higher Power at moments when you've felt a deep conviction about something or have had an intuitive flash that turns out to be quite accurate. By learning to ask your Higher Power for guidance, you'll be surprised to find that every sincere request sooner or later is answered. Furthermore, the quality of that answer generally exceeds what you could have figured out through your own conscious intellect or will.

These are some—by no means all—of the characteristics that define a close relationship with your Higher Power. All of them can contribute in a significant way to your personal recovery process. Keep in mind that there are many different paths you can take in coming into a greater awareness of your Higher Power. The particular path you choose, whether traditional or non-traditional, is up to you. The extent and sincerity of your commitment to your chosen path will determine the degree of personal healing you experience.

# Changes in Beliefs Associated with Spirituality

Developing spiritually not only leads to new experiences and changes in the way you feel, but it also can lead to a shift in your basic beliefs and assumptions about life and the world. As you develop spiritually, many of your beliefs about the meaning of life in general, and what your life is about specifically, can shift dramatically. As these basic beliefs change, your view of your condition—your personal struggle with anxiety—also begins to change.

These shifts in beliefs can lead to having more compassion and tolerance toward yourself, as well as to finding a deeper meaning in the challenges you face, instead of viewing them as arbitrary and meaningless. You may feel less like a victim who has a particular problem with anxiety. Instead, you may come to regard your condition as an *opportunity* to grow and expand who you are.

The following is a list of ten assumptions that are frequently associated with spirituality. They are not taken from any one source, tradition, or creed, but are based on my personal experience. Although they represent my own personal point of view, these ideas have been useful points of departure for discussion with a number of my clients. As you read through the ideas, give consideration to those that fit or make sense to you and feel free to discard those that do not. Each of us has a basic philosophy about life that we have to formulate for ourselves.

Some of these ideas may stimulate questions that you may want to discuss with a significant other, a trusted friend, or even a minister, priest, or rabbi. All of the ideas can lead to a more optimistic and tolerant view of life. As you adopt any of these ideas that fit for you, you may find your attitude about your condition—as well as life in general—becoming a little more positive and a little less burdensome.

### 1. Life is a school. The primary meaning and purpose of life is that it is a "classroom" for growth in consciousness.

Most people tend to define their life's meaning in terms of those people, activities, self-images, or objects to which they attach the greatest value. Whatever you value most in life—whether family, another individual, work, a particular role or self-image, your health, or material possessions—these things are probably what define your life's meaning. If you lost what you valued the most, your life might seem to lose its meaning. Think for a moment about what you value most highly in your life and what gives you the greatest satisfaction and comfort. Then imagine what your life would be like if these things were all suddenly taken away.

The truth, of course, is that everything you value most *will* eventually pass away. Nothing that you cherish lasts forever. Yet if everything you value must someday cease to be, what is the *ultimate* meaning of life? As long as you assume that there is nothing more to existence than your present life—what there is right now—then there doesn't seem to be *any* ultimate meaning. You end up saying (along with Jean-Paul Sartre and other existentialists) that the only meaning life has is what you make of it in the present moment. Apart from this, life appears to have no meaning in and of itself. Since everything, including life itself, eventually passes away, how can there be any ultimate point to any of it?

Most forms of spirituality, traditional and modern, move beyond this existential predicament. Most of them make some kind of assumption that human life is *not* all there is. Something of us persists beyond human life, and so life comes to be seen as a temporary sojourn—not the final destination. Life comes to be understood as a preparation or training ground for something else that cannot be fully understood or revealed while you are alive.

It is this particular interpretation of life's "ultimate" meaning that many people have found to be most valid and helpful. If the final meaning of life is that it is a *classroom* or *school* for growth in consciousness—for the development of wisdom and the capacity to love—then the fact that everything passes away takes on an entirely new meaning. The tasks and challenges that come up in life, and your response to them, do not have eternal repercussions. Nor do they have no meaning at all. They are more like lessons in a school, lessons to which you apply yourself and that you try to master as best you can. Each lesson is repeated until it is mastered. As you master old lessons, new ones are put before you. This "earth school" is thus a place where you learn and grow; it is not your final dwelling place. Eventually, it is time to leave this classroom and move on.

### 2. Adversity and difficult situations are lessons designed for your growth— they are not random, capricious acts of fate. In the larger scheme of things, everything happens for a purpose.

If you accept the idea that life is a classroom, then the adversity and difficulties that come into your life may be viewed as part of the curriculum—as lessons for growth. This is a very different point of view from one that sees life's misfortunes as random quirks of fate. The latter perspective leads to a sense of victimization. You can end up feeling powerless in a capricious world that appears to be completely inequitable in its treatment of people, some of whom have such good luck, while others have misfortune heaped upon them.

The view proposed here is that the difficulties of life are lessons to promote growth in wisdom, compassion, love, and other positive qualities (some religious traditions refer to "tests"). The greater the difficulty, the greater the potential for learning and growth. If you accept this idea, then the next question you may ask is this: Who establishes the curriculum or "assigns" your life lessons? Many of us may ask this question in one form or another when a given life challenge seems particularly difficult. We tend to protest and even rail against some of the misfortunes and limitations we're faced with. The question arises, "How could a loving God permit this?"

There is no easy answer to this question. None of us can fully understand how our life lessons are administered and assigned, though different spiritual traditions have different views on this matter (Eastern traditions speak of "karma," while Judeo-Christian traditions speak of "tests" and "temptations"). Each of us has to struggle with the challenges life brings without fully understanding why. What does seem apparent is that growth could not occur if the lessons were *always* easy. If the purpose of life is for us to grow in wisdom, consciousness, and compassion, then at least some of the lessons need to be difficult. This may not be an altogether consoling view, but it at least makes some sense out of the difficult situations that occur in life.

Given this view, you can stop asking, "Why did this happen to me?" and instead ask the more constructive questions: "What is this meant to teach me?" and "What can be learned from this?" You might take whatever worry or concern is bothering you the most in your life at this time and try asking the latter two questions instead of the first.

**3. Your personal limitations and flaws are the grist you have to work with for your inner growth. Sometimes you can heal and overcome them with modest effort. In other cases, they may stay with you for a long time in order to push you to evolve and develop to your fullest potential. You are not wrong or in any way to blame because of your limitations.**

Think for a moment about some of your own personal limitations—the ones you find most difficult to live with. If you are dealing with an anxiety disorder, think about your condition. You may ask why anyone should have to deal with a difficult condition such as panic disorder, agoraphobia, social phobia, or an obsessive-compulsive disorder for even a few months, let alone a longer time. Hopefully, you have utilized all of the best treatments—including medication, if necessary—and have experienced a significant and genuine recovery. In some cases, a full recovery from an anxiety disorder is certainly possible. Suppose, however, that you have received all the best treatments, worked very hard for one or two years, and have experienced a partial improvement—yet you are still dealing with your condition to a degree. Is that a reason for you to think of yourself as a failure? A reason to think that you are somehow less skillful or persistent than those people who overcame their condition quickly?

If you've worked hard on overcoming your condition but are still troubled by it, perhaps there is some significant growth experience to find in the process of having to work with your difficulty for a long time. It all depends upon the lesson you happen to be learning. Having a difficult condition that is easily dispensed with in a short time would certainly help develop your confidence in your own self-mastery—an important lesson in itself. Yet it wouldn't necessarily develop qualities of compassion or patience. It often seems that only by having to struggle with our own infirmities for a long time can we fully learn how to feel compassion or have patience with others' difficulties.

As a second example, suppose that your lesson is to learn how to let go of the excessive need for control—even more, to learn how to let go and allow your Higher Power or God to have an impact on your life. One way (not the only way) this might be learned is to have to deal with a difficult situation in which all your efforts to control it just don't work. The ability to let go of control is often fostered by those very difficulties in life that are most challenging. Some conditions and situations are so challenging that they *compel* us to let go. There is no other alternative. To struggle or fight against the condition only creates more distress and suffering. It is often at the exact moment when you fully let go of your worry or stop struggling that you may experience some kind of response or relief from your Higher Power. To let go and trust in your Higher Power should not be thought of as relinquishing responsibility for your life. Rather, it involves doing all you can to help yourself first, and then turning things over to another source of assistance.

In sum, it is a mistake to fault yourself for having any intractable condition, no matter how disabling or how long you've had it. It is there to foster and deepen certain qualities of your inner self. *How you respond to it and what you learn from it are what's important—not the condition itself.*

### 4. Your life has a creative purpose and mission. There is something creative that is yours to develop and offer.

Your life is not a random sequence of accidental events but follows a plan. This plan is *created* from a level that none of us can fully understand. Part of this plan consists of the lessons for growth in consciousness that were described in the preceding three sections.

Another very important aspect of the plan is your creative endowments, talents, or "gifts." Each of us has at least one personal form of creativity that can give our life meaning and purpose. The development and full expression of your creative talents and gifts is your "life purpose" or "life mission" spoken of earlier in this chapter.

Your life purpose is something that you feel you *need* to do in order to feel whole, complete, and fulfilled in your life. It's uniquely your own—something that can't be duplicated. Only you can do it. It comes from within, and it has nothing to do with what your parents, partner, or friends might want you to do. Generally, it moves you beyond yourself and has an impact on something or someone else.

Your purpose or mission can be a vocation or an avocation—its scope can extend to the entire world or to just one other person. Examples include raising a family, mastering a musical instrument, volunteering your services to help youth or the elderly, writing poems, speaking eloquently before groups, or tending a garden in your backyard.

Until you develop and express your creative gifts, your life will seem incomplete. You will feel more anxiety because you are not making time to do what you truly want to do, what you were, in fact, born to do. The first part of this chapter was designed to help you get in touch with your creative purpose and mission as well as design goals to achieve it. If you are not quite sure yet what it is, you may want to discuss your answers to the *Personal Values Inventory* at the beginning of this chapter with a trusted friend or counselor.

### 5. A Higher Source of support and guidance is always available.

This idea is the basis of this entire section on spirituality. Much fear and anxiety is based on the perception that you are separate and alone—or else it is based on the anticipation of rejection or loss that might eventually result in your being separate and alone. The truth is that you are not alone. Even at those times when you might find it difficult to turn to other human beings for support, there remains another source of support that can always be called on. Your Higher Power is not merely an abstract entity that created and sustains the universe. It is a force, power, or presence with which you can enter into a personal relationship. This relationship is as personal as any you could have with another human being.

In this personal relationship, you can experience both *support* and *guidance*. Support often appears in the form of inspiration or enthusiasm that can help lift and sustain you at times of low motivation and discouragement. Guidance can come in the form of clear insights and intuitions that provide discrimination and direction about what you need to do. Frequently, this type of inspired insight or realization is wiser than anything you might have figured out with your rational mind.

You may experience a dilemma about this. If you think of inspiration and intuition originating in your own subconscious mind, how do they come then from a Higher Power—from something seemingly separate from you? Certainly from the perspective of the conscious mind, everything does seem separate—you perceive yourself as separate from others, from the world, and most likely from a Higher Power. There is another level, though, that the conscious mind can't comprehend, where all things are joined. Eastern philosophy refers to this as "the One in which all things reside." The modern physicist David Bohm speaks of the "implicate order" in which everything is interconnected. In the Bible (New Testament), this idea is expressed in the statement "The Kingdom of Heaven is within you."

To receive support and guidance from your Higher Power, you simply need to ask. Nothing more is necessary. While this might seem easy enough, it may not be in practice if you believe that you're supposed to figure out and handle everything entirely on your own. Or it may not be easy if you feel that it's irrational, weak, or in some other way beneath your dignity to rely on an invisible power for support. To trust and rely on your Higher Power takes a certain willingness to let go of control as well as a certain humility—it's often humbling to come to the realization that you can't handle something completely on your own. The ability to let go and trust is something that can be learned. Often the life lessons that are the hardest—the ones that push you to your absolute limit—tend to be the ones that have the most to teach about letting go.

As you increasingly learn to allow your Higher Power (or Spirit) to assist in your life, you can grow in trusting that it is sometimes appropriate to relinquish control.

### 6. Contact with your Higher Power is directly available within your personal experience.

You can discover a personal relationship with your Higher Power within your own immediate experience. It is as personal a relationship as any you might have with another human being.

It is a two-way relationship. You can receive support, guidance, inspiration, peace of mind, inner strength, hope, and many other gifts from your Higher Power; you can also communicate your needs to Spirit through prayer and directly communicate feelings of gratitude and reverence. Such a relationship can deepen and grow to the extent that you choose to give it attention and time.

There are numerous ways in which your Higher Power can manifest in your personal experience. Some fairly common examples follow:

- Feeling supported by a loving presence.

- An inner knowing or intuitive recognition—some deep insight comes to you and you have a clear, unequivocal sense that it is true.

- After a period of stress or struggle, you suddenly feel an influx of calmness or peace. Because it comes to you without any effort on your part, there is a sense that it comes from a place beyond your personal ego.

- Feelings of awe and wonder when beholding the beauty of nature.

- Visionary experiences—actually having a visual impression within or outside of your mind of a spiritual being or presence.

- Synchronicities—something in the outside world coincidentally matches what is going on in your mind. It feels like more than just a coincidence. For example, you're obsessively worrying about something while driving and a car pulls in front of you with a personalized license plate that say, "Let Go."

- Miracles—for example, spontaneous healings that defy medical explanation.

As you read this, think about some of the ways in which you have experienced the presence of a Higher Power within your own life. There are many forms other than those listed above.

## 7. Questions sincerely asked of your Higher Power are answered.

This idea is really an extension of the previous point about your Higher Power being a source of support and guidance. The reason for making this point separately is to underscore the fact that your Higher Power's support and guidance are not only bestowed on you—you can deliberately ask for them. The famous quote of Jesus "Ask and you shall receive" is true regardless of the particular spiritual tradition or orientation you follow.

It is the assumption of all religious approaches that incorporate prayer that prayer will be answered. Perhaps you have had experiences of your prayers being answered. It often seems that the degree of earnestness of your request has something to do with how readily the prayer receives a response. A common example is when you feel overwhelmed with some situation and you almost literally cry out for help to your Higher Power. In many, if not most, cases, something about the situation improves or shifts, often within a short time.

There is actually scientific research that confirms the efficacy of prayer. Several well-controlled empirical studies of prayer are reported in the book *One Mind* by Larry Dossey, MD.

In sum, there is both anecdotal and research support for the idea that prayer is effective. This doesn't mean that whatever you pray for will come true. There are some qualifications that, in my experience, need to be kept in mind: 1) the request or plea needs to be made with genuine earnestness and sincerity, 2) the "answer" or response to prayer may not come immediately—it may take days, weeks, or months, and 3) the answer may not come all at once—instead, only a step in the direction of the answer may come (for example, if you're praying for healing from chronic pain, the answer may come in the form of a strong intuition to visit a particular doctor or healing practitioner). Prayer can be answered in many ways, and sometimes the answer may not be what you expected. It is not possible to know in advance how a particular prayer will be answered (that is where faith comes in). What can be trusted is that there will be an answer, and that answer will serve your highest good.

### 8. What you truly ask for or intend from the deepest level of yourself— from your heart—will tend to come to you.

One of the most powerful things that can foster positive change and healing is a sincerely held intention. The power of intention can promote miraculous consequences. What you believe in and commit to with your whole heart tends to come true. When the intention is for your own highest good—and when it doesn't conflict with anyone else's highest good—it is most likely to become manifest.

A deeply held intention shifts and focuses your own consciousness. It also appears to have ramifications on events in the world apart from you. Events in the outer world will tend to align with your most deeply held intention. The famous German poet and novelist Goethe summed this up in the following famous remarks:

Concerning all acts of initiative or creation,
there is one elementary truth;

The ignorance of which kills countless ideas and splendid plans:
the moment one definitely commits oneself,
then Providence moves too.

All sorts of things occur to help one
that would never otherwise have occurred.

A whole stream of events issue from the decision,
raising in one's favor
all manner of unforeseen incidents and assistance,
which no person could have dreamt
would have come their way.

**9. Love is stronger than fear. Pure, unconditional love emanates from your Higher Power (God) and is at the very center of your being and all beings. All fears can be understood as different forms of separation: separation from others, ourselves, and God—separation from the love that unites all things.**

Love is stronger than fear because it goes deeper. On a conscious level, love is the experience of feeling your heart go out toward unity with someone or something other than yourself. On a deeper level, love is the "ground state" or essential foundation of the entire universe. This is a view that is common to both Eastern and Western religions. Love is not something we either possess or do not possess, because it literally *defines* what we are at our core and in essence. Fear may go deep but never as deep as love, because fear arises only when we feel separate from the ground state of love that unifies us with everything else.

The popular phrase "We are all one" expresses the truth about love and is, on a level beyond what our conscious mind can fully comprehend, literally true.

Most of the anxiety you experience may be related to specific fears of abandonment, rejection and humiliation, loss of control, confinement, injury, or death. Fear can take on any of these forms, based on your conditioning and past experience. Yet none of these fears could ever arise if you did not experience separation. The existence of fear always points to a degree of separation—separation of your conscious mind from your innermost being, separation from others, and/or separation from God. If it is true that in essence all of us are united as one, then every fear we feel—no matter how much we believe it—is, in fact, just an illusion. If we could perceive things the way they truly are, there would be no reason to have any more fear.

Love and fear constitute perhaps the most profound duality in human existence. Yet ultimately the former can always overcome the latter.

**10. Death is not an end but a transition. Our essential nature or soul survives physical death. (To fear death as "the end" is simply an illusion.)**

This basic idea is shared by all of the world's religions. They all assume that an individual's soul continues to exist after physical death, although they differ somewhat in their conceptions about the nature of the afterlife.

Actual evidence for this view has emerged in the past twenty-five years from the widespread research on "near-death experiences." As you most likely already know, near-death experiences are based on reports of what people experienced between the time when their vital signs indicated imminent or actual death and when they were subsequently revived. These reports all share several things, such as passing through a tunnel, meeting a being of light that radiates love and understanding, witnessing a scene-by-scene review of your entire life, and sometimes meeting relatives who have already died. A smaller number of these reports describe otherworldly scenes and locales associated with the events that are experienced. Though the thousands of such reports that have been collected worldwide don't "prove" that consciousness survives death, they certainly make a strong case in that direction. Further evidence that near-death survivors get a peek into an afterlife comes from the fact that many of them lose their fear of death and become more deeply spiritual following their experience. If what they went through was simply a dream, why would it have such a deep and lasting impact?

Does fear of death come up for you or underlie other fears you might have about sickness or injury? If so, you might want to look at the literature on near-death experiences and come to your own conclusions about life after death. The classic book in the field is *Life After Life* by Raymond Moody, but there are a large number of other good books on the topic. An Amazon search of books on the topic "life after death" or "afterlife" will bring up numerous books on the topic.

## Your Concept and Relationship with Your Higher Power

The previous section presented some suggested views about spirituality. What are your own specific views? Take some time to reflect on the following questions. Write your response in the spaces provided or on a separate piece of paper.

1.  What does the idea of God or a Higher Power mean to you personally?

2.  Describe the attributes defining your notion of God, Spirit, or a Higher Power. When you think about the nature of your Higher Power, what ideas and images come to mind?

3.  Do you experience a personal, conscious connection with your Higher Power? How have you experienced this connection?

4.  What obstacles do you feel interfere with your acceptance and/or experience of a Higher Power?

5.  What would you hope to gain by developing and/or deepening your connection with a Higher Power?

# Options for Developing Your Spiritual Life

## *Exercise 1: Spirituality and Your View of Your Condition*

Go back over the ten assumptions described in the earlier section "Changes in Beliefs Associated with Spirituality" and then complete the previous section "Your Concept and Relationship with Your Higher Power."

In the light of the proposed ideas about spirituality, as well as your own ideas about a Higher Power, how do these views affect your perspective on your particular anxiety condition? Your view of life in general? On a separate sheet of paper, write down your answers to these two questions.

## *Exercise 2: Connecting with Your Higher Power*

This exercise is intended to help you get in touch with your Higher Power and obtain assistance to deal with any issue causing you worry or anxiety. Use the exercise only if it feels appropriate to you. (You may have your own methods of prayer and meditation that you prefer.) Give yourself time to get relaxed and centered first before working with the affirmations and visualization.

1.  Get comfortable in a seated position (or lie down if you prefer). Spend at least five minutes using any technique you wish to get relaxed. You can do abdominal breathing or progressive muscle relaxation, visualize going to your peaceful place, or meditate. (See chapter 4 for instructions on specific relaxation techniques.)

2.  If you're not already aware of it, bring to mind the situation, person, or whatever it is that you are worried or anxious about. Focus on this for several moments until you have it clearly in mind. If feelings of anxiety come up, allow yourself to feel them.

3.  Affirm over and over, with as much conviction as you can,

    "I turn this over to my Higher Power (or God)."

    "I release this problem to my Higher Power (or God)."

    Simply repeat these statements slowly, calmly, and with feeling as many times as you wish until you begin to feel better. While doing this, it is good to bring to mind the following ideas about your Higher Power:

    •   It is "all knowing"—in other words, it has wisdom and intelligence that go beyond your conscious capacity to perceive solutions to problems.

    •   In its greater wisdom, your Higher Power has a solution to whatever you're worried about.

    •   Even though you can't see the solution to your worry right now, you can affirm faith that there is no problem that can't be resolved through the help of your Higher Power.

4.  If you are visually inclined, imagine that you're going to meet your Higher Power. You might see yourself in a garden or a beautiful setting of your choice, and then imagine that you see a figure—your Higher Power—approaching you. It may be indistinct at first and grow gradually clearer. You may notice that this figure exudes love and wisdom. It might be a wise old man or woman, a being of light, Jesus, the supreme being in your particular religion, or any other presence that adequately represents your Higher Power.

5.  While in the presence of your Higher Power—whether you visualize it or not—simply find a way to ask for help. For example, you might say, "I ask for your help and guidance with _____." Keep repeating your request until you feel better. You may want to listen to see if your Higher Power has an immediate answer or an insight to offer you about your request. It is quite all right, though, simply to make your request and ask for help without getting an answer. The purpose of this process is to develop trust and belief in your Higher Power (what has traditionally been called "faith in God"). The key to this part of the process is an attitude of genuine humility. By asking for help from your Higher Power, you relinquish some of your conscious control of the situation and exercise a willingness to trust.

6.  *Optional:* If it feels appropriate, visualize a beam of white light going to that place in your body that feels anxious or worried. Often this might be the solar plexus region (in the middle of your torso right below the center of your rib cage) or the "pit" of your stomach. Let that area be filled with the light until the anxiety dissolves or fades away. Keep directing white light to that region until it settles down and is free of anxiety.

Give this entire process time. It may be necessary to persist with it for as long as a half hour in order to feel a genuine connection with your Higher Power and a deeply felt trust that the problem you're worried about can truly be resolved. If, after completing this process, your worry comes back the next day, simply repeat the exercise every day until you've mastered your worry.

## Exercise 3: Inventory of Your Spiritual Experiences

If you feel you already have a personal relationship with a Higher Power, how have you experienced it? As you think back over your life, you may be able to recall times when you felt inspired, in awe, moved, or uplifted beyond your everyday experience. Write your responses to the following questions in the spaces provided or on a separate piece of paper.

1.  What situations, places, persons, activities, or events give you a feeling of inspiration? A feeling of wonder or awe?

2.  Which of the following experiences do you consider to be "spiritual"? Write down an example of an inspiring experience you had in each case.

Natural beauty
(A place or an occasion in nature that filled you with awe or wonder)

Deep Insight
(Something creative you felt genuinely inspired to do)

Expression of love received or given
(Indicate when and with whom)

3.  The following experiences are commonly thought to be spiritual. Describe any of your own personal experiences that apply.

    Receiving answers to prayers

    Synchronicities (meaningful coincidences)

    Guidance

    Miracles

4. Mystical or visionary experiences—describe instances where you experienced any of the following:

Feeling supported by a loving presence

A sudden feeling of peace in the midst of turmoil

A sense of oneness of everything—or yourself being one with or part of everything

Experiencing an infusion of light that led to a feeling of peace, bliss, or joy

Witnessing a spiritual being or presence (such as angels, Jesus, or other figures within your particular spiritual tradition)

Other (any other experiences you consider to be a direct manifestation of your Higher Power)

## Your Spiritual Practices

Cultivating a relationship with your Higher Power is in some ways similar to developing a relationship with another person. The more time and energy you give to it, the closer and deeper the relationship becomes. If you're willing to give such a relationship high priority, it can develop into an important part of your everyday life. You can deepen your commitment to spirituality through any of the following practices:

*Spiritual community.* Regular participation in church or your preferred spiritually based organization. Remembering the sacred in the presence of others is a common and powerful way to experience your connection with your Higher Power. This can be through attending your preferred church, going to spiritual classes and meetings, or even sacred dance, such as Sufi dancing. You may also choose to become involved in a 12-step program that is relevant to your needs. The 12-step programs offer many people a well-conceived and effective approach for healing addictions. Although they began with Alcoholics Anonymous eighty years ago, they now include a wide range of programs, such as Emotions Anonymous, Codependents Anonymous, Overeaters Anonymous, Sex and Love Addicts Anonymous, and Workaholics Anonymous. Consult your local chapter of the National Council on Alcoholism for a list of 12-step groups in your area.

*Regular reading of inspirational literature of your preference.* It's good to do this at least once per day—upon awakening, during your lunch break, or before retiring. You can rely on traditional texts associated with your religion such as the Bible, Torah, Koran, or *Bhagavad Gita*, or more modern, contemporary books on spirituality. Some of the author's personal favorites among modern books are listed in the "Further Reading" section at the end of this chapter.

*Regular practice of meditation.* Meditation is a practice of becoming quiet to the point that you get in touch with a deeper part of your inner being: one that is nonreactive, beyond conditioning, and ultimately in tune with your Higher Power. Meditation provides a way to disidentify with self-limiting emotions and thoughts so that you can *witness rather than react* to them. For more on meditation, see chapter 19, Meditation.

*Regular practice of prayer.* Prayer is a way of actively communicating with your Higher Power, usually in the form of a request. Sometimes you may ask your Higher Power for a quality such as strength, peace, or clarity. Other times you may ask for your Higher Power to simply be present in a particular situation. Or you may relinquish a problem to your Higher Power without asking for anything in particular.

*Working with spiritual affirmations.* While prayer is an opportunity to place a request to your Higher Power, repeating spiritual affirmations is a way to reinforce your spiritual beliefs. Famous spiritual affirmations include statements such as "Let go and let God" or "My soul abides in God." Two famous self-help books on working with spiritual affirmations are *You Can Heal Your Life* by Louise Hay and *Creative Visualization* by Shakti Gawain. There is also a page-length affirmative prayer in chapter 10 of my book *Beyond Anxiety & Phobia*, entitled "An Affirmation for Restoring Wholeness," which many of my clients have found helpful. See this book for a more in-depth coverage of the topic of spirituality, including a final chapter on the nature of unconditional love, forgiveness, and compassion.

*A silent moment in nature.* If available, seek out a local place of natural beauty (preferably free of traffic noise and human noise) such as a park, an area next to a lake or river, a beach, a quiet meadow or clearing in the woods where you can witness a sunrise or sunset, or a quiet, dark-sky area where you can see the swath of the Milky Way. Then spend two or three minutes in the area in total silence, just taking in its full natural beauty, being receptive to any feelings of inspiration that arise.

*Compassionate service.* This means serving others out of a genuine motive to help. This can be volunteer work or just simple acts of kindness and compassion toward others in your day-to-day life. Helping someone else out of a dark space in their life will lighten your soul.

Having read through this partial list of spiritual practices, ask yourself whether you would like to increase your engagement or involvement in any one or more than one of them.

## A Final Caveat

Reading the previous sections may have made spirituality sound as if it were a cure-all. You might even be left with the idea that developing a relationship with your Higher Power is *all* that is necessary for you to overcome your problem with panic, phobias, or anxiety. This is very unlikely to be true. You're still going to need to draw on all of the strategies presented in this workbook to deal with your particular problem with anxiety. Relaxation, exercise, coping strategies for panic, exposure, changing self-talk and mistaken beliefs, expressing feelings, developing assertiveness, and working on self-esteem will all be necessary.

Developing your spirituality can offer you additional inspiration and hope to persist in following through with your recovery program. It can also provide you with a powerful means for breaking through to your next step forward at those times when you're feeling stuck, discouraged, or confused.

## Summary of Things to Do

1. Do you feel aware of your own unique life purpose or purposes? Use the *Personal Values Inventory* to assist you in clarifying what you would most like to do with your life.

2. Based on your values, make a list of your most important personal goals. Then develop a plan of action—a specific sequence of steps—toward attaining each of your important goals.

3. Reflect on the ten ideas presented in the section "Changes in Beliefs Associated with Spirituality" and complete exercise 1.

4. Practice the meditation "Connecting with Your Higher Power" in exercise 2 when you feel up against a personal issue that you've been unable to resolve through your own conscious efforts.

5. Among the list of options for developing your spiritual life, take some time to reflect on:

   - Experiences that you've had that left you feeling inspired, moved, or uplifted beyond your everyday awareness. Take a look at *Exercise 3: Inventory of Your Spiritual Experiences* to identify such experiences.

   - Think about any current spiritual practices you engage in. Consult the section "Your Spiritual Practices" to explore whether you would like to expand upon any of your current spiritual practices or perhaps add new ones.

# Further Reading

If you are on a traditional religious path, you probably are already familiar with a number of written sources of inspiration and guidance. The Bible has a tremendous amount of insight and wisdom to offer if you are of Christian or Jewish faith. Islamic, Buddhist, Hindu, and other traditional religions all possess a rich literature of spiritual wisdom. The books listed below are not aligned with any particular religion, but, like this chapter, speak to a universal spirituality.

Bourne, Edmund J. *Beyond Anxiety & Phobia.* Oakland, CA: New Harbinger Publications, 2001.

———. *Healing Fear.* Oakland, CA: New Harbinger Publications, 1998.

Dass, Ram. *Be Here Now.* San Cristobal, NM: Lama Foundation, 1971. (still in print).

Dossey, Larry. *One Mind.* Reprint. Carlsbad, CA: Hay House, 2014.

Forsyth, John P., and Georg H. Eifert. *The Mindfulness & Acceptance Workbook for Anxiety.* 2nd ed. Oakland, CA: New Harbinger Publications, 2016.

Gawain, Shakti. *Creative Visualization.* 40th anniversary ed. Novato, CA: Nataraj Publishing/New World Library, 2016.

———, with Laurel King. *Living in the Light.* 25th anniversary ed. Novato, CA: Nataraj Publishing/ New World Library, 2011.

Harris, Russ. *ACT Made Simple.* 2nd ed. Oakland, CA: New Harbinger Publications, 2019.

Hay, Louise. *You Can Heal Your Life.* Carlsbad, CA: Hay House, 1999. (Includes many helpful tools and affirmations for developing self-worth.)

Jampolsky, Gerald. *Love Is Letting Go of Fear.* 3rd ed. New York: Celestial Arts, 2010.

Moody, Raymond. *Life After Life.* Special anniversary ed. New York: HarperOne, 2015.

Rodegast, Pat, and Judith Stanton. *Emmanuel's Book.* New York: Bantam, 1987.

Roman, Sanaya. *Spiritual Growth.* Novato, CA: New World Library, 1992.

Tolle, Eckhart. *A New Earth: Awakening to Your Life Purpose.* 10th anniversary ed. New York: Penguin, 2008.

———. *The Power of Now.* Vancouver, BC, Canada: Namaste Publishing, 2004. (An excellent resource for going beyond the conditioned mind and developing awareness.)

Williamson, Marianne. *Illuminata.* New York: Riverhead Books, 1995. (An outstanding collection of thoughts and prayers for modern times.)

Zukav, Gary. *The Seat of the Soul.* 25th anniversary ed. New York: Simon & Schuster, 2014.

# Postscript

# A Future of Increasing Anxiety

"I'm asking you, for your good and for your nation's security, to take no unnecessary trips, to use carpools or public transportation whenever you can...and to set your thermostats to save fuel. Every act of energy conservation like this is more than just common sense, I tell you it is an act of patriotism."

—Jimmy Carter, 1980

This book has primarily focused on strategies and skills aimed to help you overcome personal anxiety disorders, such as panic attacks, phobias, or excessive worry. As an anxiety self-help book, *The Anxiety & Phobia Workbook* has mostly refrained from addressing the larger sociocultural context for anxiety that humanity is facing at the present time and going forward.

In the Introduction to this book, several drivers of anxiety at the societal level were mentioned, such as economic instability, income inequality, local and global terrorism, proliferation of nuclear weapons (particularly by rogue nations), and finally climate change, which is presently reaching a number of "tipping points" (points beyond which there can be no easy return). One of these, for example, is significant loss of ice sheets at both poles leading to discernible rises in global sea level. Another is massive deforestation—with attendant loss of biodiversity and biological habitat—as well as significant reduction in the worldwide number of trees available to help absorb carbon dioxide from the atmosphere.

Many other climate impacts might be mentioned, such as sea acidification, leading to massive loss of fish and coral bleaching, or an increasing number of cities that, during summer months, reach temperatures in excess of 120 degrees Fahrenheit, making it impossible for people to work outdoors except at night and causing increased deaths among children and elderly people, who cannot find sufficient protection from such extreme heat.

All scientific indications point toward a *future world of increasing climate threats*.

*Anxiety*, by definition, *is a natural response to a perceived or real threat*. Since the best climate science points to a future world of *increasing climate threats*, the conclusion is that we are facing a future of *greater collective anxiety*. Climate change alone leads to a future world of increasing anxiety, apart from all the other future world trends that may compromise collective security.

In the past few years, a majority of climate scientists have acknowledged that the *rate* of climate change impacts has been consistently *underestimated*: that we are likely to reach tipping points by 2030 or 2035 that, just a few years ago, had been thought unlikely to occur until 2050.

Comparisons with Pearl Harbor, the assassination of JFK, Sept. 11, 2001, and even the Black Death of the 1300s come to mind. A profound difference between these world-shaking events and the present crisis is *perceived duration*. Challenges such as Pearl Harbor or the worst of the Black Death played out in time frames lasting at most a few years. Climate change is different. Without urgent and comprehensive changes made *in the next ten years*, climate change poses increasingly catastrophic consequences for life on earth over the next fifty if not hundreds of years (short of some miraculous carbon-capture technology not yet invented or utilized). This is a future of increasing anxiety—a future it is imperative to address.

## Short List of Climate Impacts Possible in the Next Two Decades

- *Increased melting of the Greenland ice sheet as well as multiple Antarctic ice sheets.* At its worst, this process may lead to early flooding of a number of major coastal cities as well as near complete submergence of coastal portions of Bangladesh and Myanmar.

- *Increasing deforestation, most critically of the Brazilian Amazon and Indonesian forests.* Every year an average of 33 million acres of forest is cut down. Timber harvesting contributes to 1.5 billion metric tons of CO2 to the global atmosphere every year, about *20% of the total* of manmade greenhouse gas emissions. The two main objectives of rampant deforestation are lumber production and opening fields for soybean cultivation, to produce feedstock for beef cattle. If humanity were to reduce its beef consumption, fewer trees would be sacrificed.

- *Increasing average summer temperatures in a number of cities above 120 degrees Fahrenheit*, similar to the temperature of Death Valley, California. Outdoor work in such heat becomes impossible and can only be done at night when the outside temperature falls to about 90 degrees. The lives of many children and elderly are directly threatened if they can't find respite from such extreme heat. Several cities in Pakistan and India are currently experiencing such extreme temperatures continuously for up to *one or two months* during the summer, rather than just on specific days. The result is widespread heatstroke and death among vulnerable people. Other cities will join these cities if global warming continues.

- *The ocean is increasingly becoming a major "heat sink" (place for heat absorption) for global warming.* As it absorbs greater amounts of CO2, the ocean becomes increasingly acidic, decimating fish populations worldwide and bleaching out the world's largest coral reefs, such as The Great Barrier Reef off the eastern coast of Australia.

- *Increasing urban heat sink phenomena* have made major cities, particularly in Asia, unlivable in the summer without air conditioning. The *combination of high heat along with high humidity* (in excess of 60%) has proven to be especially lethal for people who can't find or afford respite from exposure. The result has been mass migration from urban centers during the summer months and substantial loss of employment.

Without further enumerating climate change impacts, the critical point is that the *rate* of change in global warming is accelerating over what it had been thought to be as recently as two or three years ago. Thus the need for mitigation is more urgent than previously thought. Many scientists use the term "climate emergency" instead of "climate change." Goals set for 2050 a few years ago are having to be recalibrated for 2030. The millions of young people demonstrating in the streets on many Fridays are there to convey this degree of urgency. Without rapid and comprehensive efforts toward mitigation of global warming, they will live to see catastrophic impacts in their lifetimes.

# A Few Proposed Solutions (many of which have been well known for more than a decade)

1. *A worldwide tax on carbon,* which gradually ramps up over time, increasing the cost to all industries, activities (such as deforestation), and vehicles that involve carbon for the amount of carbon emitted. To date, widespread use of carbon taxes has been avoided.

2. *Cap and trade systems.* A cap and trade system is a market-based strategy that gives carbon dioxide emitting companies the opportunity to set their own carbon emission limits. The "cap" part of cap and trade is usually established by a government, a region, or a state. For example, New England and California represent a region and a state, respectively, that have set a cap on allowable greenhouse gas emissions—especially aimed at energy production companies, but including all companies. Over time, the cap is gradually lowered, so that the companies need to become less carbon intensive. The "trade" part of cap and trade allows companies to purchase permits to emit greater levels of CO2 in exchange for buying "offsets" to mitigate CO2 such as reforesting an area, building solar panel systems, or installing wind-powered systems. So, a company is constrained in two ways: a cap is set on its total allowable emissions, and its opportunity to emit more than the cap must be purchased by investing in efforts that directly reduce greenhouse gas emissions.

3. *Move away from energy production based on fossil fuels (coal, oil, or natural gas) toward carbon-free forms of energy production* such as nuclear reactors (especially newer, smaller scale ones), solar cells, and wind farms. These vital changes in energy production are at best a longer-term solution, as *nearly half* the electricity produced in the U.S., China, and India still uses coal as the primary energy source.

## *Geoengineering: A Solution of Last Resort*

Reduction of the emission of greenhouse gases has been the primary goal for curtailing global warming for three decades. Yet it appears that aspirational goals, such as the goal set at the Paris Climate Agreement of 2016 to limit increases of global temperature by no more than 1.5 degrees centigrade (or failing that, at least to no more 2 degrees centigrade), have already been exceeded. At the time of the Paris Agreement, stated goals were voluntary rather than mandatory, though periodic reports by participating countries on progress were mandated. As of 2019, the average increase in global temperatures is already up *2.7 degrees centigrade.* July 2019 was the hottest month worldwide every recorded. Also, as of 2019, harmful coal emissions are still rising, including a 4.5 percent increase in coal emissions in China and a 7.1 percent increase in India over the past two years (Harvey 2018).

If all efforts to decrease greenhouse gas emissions fail, *geoengineering* provides a series of possible but untested methods of reducing sunlight input into the earth's atmosphere. The word geoengineering means exactly what it says: reengineering the environment at a global scale to reduce global warming. Below are five (by no means all) examples of geoengineering concepts (Biello 2007), some of which have been tested at a very small scale, though none of which have been seriously considered at a global scale, not only because of the efforts and/or cost involved, but because consequences to the human and animal habitat are not fully known and cannot be fully predicted:

1. *Artificially injecting aerosols, the most popular being sulfur dioxide (SO2) directly into the upper atmosphere* could have a cooling effect by blocking both heat and light from the sun. It could also bring back global rainfall averages to pre-industrial levels. The downside is that scaling up SO2 to levels that would reduce sunlight and heat globally would have an effect similar to many hundreds of concurrent volcanic eruptions (which also release sulfur dioxide). No one can predict the full effects on animal and plant species of filling the upper atmosphere with sulfites. Furthermore, if only the northern hemisphere were treated, the southern hemisphere would suffer increasingly severe climate impacts. Finally, injection of SO2 would have to continue indefinitely. If it were to stop suddenly as a result of political or economic obstacles, scientists predict a "rebound effect" of *increased rate* of global warming over initial values.

2. A second geoengineering solution is to *inject trillions of small reflective mirrors into the upper atmosphere that would literally reflect back the sun's heat and light,* cooling the earth. This particular technological alternative is more difficult to scale up to global levels than sulfate aerosol infusion and carries similar risks.

3. A third possibility *is carbon capture and storage.* This involves retrofitting all carbon emitting energy plants and other carbon-intensive companies with mechanisms for capturing and storing carbon deep underground. Though this alternative has been discussed for many years, the cost and political obstacles to doing it globally have been deemed by many scientists to be prohibitive.

4. Another longstanding proposal has been to *seed the ocean with iron filings, in order to increase phytoplankton production, since phytoplankton directly capture CO2.* As with most geoengineering alternatives, the technological, political, and economic costs of scaling up this solution to the entire planet are challenging, to say the least. No one really knows the short- or long-term effects of seeding of the world's oceans with iron might be. Some critics warn that ocean ecosystems could be upset in such a way as to result in harmful algal blooms, causing worldwide red tides and other toxic effects. While iron fertilization

of the oceans might result in lower sea acidification at higher levels, acidification could increase at deeper sea levels.

5.  Finally, the only truly *natural* form of geoengineering would involve reversing the drivers of climate change: (1) planting enormous numbers of trees, (2) blocking precipitous growth of industrialization to restore natural habitats and biodiversity, and (3) making low cost air conditioning much more widely available to residents of cities exposed to excess heat (among several other natural alternatives). This is geoengineering at its best: restoring as much as possible the resources that have stabilized the earth's climate for thousands of years. Unfortunately, this one positive option has the lowest probability of being carried out. The cost and effort to scale up such natural alternatives to levels that would make a genuine difference is truly challenging. The political will to do so is also lacking in the major countries most responsible for climate change.

## Personal Actions Each of Us Can Take

Though collective action against climate change, at global and governmental levels, will be necessary, there are also things each of us can do to mitigate climate change. Here are some actions we can personally take.

1.  *Move away from gas-consuming cars,* and their larger CO2 outputs, to hybrid gas and electric or full electric vehicles. The upside of electric vehicles is that they are carbon free. A potential downside is that the electrical grid still depends on coal-generated energy to a significant extent, though this is rapidly changing in some areas. Since the worldwide demand for cars is increasingly dramatically, the replacement of coal-based sources of electricity with solar and wind alternatives presently can't keep up.

2.  *Divest from oil companies* among stocks held (such as Exxon Mobil, Royal Dutch Shell, or British Petroleum) to companies based on renewable energy.

3.  *Eat less red meat.* Beef cattle are raised on soybeans, many of which are obtained from soybean stock grown in large deforested areas of the Amazon in Brazil as well as deforested areas of Indonesia. By eating less meat, you support maintenance of more trees on the planet, without which the world could see runaway climate change (trees absorb significant CO2). Eating meat once per day indirectly produces about 1.5 tons more greenhouse gas (CO2 and methane) per year *per person* than going vegetarian.

4.  *Move closer to work.* Reduce your travel time to a minimum. You not only gain an easier commute, but you save the planet from increased CO emissions from your car. If possible, live close enough to work to take mass transit or ride a bicycle.

5.  *Reduce jet travel to a minimum.* The kerosene burned by jet engines is a major source of carbon released into the atmosphere.

6. *Use more energy efficient "energy-star" rated appliances.* This is especially important for appliances that consume larger amounts of power such as refrigerators or air conditioners.

7. *Use LED lights.* These lights are more energy efficient than compact fluorescent lights, which in turn are more efficient than older incandescent lights.

8. *Recycle electronic waste.* Hundreds of millions of cell phones, laptops, iPads, and computer monitors end up in landfills every year. There they disintegrate over centuries, leaching out toxic metals such as lead, mercury, and lithium, which may eventually make it into the groundwater. To reverse this trend, do a google search for the nearest site in your community that takes recycled electronics. Unless you are in a remote rural area, such a site should be an easy drive away. If you wish, save up all your old, defunct electronics so that only one trip to the electronic waste recycling site is necessary.

**Note:** This is just a very partial list of actions you might take to reduce your personal "carbon footprint," i.e., the amount of carbon-based emissions you personally produce each year. For a much more complete list of things you can do toward helping the planet, see Chapter 24, "Take Action," in the author's book *Global Shift*. Also, Al Gore has produced a sequel to his iconic 2006 movie, *An Inconvenient Truth*, called *An Inconvenient Sequel, Truth to Power*, released in 2017.

# References

Biello, David. Ten Solutions for Climate Change. *Scientific American*, Nov. 26, 2007. www.scientificamerican.com/article/10-solutions-for-climate-change.

Harvey, Chelsea. "CO2 Emissions Reached an All-Time High in 2018." *Scientific American*, Dec. 6, 2018. www.scientificamerican.com/article/co2-emissions-reached-an-all-time-high-in-2018.

Bourne, Edmund. *Global Shift: How A New Worldview is Transforming Humanity*. Oakland, CA, New Harbinger Publications (in joint effort with Noetic Books of the Institute of Noetic Sciences), 2008.

# Appendix 1

# Helpful Organizations

## The Anxiety and Depression Association of America

The Anxiety and Depression Association of America (ADAA) is a nonprofit, charitable organization founded in 1980 by leaders in the field of treatment for phobias, agoraphobia, and panic/anxiety disorders. Its purpose is to promote public awareness about anxiety disorders, stimulate research and development of effective treatments, and offer assistance to sufferers and their families in gaining access to available specialists and treatment programs. In 2012, the association expanded both in name and in its resources offered to include depression.

The association's website, adaa.org, offers a "Find a Therapist" link for assistance in finding therapists in your local area who list their practice with the association. The Association prefers that you use this tool to find a therapist near where you live rather than contacting the ADAA directly.

For further information about the Anxiety and Depression Association of America, its services, publications, podcasts, and conferences, as well as how to join, please contact:

**Anxiety and Depression Association of America**

8701 Georgia Ave. #412

Silver Spring, MD 20910

1-240-485-1001

information@adaa.org

## The International OCD Foundation

The mission of the International OCD Foundation is to help individuals with obsessive-compulsive disorder (OCD) to live full and productive lives. The organization provides books and brochures, conducts research, and puts on national conferences on OCD. For comprehensive information about obsessive-compulsive disorder and a list of therapists who specialize in treating OCD, see their website, iocdf.org. You can also write or call them:

**International OCD Foundation**

PO Box 961029

Boston, MA 02196

1-617-973-5801

info@iocdf.org

## The Social Anxiety Institute

Social anxiety is the fear of being judged and evaluated negatively by other people, leading to feelings of inadequacy, embarrassment, humiliation, and depression. Presently, it is the third most common mental health problem in the anxiety disorders field. The Social Anxiety Institute offers a list of treatment providers, videos, books, and a newsletter relevant to social anxiety disorder and social phobia. For further information about their work, as well as how to become a member, contact:

**Social Anxiety Institute**

Thomas A. Richards, PhD

2058 East Topeka Drive

Phoenix, AZ 85024

1-602-230-7316

socialanxietyinstitute.org

## The National Alliance on Mental Illness (NAMI)

NAMI provides information about the full range of mental health difficulties, including anxiety disorders. It also describes a broad range of treatments for various mental health problems. NAMI is a nationwide alliance of over a thousand local affiliates in communities across the United States. For further information about NAMI, simply go to their website. To find your local affiliate group, enter your zip code and then click on the link "Find Your Local NAMI." You can also call the national information helpline. Please note that the NAMI helpline is only available Monday–Friday 10 a.m.–6 p.m. EST.

**National Alliance on Mental Illness (NAMI)**

1-800-950-6264 (helpline)

nami.org

Though speaking to a live person by phone is always more personal, in the possible instance the helpline is closed, you can text NAMI to 741741 or email them at info@NAMI.org.

**Note:** If you or someone you know is in serious crisis—whether considering suicide or not—please call the toll-free Lifeline at 1-800-273-8255 to speak with a trained crisis counselor 24/7.

# Appendix 2

# Resources for Relaxation

There is a wide variety of resources for training yourself to achieve a deep state of relaxation, available either in CD format or as downloads to your computer or smartphone.

## Relaxation and Visualization

*Deep Relaxation*

A large variety of CDs and audio downloads that facilitate deep relaxation can be found at Sounds True (soundstrue.com). Click on the link "Meditation."

*Guided Visualizations*

A good resource for CDs, downloads, and books that can facilitate anxiety reduction and deep relaxation is the website of Dr. Emmett Miller: drmiller.com.

You may also want to do an Amazon search for "visualizations for relaxation."

## Music

*Calm, Peaceful*

Go to amazon.com/music and do a search using the keyword "Relaxation" to find peaceful, calming music.

*Classical*

For classical enthusiasts, see *The Most Relaxing Classical Album in the World...Ever!* (Virgin Records).

*Compilations*

In general, compilations of music by Windham Hill and Narada are usually conducive to relaxation. Go to amazon.com/music and do a search for either "Windham Hill" or "Narada."

# Appendix 3

# How to Stop Obsessive Thoughts

Obsessive thoughts can become a *negative spiral*. The longer you spend time with them, the deeper into them you may get. Obsessive thoughts are generally fearful and tend to leave you with doubt, for example: "What if I forgot to turn off the gas stove before I left home" or "What if I became contaminated from touching the public toilet flush lever, even though I washed my hands." This doubt, in turn, leads you to revisit the fearful thought again and again in an effort to assuage the doubt. It may also be viewed as a form of trance. The more you induce it by repetition, the more entranced you get, and the more difficult it may be to "break the spell."

*It takes a deliberate act of will to stop obsessive thoughts.* You need to make a deliberate effort to move away from circular mental activity and *get out of your head* by "shifting gears" to another modality of experience. Some examples are engaging in physical activity, calling a good friend, watching a funny movie, or solving puzzles (a kind of alternative "positive" obsessive focus).

The downward pull of an obsessive spiral can be very compelling. Following the path of least resistance is likely to keep your mind going round and round. Although deliberately choosing to break out of the obsessive thinking may be difficult at first (especially if you're highly anxious), with practice it will get easier.

Below are some examples of alternative activities and experiences that can help you shift out of your mind and away from obsessive thinking.

1. *Do physical exercise.* This can be your favorite outdoor or indoor exercise, dancing, or just household chores.

2. *Do progressive muscle relaxation alone or in combination with abdominal breathing.* See chapter 4 for more detail. Keep this up for five to ten minutes until you feel fully relaxed and freer from obsessive thoughts.

3. *Use evocative music to release repressed feelings.* Such feelings—usually sadness or anger—may underlie and "drive" worry or obsessive thinking.

4. *Talk to someone.* Converse about something other than the worry, unless you want to express your feelings about it, as in point 3.

5. *Use visual distractions.* This can be TV, movies, video games, your computer, uplifting reading, or even a rock garden.

6. *Use sensory-motor distraction.* Try doing arts and crafts, repairing something, or gardening.

7.  *Find an alternative, "positive obsession."* For example, work out a crossword or jigsaw puzzle.

8.  *Practice healthy rituals.* Combine abdominal breathing with a positive affirmation that has personal significance. Keep this up for five to ten minutes, or until you're fully relaxed.

| *Examples of Affirmations:* | *For the Spiritually Inclined:* |
|---|---|
| "Let it go." | "Let go and let God." |
| "These are just thoughts— they're fading away." | "I abide in Spirit (God)." |
| "I'm whole, relaxed, and free of worry." | "I release this negativity to God." |

# Appendix 4

# Affirmations for Overcoming Anxiety

The following affirmations are intended to help you change your attitude and respond constructively to the kinds of negative self-talk that can feed anxiety. Reading through them once or twice probably won't make much difference. Rehearsing some or all of them daily for a few weeks or months will begin to help you change your basic outlook about fear in a constructive direction. One way to do this is to read through one of the two sections below slowly, once or twice each day, giving yourself time to reflect on each affirmation. Even better, record one or both sections, leaving a few seconds of silence between each affirmation. Then listen to the recording once daily, when relaxed, to reinforce a more positive and confident attitude about mastering your anxiety.

## Negative Thoughts and Positive Affirmations to Combat Them

(Use only the affirmations, if you're making a recording.)

| | |
|---|---|
| *This is unbearable.* | I can learn how to cope better with this. |
| *What if this goes on without letting up?* | I'll deal with this one day at a time. I don't have to project into the future. |
| *I feel damaged, inadequate relative to others.* | Some of us have steeper paths to walk than others. That doesn't make me less valuable as a human being—even if I accomplish less in the outer world. |
| *Why do I have to deal with this? Other people seem freer to enjoy their lives.* | Life is a school. For whatever reasons, at least for now, I've been given a steeper path—a tougher curriculum. That doesn't make me wrong. In fact, adversity develops qualities of strength and compassion. |
| *Having this condition seems unfair.* | Life can appear unfair from a human perspective. If we could see the bigger picture, we'd see that everything is proceeding according to plan. |
| *I don't know how to cope with this.* | I can *learn* to cope better—with this and any difficulty life brings. |

| | |
|---|---|
| *I feel so inadequate relative to others.* | Let people do what they do in the outer world. I'm following a path of inner growth and transformation, which is at least equally valuable. Finding peace in myself can be a gift to others. |
| *Each day seems like a major challenge.* | I'm learning to take things more slowly. I'm making time to take care of myself. |
| *I don't understand why I'm this way—why this happened to me.* | The causes for my anxiety are many, including heredity, early environment, and cumulative stress. Understanding causes satisfies the intellect, but it's not what heals. |
| *I feel like I'm going crazy.* | When anxiety is high, I may *feel* like I'm losing control. But that feeling has nothing to do with going crazy. Anxiety disorders are a long way from the category of disorders labeled "crazy." |
| *I have to really fight this.* | Struggling with a problem won't help as much as making more time in my life to better care for myself. |
| *I shouldn't have let this happen to me.* | The long-term causes of this problem lie in heredity and childhood environment, so I didn't cause this condition. I *can* now take responsibility for getting better. |

## Antianxiety Affirmations

Choose your favorite affirmations from the following list. Your list might contain five to ten key affirmations (or more if you prefer). Then read through the list slowly, or record your list, reading slowly, and play it back once each day.

- I am learning to let go of worry.

- Each day I'm growing in my capacity to master worry and anxiety.

- I am learning not to feed my worries—to choose peace over fear.

- I am learning to consciously choose what I think, and I choose thoughts that are supportive and beneficial for me.

- When anxious thoughts come up, I can slow down, breathe, and let them go.

- When anxious thoughts come up, I can make time to relax and release them.

- Deep relaxation gives me the freedom of choice to move out of fear.

- Anxiety is made of illusory thoughts—thoughts I can let go of.

- When I see most situations as they truly are, there is nothing to be afraid of.

- Fearful thoughts are usually exaggerated, and I'm growing in my ability to turn them off at will.

- The true risk I face in most situations is actually very small.

- Every worry involves overestimating the risk of danger—and underestimating my ability to cope.

- More and more, it's becoming easier to relax and talk myself out of anxiety.

- I keep my mind too busy thinking positive and constructive thoughts to have much time for worry.

- I'm learning to handle my mind and choose the thoughts that I prefer to think.

- I am gaining more confidence in myself, knowing I can handle any situation that comes along.

- Fear is dissolving and vanishing from my life. I am calm, confident, and secure.

- As I take life more slowly and easily, I have more ease and peace in my life.

- As I grow in my ability to relax and feel secure, I realize that there is truly nothing to fear.

For a more complete discussion of both visualizations and affirmations, see chapter 10, "Create Your Vision," in the author's book *Beyond Anxiety & Phobia*.

**Edmund J. Bourne, PhD,** has specialized in the treatment of anxiety, phobias, and other stress-related disorders for over two decades. His self-help books have helped over a million people and have been translated into numerous languages. He currently resides in Florida and California.

Phone counseling for problems with panic attackse, phobias, and other anxiety difficulties is available with Edmund Bourne. For information, please call 1-415-686-7516. For resources in your local area, please see Appendix 1. Further information about Bourne's work in the anxiety disorders field may be found at **helpforanxiety.com**.

For Edmund Bourne's work outside the field of anxiety disorders, please see his website, **journeysofthemind.net**.

# How to Access Resources for
## *The Anxiety & Phobia Workbook*

You can register your copy of The Anxiety & Phobia Workbook, 7th edition—whether you bought the book or borrowed it, and whether your book is in print or electronic format—to download the resources listed below.

Just visit newharbinger.com/44833 and follow the prompts that appear. They'll guide you through the process of creating a NewHarbinger.com account and registering your book there. If you need help with this, please visit newharbinger.com/accessories.

**Audio Files, Handouts, and Worksheets/Exercises**
The titles below are listed by chapter in the order in which they appear in that chapter. The icon in front of the title indicates whether it is an audio file, handout, or worksheet/exercise:

 ⁓ℂ = audio file          ▤ = handout          ✎ = worksheet/exercise

**Chapter 3—Recovery: A Comprehensive Approach**
✎ Weekly Practice Record

**Chapter 4—Relaxation**
⁓ℂ Abdominal Breathing Exercise
⁓ℂ Calming Breath Exercise
⁓ℂ Progressive Muscle Relaxation
⁓ℂ Passive Muscle Relaxation
⁓ℂ Peaceful Scene

**Chapter 5—Physical Exercise**
✎ Daily Record of Exercise

**Chapter 6—Coping with Panic Attacks**
✎ Panic Attack Worksheet 1: Basic Symptoms
✎ Panic Attack Worksheet 2: Catastrophic Thoughts
✎ Connecting Bodily Symptoms and Catastrophic Thoughts
✎ Panic Attack Record

**Chapter 7—Exposure for Phobias**
✎ Hierarchy Worksheet

**Chapter 8—Self-Talk**
✎ Subpersonality Worksheets: The Worrier, The Critic, The Victim, The Perfectionist
✎ Countering Self-Talk Worksheet

**Chapter 10—Overcoming Worry**
✎ Exercise: Make a Plan to Deal with Your Worry

**Chapter 11—Personality Styles That Perpetuate Anxiety**
✎ Checklist for Symptoms of Stress

**Chapter 14—Being Assertive**
▤ Personal Bill of Rights
✎ Exercise: Write Out Assertive Requests for Real-Life Situations

**Chapter 16—Nutrition**
✎ Food Diary

**Chapter 19—Meditation**
⁓ℂ Basic Meditation Exercise
⁓ℂ Sensing Your Body During Meditation
⁓ℂ Witnessing Thoughts and Feelings

**Chapter 21—Personal Meaning**
✎ Plan of Action: Steps Toward Your Goal
⁓ℂ Connecting with Your Higher Power

# MORE BOOKS *from*
# NEW HARBINGER PUBLICATIONS

Register your **new harbinger** titles for additional benefits!

When you register your **new harbinger** title—purchased in any format, from any source—you get access to benefits like the following:

- Downloadable accessories like printable worksheets and extra content
- Instructional videos and audio files
- Information about updates, corrections, and new editions

Not every title has accessories, but we're adding new material all the time.

Access free accessories in 3 easy steps:

**1.** Sign in at NewHarbinger.com (or **register** to create an account).

**2.** Click on **register a book**. Search for your title and click the **register** button when it appears.

**3.** Click on the **book cover or title** to go to its details page. Click on **accessories** to view and access files.

That's all there is to it!

If you need help, visit:

NewHarbinger.com/accessories

**new harbinger**
CELEBRATING
**40** YEARS